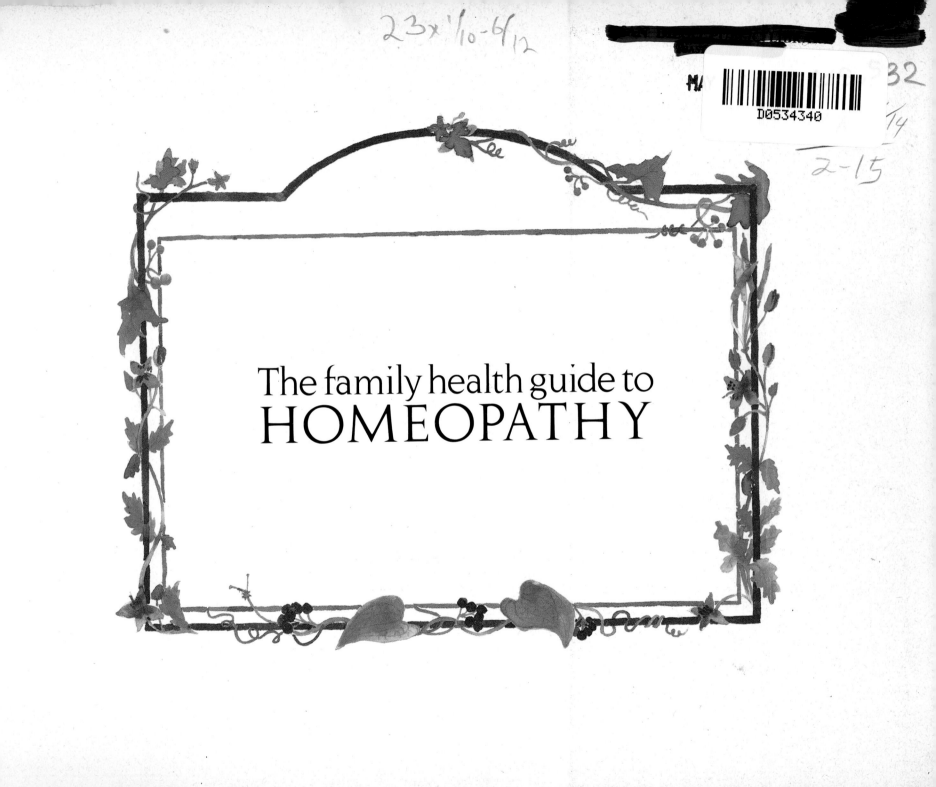

The family health guide to
HOMEOPATHY

The family health guide to
HOMEOPATHY

DR BARRY ROSE

Foreword by Lord Yehudi Menuhin

CELESTIALARTS
Berkeley, California

First published by Dragon's World Ltd, G.B., 1992
First published by Celestial Arts, U.S.A., 1993

For information write:
Celestial Arts Publishing
P.O. Box 7327
Berkeley, California 94707

Printed in Italy

Editor: Patricia Burgess
Art Editor: Judith Robertson
Editorial Director: Pippa Rubinstein

Typeset by Bookworm Typesetting

Library of Congress Cataloging-in-Publication Data
Rose, Barry, Dr.
    The family guide to homeopathy / Barry Rose : foreword by
Yehudi Menuhin.
       p.   cm.
    ISBN 0–89087–695–9 : $32.95
    1. Homeopathy—Popular works.   I. Title.
Rx76.R75   1991
615.5'32—dc20   93–3586
                        CIP

1 2 3 4 5 6 7 / 99 98 97 96 95 94 93

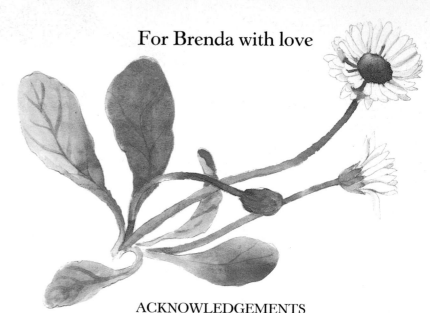

For Brenda with love

ACKNOWLEDGEMENTS

I owe a debt of gratitude to the late Dr Marjory Blackie, Homeopathic Physician to Her Majesty Queen Elizabeth, for introducing me to the fascinating study of homeopathic medicine. Since those early days I have sat at the feet of many great and learned homeopathic doctors and to them too I am grateful for the knowledge they have imparted.

My editor, Trish Burgess, has been a pleasure to work with. She has led me carefully round many possible hazards and has always been helpful, tactful and instructive. Judith Robertson, the designer, has been no less considerate, and to both of them many thanks.

The publishers gratefully acknowledge the help of Ainsworths' Homeopathic Pharmacy, London, who generously lent props for the cover photograph. Thanks also to Jay Borneman of Standard Homeopathic Company, Philadelphia, and Dana Ullman of Homeopathic Educational Services, California, who both provided useful information about homeopathy in the United States.

CONTENTS

Foreword 7

Introduction 8

How to Use This Book 12

TREATMENT SECTION 14

Emergencies and First Aid 15

Children's Ailments 28

Infectious Diseases 44

Emotional and Nervous Disorders 50

The Head, Scalp and Face 71

The Eye 79

The Ear 86

The Nose and Sinuses 93

The Mouth, Tongue and Lips 103

The Teeth and Gums 109

The Throat 113

The Circulatory System 119

The Respiratory System 127

The Digestive System 137

The Rectum and Anus 148

The Urinary System 155

Female Health 160

Pregnancy 173

Male Health 182

The Back and Limbs 187

The Skin 203

Holiday Remedies 213

MATERIA MEDICA 217

including How to Take Homeopathic Medicines

Bibliography 306

Further Reading 307

Useful Addresses 308

Index 310

Health Records 320

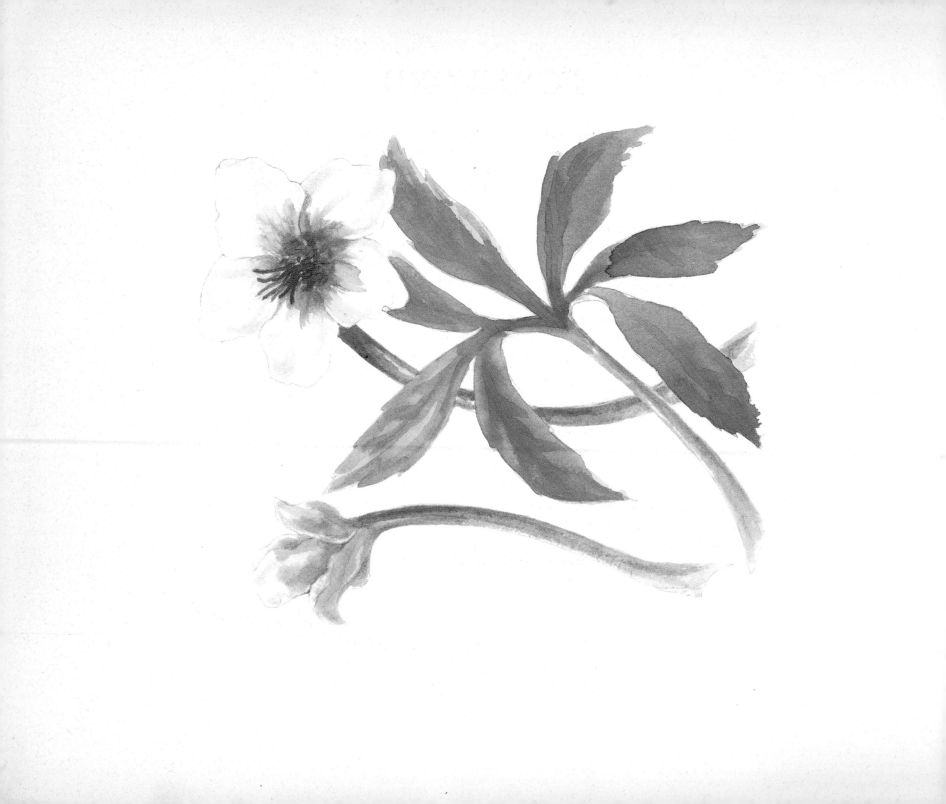

FOREWORD

*I*n the 150 years since Samuel Hahnemann discovered the system of medical treatment known as homeopathy, the world has undergone many changes. In fact, so much is different that Hahnemann might be surprised that his marvellous discoveries have not been superseded. But how can you improve on something that is safe, natural and effective?

Homeopathy is concerned with the whole person, treating each and every one of us as unique individuals. Remedies are selected on the basis of symptoms, factors which make them better or worse, disposition and appearance. Thus, a thin, nervous woman suffering from migraine might require a different medicine than a portly, aggressive woman suffering from the same ailment.

The efficacy of homeopathic remedies perplexes many people who are used to the ways of orthodox medicine. Instead of suppressing symptoms, and thus allowing the possibility of their recurring, homeopathy gets to the root cause, removing symptoms in the order in which they appeared, and thus paves the way for a complete cure. Indeed, sufferers from chronic complaints like asthma and eczema can, with time and patience, be returned to full health.

In the current age of technology, where so much of modern medicine seems to depend on harsh drugs and radical surgery, natural and gentle alternatives can arouse scepticism. However, there is no medical practice in the world as benign and safe as homeopathy. As a musician, what I particularly love about it is the great effect of subtlety – the enormous response to an infinitesimal but crucial intervention. Too long have we put our faith in quantity and massive attack. It is high time humanity learned the extreme value of the minute and the minimal. May this book make known to the wider public the value of homeopathy.

Yehudi Menuhin

Lord Yehudi Menuhin

INTRODUCTION

Homeopathy is a system of medical treatment which looks at the whole person, not just the illness from which he or she is suffering. If this seems a strange idea, a simple example will illustrate the point. Suppose both Mrs Smith and Mrs Jones have rheumatism and both complain of pain and stiffness. Mrs Smith, although bad on first movement, becomes much easier as she moves around and a warm bed makes the joint feel much more comfortable. In contrast, Mrs Jones finds any movement absolute agony and therefore keeps as still as possible. She might even bandage the affected joint to keep it perfectly still. Warmth most certainly does not relieve her discomfort – in fact, it makes it worse.

From this example you can see that the same ailment can affect two people very differently. As a result, homeopathy may recommend several different remedies for any one illness. The information given in this book will enable you to confirm your ailment and choose the medicine which most closely resembles your symptoms.

For ease of reference this book has been divided into two main sections. The Treatment Section, designed to help you diagnose ailments and treat them yourself, is devoted to descriptions of common illnesses and lists the remedies that may prove useful, including advice on dosage. While many common ailments can be self-diagnosed and treated successfully at home, others may require expert medical advice. Such cases are pointed out in the text.

Certain illnesses, such as cancer, are not included for obvious reasons. Although sufferers may be helped by homeopathic treatment, it should always be given under the guidance of a doctor or to complement whatever orthodox treatment may already have been prescribed.

The second major part of the book is the *materia medica*, which describes 100 homeopathic remedies and lists the illnesses and symptoms for which they are used. It also advises which remedies you might keep in your home medicine cabinet, how to obtain them and how to store them.

At the end of the book are lists of further reading and useful addresses.

THE DISCOVERY OF HOMEOPATHY

In the late eighteenth century prescriptions for medicines often contained a multitude of ingredients. Blood-letting and leeching, believed to remove impurities from the system, were commonplace, while surgery was crude and often fatal. If the twentieth century can be described as the age of scientific medicine, the eighteenth century was surely just the opposite.

Into this medical free-for-all came Dr Samuel Hahnemann (1755–1843), a recent graduate of Leipzig University, who was eager to help the sick. Sadly, he soon became disillusioned as he found the then current methods of treatment unacceptable, sometimes inappropriate and occasionally even wrong.

This state of affairs might well have continued had Hahnemann not also been a brilliant linguist (at the age of twenty-two he was said to be fluent in eight languages). Undertaking translation work to supplement his income, he was one day working on a medical text by Professor Cullen of Edinburgh University when he came across some information that he felt to be wrong. Cullen was writing about the use of a substance called Cinchona in treating the ague. (We now know the medicine as Quinine and the illness as malaria.)

Hahnemann did the only thing possible to help him resolve his doubts: he took several doses of Cinchona over the next few days, observing and recording the effects of the substance on himself. To his considerable surprise the medicine produced the very same symptoms that Cullen said it was used to treat.

Hahnemann used his findings to open up a whole new world of medical treatment. He observed that a substance which produced certain symptoms in a healthy person could be used to treat those same symptoms when they occurred in an ill person. He encapsulated his theory in the maxim, 'Similia similibus curentur' (Let like be treated by like).

Over the next few years he worked slavishly to add to his knowledge of the effects of drugs. In his experiments, called provings, he tested the effects of several commonly used medicines on healthy people. Hahnemann correlated all this information, publishing his findings in 1796. Thus was homeopathy born – but perhaps 'reborn' would be more accurate, as research has since shown that Hippocrates, the Greek 'Father of Medicine', had used the same principle of similars centuries earlier.

Since Hahnemann's original work, many more substances have been tested. Indeed, provings are still being carried out and new substances continually being added to the *materia medica*.

Early practitioners of the science soon discovered another feature of homeopathy, namely its greater effectiveness in minute quantities. Conventional scientists were to take another 150 years to discover this fact, but the efficacy of the 'mini-dose' is now widely accepted. Fluoride, for example, is particularly effective against tooth decay when diluted to twelve parts in a million. Similarly, immunization uses minute doses of dead bacteria to stimulate the body into producing antibodies which can fight off specific illnesses – a pure homeopathic response, if you think about it!

However, the tiny doses employed in homeopathic medicine have led to more confusion and doubts in the minds of orthodox medical practitioners than any other feature of homeopathy. But let it be quite clear: homeopathic doctors do *not* use smaller doses of the drugs prescribed by orthodox doctors. They use substances that are homeopathically related to the illness and its many facets.

Consider a viral throat infection, for example, a common illness displaying symptoms that are easily recognized. Apart from a painful sore throat, the patient would be very hot and red-faced, the pupils of the eyes might be dilated, there might be a headache and the patient might even be delirious and hallucinating. Orthodox treatment would only alleviate the symptoms by using paracetamol or a similar painkiller. Homeopathic treatment would be with Belladonna.

Why this particular remedy? Because it is known that Belladonna, if taken in too high a dose, will produce a hot, red face, dilated pupils, a headache and possibly even hallucinations. In other words, if given to a healthy person, it causes the very symptoms that the patient with the throat infection is suffering from. The normally poisonous substance is rendered safe by administering it in a minute dose prepared in the homeopathic manner (see p. 218).

HOMEOPATHY AND ORTHODOX MEDICINE

One of the great disadvantages of orthodox medicine is its strength; it is, if you like, too good. It is certainly too powerful. Not only does it treat the illness for which it has been prescribed, it may also produce alarming side-effects. A recent assessment of hospital admissions revealed the astounding information that nearly 20 per cent of all hospital admissions were the result of previous treatment. Perhaps, on reflection, this is not so surprising; for example, many people get a sore mouth and possibly diarrhoea after taking an antibiotic, while antihistamines can cause drowsiness. Such side-effects are common enough to be accepted as inevitable. In addition, much of modern orthodox medicine is suppressive rather than curative, so once treatment is stopped, the ailment recurs.

So what are the advantages of homeopathic medicine and how does it mix with orthodox treatment? First it must be said that there is no clash between the two systems of treatment and they can, if essential, be taken at the same time. Indeed, practitioners prefer to think of homeopathic medicine as complementary, not alternative, to orthodox medicine. Although there are some drugs which slow down the homeopathic response, none appear to stop it.

Homeopathic remedies are easy to administer, usually in the form of powders, granules, tablets or pills. They have a neutral or sweetish taste which makes them easy to take, especially by children. Injections are rarely used. In acute illnesses, such as tonsillitis, the response to a homeopathic remedy can be astonishingly quick. The Belladonna referred to earlier can, for example, start to lower the temperature in a few minutes. In the treatment of chronic disease a cure may take longer to effect since the disease has probably caused many bodily changes and these may need to be dealt with as the treatment progresses. This process is called constitutional treatment and has been likened to peeling an onion – removing one layer (symptom) after another until the centre (root cause) is reached.

A further advantage of homeopathic treatment is that no side-effects occur. On fairly rare occasions it is possible that a patient's symptoms may worsen for a short while, but if an improvement soon follows, the aggravation is an indication that the remedy is the correct one. A patient who continues to deteriorate, demonstrating no sign of improvement, has simply been prescribed the wrong treatment. Among the homeopathic profession it is becoming increasingly accepted that true aggravations are much less frequent than previously imagined.

Thanks to the manner of their action and their high dilution, homeopathic medicines are extremely safe; in fact, it is impossible to take an overdose. To do this it would be necessary to swallow about 12 million tablets at one go.

In addition to being safe, easy to give, free of side-effects and often quick-acting in acute illness, homeopathic medicines are cheap. An average course of treatment costs very little in comparison with some modern drug regimes.

RESEARCH IN HOMEOPATHY

One of the most frequent but totally inaccurate misconceptions about homeopathy is that the success of its remedies is entirely a placebo response. In other words, any improvement is psychological. Such views are absolute nonsense, as has been proved by work done at the Glasgow Homeopathic Hospital by Dr D. T. Reilly and his associates. A 1986 study into the effects of homeopathic medicine on hay fever emphatically showed that no placebo response was involved. As a bonus, it also revealed that homeopathic treatment for hay fever was more successful than conventional drugs.

Another nail in the coffin of placebo response is the value that homeopathy has in treating animals. As with humans, it has become quite clear that homeopathy not only works, but that it often works many times better than orthodox treatment.

HOMEOPATHY AROUND THE WORLD

There must be very few countries in the world in which it is not possible to consult a homeopath. Western Europe, North and South

America, Asia, Australia, South Africa and even the USSR all have a flourishing interest in homeopathy, but this has not always been the case. In fact, the changing fortune of homeopathy in the United States is particularly noteworthy.

In 1844 the American Institute of Homeopathy was created, homeopathy having been introduced to the country around 1825. It very soon found itself in conflict with the American Medical Association (AMA), an organization which, it is said, was created largely to slow the growth of homeopathy, the success of which was threatening the livelihood of orthodox physicians. In spite of this opposition, homeopathy flourished and by 1900 boasted over 100 hospitals and twenty-two medical colleges.

Unfortunately, the AMA's efforts at discrediting and suppressing homeopathy eventually began to take effect, no doubt aided by the apparent disagreement among homeopaths themselves as to the type of homeopathy to practise. (Classical homeopathy, based largely on the teachings of Hahnemann, administers one remedy at a time. Complex homeopathy, as practised particularly in France and Germany, gives several remedies at the same time, and may also involve the use of electrical devices to make diagnoses and select treatment.) By 1950 all homeopathic colleges in the United States were closed and fewer than 150 homeopathic physicians remained in practice.

After a long time in the doldrums, a renaissance in American homeopathy began to take place. Public interest has burgeoned in recent years and by the 1980s it was estimated that the USA had approximately 1000 physicians specializing in homeopathy – a good sign for the future.

The establishment of homeopathy in Great Britain came about through the efforts of Dr Frederick Quinn, a graduate of Edinburgh University who worked for a short time with Hahnemann himself.

Founder and first president of the British Homeopathic Society, he also founded the first London Homeopathic Hospital in 1849 (it was granted the prefix 'royal' 100 years later).

The Royal Family's interest in homeopathy continues to this day. The Queen has a homeopathic physician, the Queen Mother is patron of the British Homeopathic Association and several family members use homeopathic remedies in their own home treatment of minor illnesses and injuries.

When the National Health Service was started in 1948, the then minister of health gave assurances that homeopathy would remain available within it. Today there are five NHS hospitals in Great Britain – London, Glasgow, Bristol, Liverpool and Tunbridge Wells. A letter of referral from your GP is needed in order to obtain treatment at these places.

Although the NHS charter allows GPs to practise homeopathy and issue prescriptions for homeopathic medicines, few actually do so. Most people have to seek treatment privately. Always look for the letters MFHom or FFHom after a practitioner's name. A list of homeopathic doctors practising in your region may be obtained from the Faculty of Homeopathy (see Useful Addresses, p. 308).

Public interest in homeopathy and other forms of complementary medicine is being mirrored to some extent by the orthodox medical profession. A survey reported in the *British Medical Journal* in June 1986 showed that over 40 per cent of doctors had at some time referred patients to homeopathic physicians.

The Faculty of Homeopathy is responsible for the teaching and advancement of homeopathy throughout Great Britain. In recent years it has seen a doubling in the number of doctors studying under its aegis and it is hoped that before long homeopathy will be taught in all university medical schools so that every doctor will have some knowledge of it by the time he or she qualifies.

HOW TO USE THIS BOOK

The following case history shows you how to choose the correct homeopathic remedy for an illness.

Imagine your sixteen-year-old son, who has occasionally suffered from styes, develops one on his left lower eyelid. When you look at the eye the lids appear swollen and red. He tells you that the tears seem to burn and sting the eye. In fact, the eye is so sore that he cannot bear the slightest touch and describes the pain as sharp and piercing. He is a somewhat clumsy type, forever dropping things. At times you find him rather apathetic and indifferent but put this down to his age.

Details such as these, which you should not find difficult to put together about your own illness or that of a family member, are essential in selecting a remedy. The next step is to consider the following aspects of the ailment in the order given.

1. What part of the body is the illness in? The eye.
2. Turn to the eye section of the book and find the treatment of styes.
3. Read the description of a stye to makes sure you are treating the correct condition.
4. Under Treatment you will see that there are seven remedies.
5. Read the Key Features of each remedy and you will find that the description of Apis fits your son's case best.
6. Now look under Dosage and give the remedy as directed.
7. If you wish to make a final check that you have selected the correct remedy, turn to the description of Apis in the Materia Medica section.
8. The general description confirms that you have chosen a remedy that suits your son's temperament.

9. Main Medical Uses shows that Apis is used for styes.
10. In Major Symptoms the subsection Eyes describes symptoms that are similar to your son's.

Thus, in ten simple steps you have found and confirmed the correct homeopathic treatment for a particular case.

USING THE MATERIA MEDICA

Information on 100 remedies appears in the Materia Medica. Each is listed by its common name (usually abbreviated), with its Latin name underneath. This is followed by a general description, which will help you to match the remedy to the temperament of a particular patient. The conditions for which it is best suited are listed

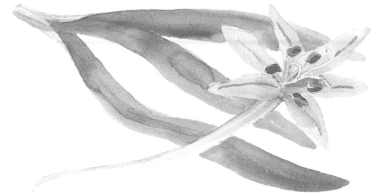

under Main Medical Uses, and more detailed information about its applications appear under Major Symptoms. (Although several symptoms may be listed for each part of the body mentioned, your patient may not exhibit all of them.) Situations that tend to improve or exacerbate a patient's condition appear under the headings Better and Worse.

REFERRING ILLNESSES TO YOUR FAMILY DOCTOR

Very infrequently certain symptoms may be the early signs of a more serious underlying illness. You may feel more secure therefore in using homeopathic medicine after first visiting your family doctor to confirm your diagnosis of what is wrong with you or your child.

Doctors sympathetic to homeopathy (and you'll be pleased to know that many are, and indeed their numbers are growing) will possibly suggest that you try homeopathic treatment first, but if there is no response within a certain period of time, which of course will vary from illness to illness, you make use of the prescription he has given you for a customary medicine. As you grow more confident in the use of homeopathy, you will find that the occasions when you need the conventional medication grow less and less.

Remember, however, that if you do initially use homeopathy successfully, you will be confirming what all homeopaths already know – that homeopathy really works. You will then feel more comfortable in using it again and again when necessary.

The inclusion of an illness in either the treatment section or materia medica section of this book does not necessarily mean that it is suitable for home treatment without expert medical advice. There is no reason, however, why homeopathic and conventional treatment should not be given at the same time. Even when a patient is receiving orthodox treatment, the addition of a homeopathic remedy may help the case, but do first obtain your doctor's approval for this. Showing him this short statement may be helpful.

With regard to homeopathic constitutional treatment for chronic (long-standing) conditions, remedies should be selected and used only under the supervision of a qualified homeopathic doctor, or after initial diagnosis by a trained professional homeopath.

TREATMENT SECTION

EMERGENCIES AND FIRST AID

CONTENTS

Abrasions and Grazes	16
Bleeding, Heavy	16
Bruises	18
Burns and Scalds, including Sunburn	18
Cuts, Lacerations and Incised Wounds	19
Fainting	19
Fits, Temperature	20
Fractures	21
Head Injuries, including Concussion	21
Heart Attack	22
Heatstroke	23
Insect Bites and Stings	23
Panic Attacks	24
Punctured Wounds	24
Shock and Collapse	25
Sprains and Strains	26
Stroke	26
Suffocation	27

*H*omeopathic medicines are of special value in the treatment of unexpected medical emergencies, and as first-aid treatment for many of the minor, and sometimes major, injuries that occur in everyday life. Some of the conditions in this section are serious and acute medical emergencies, such as heart attacks and strokes. It is not expected that you will treat such conditions on your own, but homeopathic remedies can be used as very valuable first-aid measures while waiting for the doctor or ambulance to arrive.

It is generally accepted that homeopathic remedies are best taken between meals and not too close to eating, drinking, smoking (shame on you if you still do!) or cleaning the teeth. Quite obviously, this rule does not apply if a person has a heart attack in the middle of eating a large meal. Get the homeopathic remedy into the patient's mouth as soon as possible and use it according to the dosage instructions you will find with the treatment advice for each emergency condition mentioned in this section.

If you are very new to homeopathy and have not yet acquired a stock of homeopathic medicines, one remedy above all others should be obtained because of its almost universal value in the treatment of injuries. This remedy is called Arnica and it is used for any condition where there is bruising – either physical bruising after suffering an injury, or mental bruising such as one might experience when undertaking a lengthy journey, or after a difficult interview.

Do remember that homeopathic remedies can be used at the same time as conventional medicine. Indeed, your doctor's recommended treatment may be greatly enhanced by the addition of a homeopathic remedy and the recovery time from the emergency or accident greatly reduced. However, do discuss such a course of action with your doctor first.

Occasionally it is found that some symptoms occur a long time after an accident. By using the appropriate homeopathic remedy that you *would* have used at the time, such symptoms can be removed. For example, you may begin to suffer from headaches which start for no apparent reason and for which your doctor can find no cause. Looking back you remember a blow to the head some years previously but which caused no problem at the time. By using the homeopathic remedy Natrum sulph, which is used for head injuries, it is possible to stop the headaches because at last you have treated the root cause of the problem.

ABRASIONS AND GRAZES

When the skin surface becomes damaged by scraping or rubbing, the resulting injury is known as an abrasion or graze. It most often occurs from a sliding fall and the raw area produced will then be dirty and may have grit embedded in it. The wound should be carefully cleaned with warm water and any dirt or grit removed before using Calendula or Hypericum lotion as outlined below. A ready-mixed lotion of Calendula and Hypericum, known as Hypercal, is available from homeopathic pharmacies.

Dirty wounds require a tetanus injection.

KEY FEATURES	TREATMENT
Use first to lessen the risk of infection	CALENDULA 6 three times a day for five days.
Very painful and sensitive graze	CALENDULA LOTION (15 drops of the mother tincture in 8 fl oz (250 ml) of cool, previously boiled water) can be applied after cleaning the area with water. HYPERICUM 6 three times a day for three days. HYPERICUM LOTION (15 drops of the mother tincture in 8 fl oz (250 ml) of water) can be applied as a moist dressing.
If the wound becomes infected	HEPAR SULPH 30 three times a day for four days.

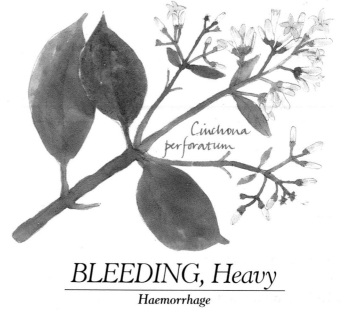

Cinchona perforatum

BLEEDING, *Heavy*
Haemorrhage

When a blood vessel is cut, blood runs out. If the vessel is an artery, the blood is bright red and pumps out with each heartbeat; if it is a vein, the blood is darker, runs out more evenly and under less pressure. Fortunately, the body has ways of slowing down or even stopping bleeding – the blood vessel ends contract and a clot forms which plugs the opening. Bleeding from surface blood vessels is usually due to a direct injury such as a cut, but it can also occur within many organs of the body. For example, it may occur in the stomach from an ulcer or in the bladder from inflammation or a growth. For treatment of nosebleeds see p. 41.

As well as using homeopathic treatment, the necessary first-aid procedures should be carried out while waiting for medical assistance.

Unexplained bleeding anywhere in the body requires medical attention and, possibly, investigation.

KEY FEATURES	TREATMENT
Sense of panic and great restlessness Desire for ice-cold drinks	ACONITE
After any form of injury, especially when bruising may be present	ARNICA
Restlessness with anxiety and marked exhaustion	ARS ALB
Loss of bright red blood which clots easily The head is hot, the face red	BELLADONNA
Signs of collapse with cold, clammy sweat and air hunger Steady seepage of dark blood	CARBO VEG
Faintness and weakness with ringing in the ears The blood is dark, almost brown Post-partum haemorrhage (bleeding after childbirth)	CHINA
The blood is profuse, bright red and clots easily Nosebleeds	FERRUM PHOS
Slow but steady flow of dark blood Feeling of exhaustion but no anxiety Bleeding from piles	HAMAMELIS
The blood is bright red Persistent bleeding, but in fits and starts Feeling of emptiness in the stomach Desire for ice-cold drinks Bleeding from polyps and fibroids	PHOSPHORUS
Brisk flow of blood with dark clots With pelvic pain Bleeding from a miscarriage	SABINA
Intestinal haemorrhage with severe collapse	VERATRUM ALB

DOSAGE

The selected remedy should be taken in the 30 potency and repeated at five-minute intervals until an improvement is maintained.

BRUISES

When a blood vessel becomes damaged by an injury and a seepage of blood occurs, this will show as a blue-purple discoloration under the skin that is known as a bruise. If the area involved is large, there may be considerable pain and swelling.

KEY FEATURES	TREATMENT
Use first for all bruises	ARNICA 30 three times a day for two or three days, depending on the severity and extent of the bruising.
Only if the skin is unbroken	ARNICA LOTION (5 drops of the mother tincture in 8 fl oz (250 ml) water) may be used as a compress for about fifteen minutes.
If the bruise is slow to subside	LEDUM 12 twice a day for five days.

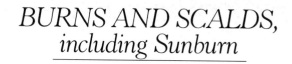

Calendula officinalis

BURNS AND SCALDS,
including Sunburn

Burns are injuries caused by heat, certain chemicals, electricity, extreme cold and radiation. When the heat is 'dry' we refer to the injury as a burn; if it is 'moist' heat, as for example from steam, it becomes known as a scald. The seriousness of the injury depends upon the size and depth of the burn or scald. A burn more than 1 inch (2 cm) square which goes deeper than the very surface of the skin needs medical attention.

All but very small and minor burns and scalds require medical attention after immediate first aid.

KEY FEATURES	TREATMENT
As there is always fright and shock, first give	ACONITE 200 one dose.
In severe cases follow Aconite with	CANTHARIS 30 at fifteen-minute intervals until there is pain relief.
Minor redness of the skin	URTICA 30 at thirty-minute intervals until there is relief.

Moist dressings of Urtica lotion (15 drops of mother tincture to 8 fl oz (250 ml) of cold, previously boiled water) should be placed on the area involved. Once on they should be kept moist and left undisturbed.

CONCUSSION

(see Head Injuries, p. 21)

CUTS, LACERATIONS AND INCISED WOUNDS

If the skin becomes damaged by being torn open, treatment to some extent depends upon the type of damage produced. A cut from a sharp knife or razor blade is known as an incised wound and it may bleed very freely because the damaged blood vessels cannot shut down easily. Wounds with irregular edges are called lacerations. These tend to bleed less freely but are more likely to become infected. Firm pressure or squeezing the edge of the wound together will usually stop the bleeding. A firm, clean dressing may then be put over the site.

As tetanus spores thrive in dirt, it is advisable to get a tetanus injection for all wounds that occur in dirty situations. The same applies to animal bites that draw blood.

KEY FEATURES	TREATMENT
For immediate shock	ACONITE 200 one dose.
With much bruising	ARNICA 30 half an hour later.
If the wound is deep and/or extensive, with much pain	HYPERICUM 30 three times a day for three to four days.
With much bleeding and if infection is likely	CALENDULA 30 three times a day for four to five days.
Cuts from a sharp instrument	STAPHISAGRIA 30 one dose. Then apply a dressing moistened with CALENDULA and HYPERICUM lotions (5 drops of each tincture in 8 fl oz (250 ml) of cooled, previously boiled water). To assist healing, follow with CALENDULA 12 twice a day for three days.

FAINTING

Fainting is due to a temporary lack of oxygen to the brain. It can follow any sort of emotional upset or disturbance.

Frequent or repeated fainting attacks require expert medical investigation.

KEY FEATURES	TREATMENT
After a fright or with severe pain	ACONITE
With anaemia	ACETIC ACID
From overeating	ANT TART
From fear, shortage of breath and stomach-ache	ARS ALB
On sitting up after lying down	BRYONIA

19

Due to stooping	ELAPS
After exertion	GLONOINE
From wearing tight clothes	LACHESIS
In a warm room	LILIUM TIG
With hysteria and while eating	MOSCHUS

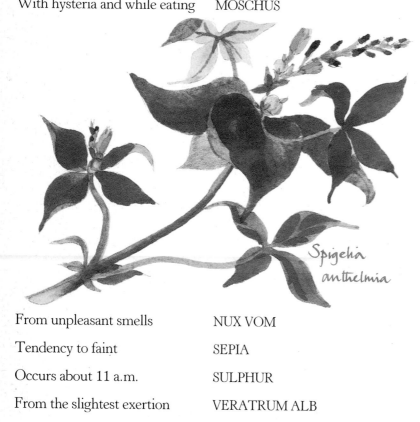

Spigelia anthelmia

From unpleasant smells	NUX VOM
Tendency to faint	SEPIA
Occurs about 11 a.m.	SULPHUR
From the slightest exertion	VERATRUM ALB

DOSAGE

The selected remedy should be taken in the 200 potency, if it is available, otherwise use the potency nearest to this. Crush a tablet and place a few grains on the patient's tongue. In view of the temporary nature of a faint, one such dose should be sufficient.

FITS, TEMPERATURE
Febrile convulsions

As these are purely due to a raised temperature, cooling the patient (usually a child) may be of considerable benefit. The temperature control mechanism in very young children is not fully developed, so very high temperatures may develop quite quickly and it is these that lead to fits. As the child ages, the chance of these convulsions occurring diminishes almost totally. Although they may not be related to epileptic fits, convulsions in children or adults need hospital investigation.

First-aid procedures should be carried out while waiting for medical assistance. Homeopathic remedies may be administered once the patient is calm.

KEY FEATURES	TREATMENT
Sudden onset of fever Bright red head and body Hot sweat on the body With delirium Much sensitivity to noise and light Dilated pupils	BELLADONNA
While teething The child is very restless and cries incessantly One cheek is red, the other pale	CHAMOMILLA
After too much sun The head is hot and congested The face is dusky red	GLONOINE

Fits during infectious diseases
The head rolls from side to side
The feet are restless and the
  legs jerk while asleep   ZINC MET

DOSAGE

The selected remedy should be taken in the 30 potency if possible, otherwise use the highest potency you have. Crush one tablet and place a few grains on the patient's tongue. Repeat every few minutes until an improvement occurs.

FRACTURES

A fracture is a broken bone. Depending on the site of the injury, there is usually pain, which is increased by attempting to move the part. Swelling and tenderness develop and in a bad fracture the affected part may appear deformed. First-aid treatment should be given to prevent any movement of the fractured bone ends as this can lead to further damage and cause considerable pain and shock.

All fractures require hospital attention. Use first-aid procedures and initial homeopathic treatment as soon as possible after the injury is sustained.

KEY FEATURES	TREATMENT
For shock and pain first give	ACONITE 200 one dose.
For bruising and soft tissue damage follow with	ARNICA 200 one dose followed by ARNICA 30 three times a day for four days.

After this and to aid bony union	SYMPHYTUM 12 twice a day for two weeks.
If healing and union are slow, as in the elderly	CALC PHOS 12 twice a day for a further four to eight weeks.

HEAD INJURIES, including Concussion

Any blow to the head should be considered potentially dangerous. Children are particularly prone to these injuries, but fortunately, serious damage is rare. However, any injury that leads to a concussion (a loss of consciousness, even momentary), should be regarded as serious.

All but the minor bumps and bangs, which may produce local tenderness and bruising, require medical attention. Immediate first-aid procedures should always be carried out.

KEY FEATURES	TREATMENT
First give	ARNICA 30 and repeat half-hourly for six doses.
If there are signs of brain irritation, i.e. confusion, muscular twitching and spasms, dilated pupils	CICUTA 30 three times a day until improvement occurs.
For persistent headaches after a head injury	NAT SULPH 30 three times a day until relief is obtained.

HEART ATTACK

Coronary thrombosis/Myocardial infarction

The symptoms are a sudden, agonizing, constricting chest pain which may radiate to the neck, jaw or arms, mainly the left. The patient is usually in shock – cold and sweaty with a grey complexion and a shallow, rapid pulse. The pain does not pass off with rest.

Sudden severe chest pain for which there is no apparent cause requires urgent diagnosis by a doctor. Homeopathic treatment and first-aid procedures should be used while waiting for medical assistance.

KEY FEATURES	TREATMENT
Great anxiety with difficulty in breathing, plus numbness and tingling in the fingers	ACONITE
The patient feels better sitting up	
Chest pain after exertion or fatigue	ARNICA
The chest feels sore and bruised	
The heart feels as if grasped in a fist	CACTUS
The lower part of the chest feels tied down and the pain makes the patient cry out	
Weakness and numbness in the left arm	DIGITALIS
The skin has a blue tinge	
The patient fears the heart will stop if he moves about	
The patient wakes from sleep feeling smothered and unable to lie flat	LACHESIS
Violent chest and left-arm pain, the pulse is very rapid and the patient has great difficulty in breathing	LATRODECTUS
The pain wakes the patient with the heart feeling as if trapped in a vice	LILIUM TIG
The patient has to bend double to try to ease the pain	
Palpitations, irregular pulse with paroxysms of suffocation and tightness across the upper chest	TABACUM

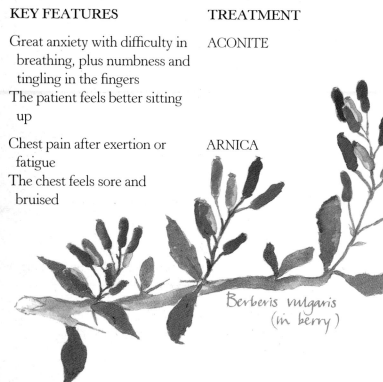

Berberis vulgaris (in berry)

DOSAGE

Use the selected remedy in the highest potency you have and repeat at five-minute intervals until relief is obtained.

HEATSTROKE

Exposure to high temperatures, particularly with high humidity, may lead to this condition. Early symptoms are headache, dizziness, nausea and lassitude. These may quickly lead on to muscle cramps, convulsions, collapse and coma.

Medical help is required. As well as using homeopathic treatment, first-aid procedures to cool the patient should be carried out.

KEY FEATURES	TREATMENT
Of sudden onset, with burning, hot, dry skin, dilated pupils and delirium	BELLADONNA 30
Severe headache, worse on attempting to move or even sit up	BRYONIA 30
With severe muscle cramps	CUPRUM MET 30
Throbbing headache with a hot red face and generalized sweating	GLONOINE 30

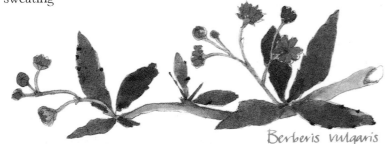

Berberis vulgaris

DOSAGE

The selected remedy should be repeated at two-hourly intervals until an improvement is maintained.

INSECT BITES AND STINGS

If the sting is left in the skin, try to remove it carefully with tweezers but do not squeeze the sting as its poison will be forced out into the skin. If a sting occurs in the mouth, or if there are multiple stings, the patient should be taken to a hospital.

KEY FEATURES	TREATMENT
In all cases use first	LEDUM 30 every hour for four doses.
If there is a lot of burning, stinging and rapid swelling	APIS 30 every hour for four doses.
If the area is red, hot and angry-looking	CANTHARIS 30 three times a day for four days.
Bee sting	CARBOLIC ACID 30 every hour for three doses. URTICA mother tincture dabbed on the sting will soothe it.
Gnat, Sandfly or Marchfly bites	HYPERICUM mother tincture dabbed on the bites will soothe them.
Wasp sting	LEDUM mother tincture dabbed on the sting will soothe it.
If the area remains cold, numb and very sensitive, but better after a cold dressing	LEDUM 30 three times a day for four days.

If the area is hot and blue	TARENTULA 30 three times a day for three days.
With an itchy, blotchy allergic type of skin reaction	URTICA 30 every hour until relief is obtained.

PANIC ATTACKS

This is a distressing condition which is often totally irrational. Homeopathic treatment induces calm and confidence.

KEY FEATURES	TREATMENT
After a severe fright The patient is impatient and difficult to calm Arising after an accident	ACONITE 30
Great apprehension and panic in a crowded place Fear of heights Before exams or interviews	ARG NIT 30
Restless with great anxiety and unease Irrational fears develop Symptoms worsen if the patient is alone	ARS ALB 30
Trembling and shaking; the patient feels unable to move and needs to be held firmly	GELSEMIUM 30
After a violent shock or shattering experience	OPIUM 30 *(prescription required in US)*

DOSAGE

The selected remedy should be taken every thirty minutes until an improvement is maintained.

PUNCTURED WOUNDS

Any sharp object such as a nail, needle or garden fork can produce a puncture wound. If it is deep, there is considerable risk of infection having been introduced by the sharp object, and injury to deeper tissues may also have been caused.

Punctured wounds require a tetanus injection.

KEY FEATURES	TREATMENT
Immediately after injury	LEDUM 30 three times a day for two to three days.
If the wound remains painful after this	HYPERICUM 6 three times a day for three to four days.
If the area remains cold and numb, and is sensitive to touch, getting relief from cold applications	LEDUM 6 four times a day for four days.
If a splinter remains in the wound	SILICA 12 four times a day until it becomes removable.
If the area becomes infected, hot, red swollen and painful	HEPAR SULPH 30 three times a day for four days.

SHOCK AND COLLAPSE

Shock occurs after severe injuries, bleeding or burns and is due to the reduced blood volume and blood pressure that these conditions can produce. It may follow a nervous shock, such as a severe fright or the receipt of bad news. Symptoms occur because insufficient oxygen gets to the nervous system and other tissues. The patient will have pale, cold, clammy, grey-coloured skin, shallow breathing, a weak pulse and appear restless. In lesser shock the patient may just feel shaky for a few minutes, or go into a faint.

As well as using homeopathic treatment, first-aid procedures should be carried out while waiting for medical assistance.

KEY FEATURES	TREATMENT
From sudden fright or shattering experience Extreme terror, restlessness, rapid pulse and soaking sweat	ACONITE
From trauma The patient is pale, panting and pulseless, and either belittles the situation or feels that death is imminent	ARNICA
Great restlessness and anxiety with a worried or even terrified expression The pulse is weak or irregular The lower eyelids are puffy	ARS ALB
Icy coldness with blueish, shrivelled-looking skin The lips become drawn back, showing the teeth, the voice high-pitched or husky The patient throws off the bedclothes The eyes are upturned or closed	CAMPHOR
Air hunger with cold breath; the patient wants to be fanned Feeling of coldness, particularly around the knees	CARBO VEG
After haemorrhage	CHINA
The skin is cold and resembles marble Beads of cold sweat appear on the forehead Pale, drawn and sunken face Weak barely perceptible pulse Watery saliva dribbles from the mouth The lips, hands and nails are blue Death is imminent	VERATRUM ALB

DOSAGE

Use the selected remedy in the highest potency you have. Crush a tablet and place a few grains on the patient's tongue. Repeat every few minutes until an improvement occurs.

SPRAINS AND STRAINS

A sprain occurs if the tissues around a joint are suddenly stretched or torn. There will be pain, tenderness and swelling, which are all increased by movement of the joint. A cold compress applied as soon as possible after the injury will be helpful in reducing the amount of swelling that occurs.
A strain develops when a muscle is overstretched or torn by a sudden violent movement and is diagnosed by the occurrence of a sudden sharp pain and swelling at the injury site. Sprains and strains are sometimes difficult to distinguish from a fracture because of the large amount of damage caused. In these circumstances they should be treated as a fracture and the patient taken to a hospital.

All but minor sprains should have medical attention if they fail to improve after twenty-four hours or if the diagnosis is in doubt.

KEY FEATURES	TREATMENT
For the initial bruising, swelling, pain and shock	ARNICA 30 every hour for four doses.
Followed with	RHUS TOX 6 four times a day until the symptoms are relieved, or
If the injury is close to a bony surface which is sore, use instead of Rhus tox	RUTA 6 four times a day until the symptoms are relieved.
If the injury is close to a joint which becomes swollen and painful on movement	BRYONIA 30 three times a day for three days followed by RHUS TOX 6 as above.

STROKE

Apoplexy/Cerebral haemorrhage/Cerebral thrombosis

This is caused by a sudden cutting off of the blood supply to part of the brain. The symptoms will vary according to the area involved and the amount of damage to the brain tissue, and can be anything from loss or diminution of muscle power in the affected part of the body to total coma and eventual death.

As well as using homeopathic treatment, first-aid procedures should be carried out while waiting for medical assistance.

KEY FEATURES	TREATMENT
Anxiety in the early stage of a minor stroke	ACONITE 30 one dose should be given as soon after the event as possible.
After taking Aconite, for the first few days	ARNICA 30 one dose three times a day for three days.
For an unconscious patient	ARNICA 200 one crushed tablet should be placed under or on the tongue.
Dusky, flushed, collapsed patient with a slow pulse and dilated pupils	OPIUM 200 one crushed tablet should be placed under or on the tongue.
In a patient with known high blood pressure	STRYCHNINUM 200 one crushed tablet should be placed under or on the tongue.

SUFFOCATION

Asphyxia

This condition occurs when the blood is unable to obtain sufficient oxygen due to some interference with respiration. The skin will have a purplish appearance and breathing may be irregular, eventually ceasing altogether. Possible causes include: obstruction of the air passages after choking or drowning; the tongue being swallowed while unconscious; the effects of drugs or electric shock; injuries to the chest wall; poisoning by carbon monoxide from household gas or car exhaust fumes.

First-aid procedures should be carried out while waiting for medical help. Once consciousness has been regained, homeopathic remedies may be administered.

KEY FEATURES	TREATMENT
The face is cold, blue, pale and covered with cold sweat The chin and lower jaw quiver Coughing and gasping occur alternately	ANT TART
Due to swelling of the tongue or throat	APIS
Due to gas or charcoal fumes	BOVISTA
The face is puffy, pale, blue or mottled and covered in cold sweat The patient cannot get enough air (air hunger) and feels ice cold	CARBO VEG
The pulse is weak Collapse due to loss of body fluids through diarrhoea, vomiting or bleeding, drugs, or chronic illness	
The face is cold and blue The patient gasps for breath and clutches the heart	LAUROCERASUS
Irregular noisy breathing with long pauses between breaths The face is red and bloated with contracted pupils, and the patient stuporous or comatose	OPIUM *(prescription required in US)*

DOSAGE

The selected remedy should be used in the highest potency you possess. Crush a tablet and place a few grains on the patient's tongue. Repeat every few minutes until an improvement occurs.

Bryonia alba

SUNBURN

(see Burns and Scalds, p. 18)

27

CHILDREN'S AILMENTS

CONTENTS

Bed-wetting	28
Colds and Influenza	29
Colic	30
Constipation	31
Coughs	32
Croup	33
Diarrhoea	34
Digestive Upsets	35
Earache with Discharge	36
Earache without Discharge	37
Eczema	37
Feeding Problems	38
Headache	39
Nappy (Diaper) Rash	40
Nightmares	40
Nosebleeds	41
Sleep Problems	41
Throat, Sore	42
Toothache and Teething Problems	42
Vomiting	43

Children respond particularly well to homeopathic medicine. Of its many advantages, three in particular stand out: it is pleasant to the taste, so easy to take; it is painless (injections are rarely used); it is safe enough to use even with a new born baby.

The remedy is best given as a powder. This can be obtained from the chemist, or made at home by crushing a tablet or pill between two clean, dry spoons. It may then be given directly into the mouth or dissolved in water first.

BED-WETTING
Nocturnal enuresis

As this problem is very occasionally caused by an infection or a defect in the urinary tract, it is advisable to consult your doctor before starting to use homeopathic treatment.

KEY FEATURES	TREATMENT
Restless sleep in nervous, excitable children who pass frequent but small amounts of urine	BELLADONNA 30
Highly coloured urine smelling strongly of ammonia	BENZOIC ACID 30
The urine is passed in the first sleep After excitement during the day In weak children with dark shadows under the eyes	CAUSTICUM 30
Constant nightly wetting and the urine looks cloudy	EQUISETUM 30

In heavy sleepers who wet in the first sleep — KREOSOTE 30

In girls who wet during the day as well as at night

Profuse, pale watery urine — PULSATILLA 30

DOSAGE

The selected remedy should be taken one hour before bedtime, with a second dose at bedtime.

COLDS AND INFLUENZA

The common cold is an infection caused by a very widespread virus. Symptoms include a runny nose, which can cause problems with breathing through the nose and with feeding in young children and babies, headache, sore throat, cough, generalized aching and malaise. The temperature is raised, but the whole illness is usually over within a few days. Influenza produces virtually the same symptoms, but they tend to be more severe and last for a longer period.

Atropa belladonna

KEY FEATURES	TREATMENT
After exposure to cold, dry weather or to winds and draughts Chilliness followed by fever, the nose is dry and feels blocked Bouts of sneezing	ACONITE 30 three doses over 6 hours
The nose is sore from an acrid, burning discharge, worse in a warm room Profuse, bland watering of the eyes Prolonged sneezing	ALLIUM CEPA 30
A thin, watery nasal discharge makes the upper lip sore The patient is very chilly The eyes water Much sneezing occurs Thirst for cold drinks	ARS ALB 30
Blocked nose with yellow nasal catarrh The nostrils become sore	ARUM TRIPH 30
Shivering and sneezing Great chilliness, or the patient feels hot and cold alternately	DULCAMARA 30
Catarrhal snuffles in children when the nose seems blocked	ELAPS 30
A cold of slow onset with general malaise and body ache The head is hot and feels full The patient is very chilly Sneezing accompanied by a bland, watery nasal discharge Colds in mild, damp weather Sore throat	GELSEMIUM 30

Violent sneezing	MERCURIUS 30
The nose drips a green-yellow, offensive discharge	
Sore throat, hoarse voice, and tickly dry cough, with bad breath and profuse sweating	
The patient feels chilly and shaky	
In cold, dry weather	NUX VOM 30
The nose is alternately blocked and running, blocked at night, running during the day	
Much sneezing and the throat feels scraped	
The patient is unable to get warm	
Persistent cold with a thick, bland, yellow nasal discharge	PULSATILLA 30
The lips are chapped and sore	
Pain in the face and nose which feels stuffed at night, but runs in the morning and out of doors	
Better in fresh air	

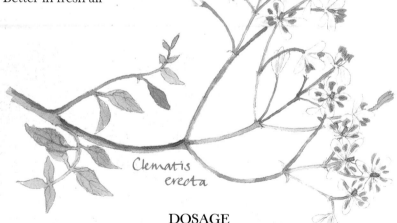

Clematis
erecta

DOSAGE

With the exception of Aconite, which, if taken early enough in an attack, will prevent it becoming a full-blown cold, the selected remedy should be taken four times a day until there is an improvement. It may then be stopped.

COLIC

This may occur frequently during the first few months of life. The child is usually restless and cries, drawing up its legs with the spasmodic abdominal pain. Wind may be passed but this gives only temporary relief. Older children may also suffer from colic but this is usually associated with constipation, flatulence and dietary indiscretions.

If the baby sleeps between pain spasms, screams with the pain, is pale, looks shocked and passes a loose, blood-stained stool (like redcurrant jelly), a doctor should be called immediately.

KEY FEATURES	TREATMENT
Colic with flatulence, but passing wind does not relieve the pain	CHAMOMILLA 12
The abdomen is distended and sensitive to touch	
The child is irritable and calms only for a few minutes if carried	
Local warmth helps the pain	
Extreme restlessness with moaning between spasms, twisting and doubling up the body to try to relieve the pain	COLOCYNTH 12
Relief from warmth and gentle pressure	MAG PHOS 12
Flatulence and constipation in an irritable and angry child	NUX VOM 12
Colic from overfeeding	
Violent colic with abdominal rumbling and obstinate constipation	PLUMBUM 12

Flatulent colic with vomiting in a child who stops crying if picked up — PULSATILLA 12

DOSAGE

The selected remedy should be taken every thirty minutes until the child gains some relief. No more than three doses should be taken. If by then there is no improvement *a doctor should be consulted.*

CONSTIPATION

In this condition, the bowel is opened less frequently than normal. The stool may be hard, and painful and difficult to pass. Often due to wrong feeding, it may produce quite severe colicky abdominal pain. Giving the child more to drink and increasing the fibre in the diet may be all that is required to cure this condition.

KEY FEATURES	TREATMENT
A soft, sticky or hard, dry stool, both difficult to pass	ALUMINA 6
A hard, dry, dark, lumpy stool makes defaecation difficult due to a lack of urge	BRYONIA 6
A large, smelly stool of many lumps stuck together with mucus No real urge to defaecate and the stool is painful to pass	GRAPHITES 6
A hard, dry stool which is painful to pass	LYCOPODIUM 6
Light-coloured and crumbly stools	MAG MUR 6

Frequent, ineffectual urging and only an incomplete stool is passed, so the rectum feels unemptied
The patient is chilly and irritable — NUX VOM 6

Complete lack of desire
The stool is composed of hard little balls
The appetite is very poor — OPIUM 6 *(prescription required in US)*

Hard stools which may slip back when partially expelled — SILICA 6

The stool is hard, dry, black and smelly
Anal irritation with pain and burning on defaecation
Reluctance to defaecate because of the pain — SULPHUR 6

DOSAGE

The selected remedy should be taken three times a day until an improvement occurs. It may then be reduced to twice a day for three days, once a day for three days and then stopped.

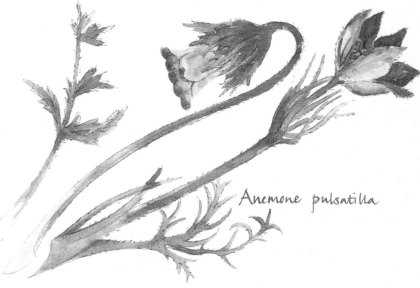

Anemone pulsatilla

CONVULSIONS

(see Fits, p. 20)

COUGHS

Most coughing in young children and babies is due to catarrh in the upper part of the respiratory tract. It is often worse during the night when a 'post-nasal drip' develops; catarrh runs down the throat from the back of the nose causing irritation and coughing.

If the illness appears to worsen, if the breathing becomes difficult or laboured and if the temperature remains raised, medical advice should be sought.

KEY FEATURES	TREATMENT
A hard, dry, barking cough with little or no expectoration The illness has a sudden onset, after being in cold, dry weather With a slight fever The child is anxious and restless	ACONITE 30
A persistent cough with whistling and rattling respiration The cough sounds loose but it is difficult to get phlegm up The patient needs to sit up to avoid a sense of suffocation when lying down *All these symptoms require urgent medical help.* *Use Ant tart while waiting.*	ANT TART 30
A dry, tickly cough with violent, painful bursts of coughing that make the child cry	BELLADONNA 30
A hard, dry, spasmodic cough The chest is painful on coughing and a headache is often present as well The patient wants long, cold drinks All movement is painful	BRYONIA 30
A crowing cough relieved by drinking cold water	CUPRUM MET 30

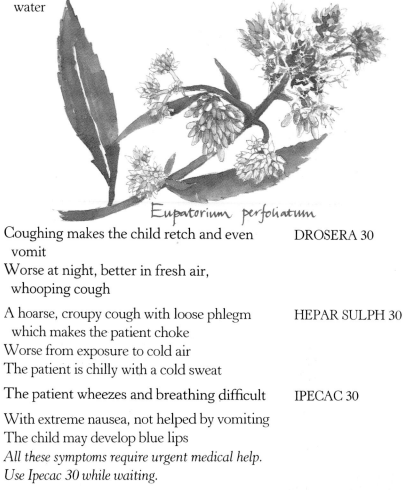

Eupatorium perfoliatum

Coughing makes the child retch and even vomit Worse at night, better in fresh air, whooping cough	DROSERA 30
A hoarse, croupy cough with loose phlegm which makes the patient choke Worse from exposure to cold air The patient is chilly with a cold sweat	HEPAR SULPH 30
The patient wheezes and breathing difficult With extreme nausea, not helped by vomiting The child may develop blue lips *All these symptoms require urgent medical help.* *Use Ipecac 30 while waiting.*	IPECAC 30

A hard barking cough which seems to start in the stomach	KALI BICH 30
Yellow, stringy phlegm which is difficult to get up	
A dry, hard, tickly cough with rawness in the larynx and below the breastbone	PHOSPHORUS 30
The patient has to hold his chest to prevent it hurting while coughing	
The amount of coughing produces a headache	
Any temperature change makes the cough worse	
A persistent choking cough with thick, yellow, loose phlegm	PULSATILLA 30
The cough is worse in a warm room and in the evening	
The patient is neither hungry nor thirsty and prefers the window to be open	
A hard, dry, barking, almost croupy cough, worse at night	STICTA 30
Little or no phlegm	
A hard, ringing, metallic-sounding cough, worse for deep breathing and helped by warm or hot drinks	SPONGIA 30

DOSAGE

In treating coughs the chosen remedy should be taken four times a day for three days and then less frequently, depending upon the response from the patient.

CROUP

This condition can occur during a cold or cough but may also start for no apparent reason. It may come on quite quickly and last for several hours. There is spasm of the vocal cords which makes breathing in difficult and causes a crowing noise to be produced. A barking cough frequently occurs at the same time. Croup will improve in a warm, moist atmosphere, which may be produced by boiling a kettle in the patient's room while starting the homeopathic treatment.

Croup is a serious condition. If there is no improvement within half an hour of starting homeopathic treatment, or if the symptoms become worse and/or the child develops blue lips, a doctor should be called immediately.

Three homeopathic remedies are used to treat croup. They are taken one at a time in the following order, leaving ten minutes between each dose:

ACONITE 30 – HEPAR SULPH 30 – SPONGIA 30

After this, take the following remedies alternately at fifteen-minute intervals until an improvement occurs and is maintained:

HEPAR SULPH 30 – SPONGIA 30

DIAPER RASH

(see Nappy Rash, p. 40)

DIARRHOEA

Simple diarrhoea in children is usually a self-limiting condition, the only treatment required being a good intake of fluid to replace that lost and to prevent dehydration, particularly in very young children. This is much more likely to occur in very hot weather. Homeopathic treatment will shorten the length of the illness, so may be used even if a 'fluids only' regime is recommended by your doctor. Nervous diarrhoea is also a problem in children and responds well to homeopathic medicines.

If dehydration is suspected expert medical help must be sought.

KEY FEATURES	TREATMENT
After exposure to cold dry winds or as a result of a fright Brought on by cold drinks	ACONITE 12
From food poisoning With vomiting, often at the same time With restlessness and anxiety Worse during the night The rectum feels burnt by the watery diarrhoea Thirst for small quantities of warm drinks	ARS ALB 12
With teething The child is peevish and fretful, worse in the evening The stool is frothy, offensive and greenish	CHAMOMILLA 12
Painless, watery, offensive, yellow stools The patient shows extreme weakness After eating too much fruit	CHINA 12
Painful, cramping colic relieved by pressure or bending double Thin, spluttery, copious, yellow stools immediately after eating	COLOCYNTH 12

Paris quadrifolia

Painless, profuse, watery stools containing undigested food Of nervous origin	PHOS ACID 12
Profuse, spluttery, watery, 'pea-soup'-like diarrhoea Worse in the early morning and often preceded by painful colic The stool is extremely offensive The diarrhoea is followed by a feeling of great weakness	PODOPHYLLUM 12
Diarrhoea and vomiting occur together The patient is icy cold with a cold sweat, asks for cold water and wants to be in the cold, fresh air Faintness	VERATRUM ALB 12

DOSAGE

The selected remedy should be taken hourly until an improvement is maintained.

DIGESTIVE UPSETS/NAUSEA

Children can suffer from indigestion and this may show itself by a change in appetite, nausea and/or vomiting, or even an alteration in bowel habit, producing either constipation or diarrhoea. The sensation felt by the patient, usually in the 'pit' (upper middle part) of the stomach, is best described as a discomfort rather than a pain.

Children also often complain of nausea. This may be due to an emotional cause, such as the stress of attending school for the first time, or it can be an early symptom of another illness, such as one of the infectious diseases. As it can also precede disorders of the alimentary tract, such as appendicitis, it is always wise to obtain a medical opinion for unexplained nausea, but do remember that a common cause is over-indulgence in sweets or ice-cream.

KEY FEATURES	TREATMENT
Nausea and/or vomiting straight after eating The tongue is white-coated Nausea and loss of appetite Distension from overeating	ANT CRUD 30
Craving for sweet things which produce much flatulence Discomfort relieved by pressure on the abdomen, or by bending double Often related to nervous apprehension	ARG NIT 30
Burning pain soon after eating Sensation of a stone in the stomach	ARS ALB 30
Better after a warm drink or after vomiting Loss of appetite Nausea comes on after midnight	
Tenderness in the pit of the stomach radiates to the chest and back Bloating with offensive, sour-tasting wind Belching gives temporary relief Worse for even the simplest food	CARBO VEG 30
Stomach upsets in weakly children who are often sleepy while eating With excessive flatulence Nausea from over-excitement	KALI CARB 30
Ravenous hunger which, if not satisfied, causes headache Sour taste, sour belching, and sour vomiting	LYCOPODIUM 30
Discomfort about an hour after eating makes the patient bad-tempered Nausea with empty retching Excessive hunger From too rich a diet; symptoms are worse in the morning	NUX VOM 30
Flatulence relieved by belching The tongue is coated and white After eating rich, fatty or very cold food Nausea caused by excess catarrh Worse in the evening	PULSATILLA 30

DOSAGE

The selected remedy should be taken three times a day for three days

EARACHE with Discharge

Untreated inflammation of the ear, leading to an accumulation of pus (see p. 37) may eventually cause the eardrum to burst and release a pus-like discharge into the outer ear passage. With its release, the pressure on the drum and the accompanying pain are both relieved. The perforation thus caused will usually heal over and the hearing eventually return to normal.
Earache with discharge may also arise from infection of the outer ear canal, and from conditions such as eczema and dermatitis. These causes are usually pain-free.

This condition requires medical attention if it does not respond quickly to homeopathic treatment.

KEY FEATURES	TREATMENT
The skin around the ear is raw and burning Thin, offensive, burning, acrid discharge A roaring noise with each bout of pain	ARS ALB 30
Of sudden onset, with violent burning and throbbing pain The patient is very hot and red-faced Thin and burning discharge With delirium	BELLADONNA 30
Violent, unbearable pain with restlessness, and a very fretful child	CHAMOMILLA 30
Throbbing, pulsating pain and cracking noises in the ear Discharge of mucus and pus Hearing becomes affected	CALC CARB 30
Paroxysms of throbbing pain with noises in the ear and a discharge of mucus and pus which may be blood-stained	FERRUM PHOS 30
Smelly discharge, throbbing noises in the ear and diminished hearing	HEPAR SULPH 12
A thick, yellow, stringy discharge, with swelling, usually of the left ear, and tearing pain	KALI BICH 12
The discharge has an offensive odour like rotten meat	PSORINUM 30
The ear is hot, red and swollen, with darting pain, worse at night A profuse, thick, yellow-green discharge Ringing in the ears	PULSATILLA 30
Smelly discharge Sensitivity to noise with roaring in the ears	SILICA 12
Chronic inflammation with a thin, acrid, offensive discharge The ear canal is very sensitive to touch	TELLURIUM 12

DOSAGE

Chamomilla 30 should be taken every fifteen minutes until relief is maintained.
Other remedies in the 30 potency should be taken four times a day until relief is maintained.
Remedies in the 12 potency may be used twice a day for one week.

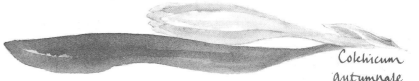

Colchicum
autumnale

EARACHE *without Discharge*

Pain in the ear may become quite severe in children; it is more common in the first five years of life and is often a complication of a cold or other throat or nasal infection. The infection may spread behind the ear drum, which becomes red, inflamed and painful, and bulges outwards from the pus which forms behind it. These symptoms are accompanied by a high temperature and the child is quite unwell.

Any of the following symptoms, if not treated, may lead to a discharge. The remedy may then need to be changed.

KEY FEATURES	TREATMENT
The external ear is hot and red Stinging, cutting or throbbing pain after exposure to cold, dry wind, worse at night	ACONITE 30
Pain shoots up from the throat	ALLIUM CEPA 30
The external ear is red and sore with stinging pain	APIS 30
Shooting pain from the throat and swollen tonsils	GELSEMIUM 30
Severe neuralgic pain, worse behind the right ear and worse in cold air	MAG PHOS 30
Shooting pains from the throat, worse on swallowing	PHYTOLACCA 30
With toothache The hearing becomes very acute Pain appears to go from ear to ear	PLANTAGO 30

DOSAGE

Remedies should be taken four times a day until an improvement is maintained.

ECZEMA

This sometimes distressing condition can take many forms, varying from a small dry patch of skin to a moist, extremely itchy, cracked and bleeding eruption involving most of the body. When the rash is extensive there is an added risk of it becoming infected.

There is often a family history of allergy, hay fever, asthma or skin disorder and the patient himself may have an allergy. In infantile eczema the allergy may be to cow's milk. Stress is another factor that has to be considered, but it must be realized that the irritation of the condition itself may cause tension in the patient, especially if the sleep is disturbed by it. Constitutional treatment from a medical homeopath should also be sought.

KEY FEATURES	TREATMENT
In the scalp and behind the ears Clear, honey-like discharge	GRAPHITES 6
Moist, with extreme itching The secretion quickly dries, producing thick scabs which ooze pus	MEZEREUM 6
With deep cracks and fissures, mainly of the fingertips and hands	PETROLEUM 6

The skin appears dirty, grey and greasy — PSORINUM 6
The irritation is worse from cold
In the bends of the knees and elbows

Dry, red, itchy blisters on the hands and wrists — RHUS TOX 6
Extreme irritation better for warmth and worse
  in cold, damp weather

Dry, rough, red, irritable skin which often — SULPHUR 6
  becomes infected
Worse after washing and from the heat of the
  bed

DOSAGE

The selected remedy should be taken three times a day until there is a change in the condition (better *or* worse), then stopped until the reaction setles or an improvement becomes established.
Treatment is then stopped and not recommenced unless the eczema deteriorates. Approximately one in four patients will note intensification of itching on Sulphur. If so, stop the remedy and improvement will follow.

FEEDING PROBLEMS

The cause of difficulties with feeding is seldom the food itself, although intolerance to formula milk undoubtedly exists and may lead to infantile eczema and asthma in susceptible infants.
The main causes of feeding problems are insufficient or poor quality breast milk; the bottle teat hole is too small; the baby is swallowing air instead of milk; the baby's wind is not brought up adequately.

Babies who fail to gain weight or thrive need medical attention.

KEY FEATURES — **TREATMENT**

Milk intolerance makes the child vomit, then — AETHUSA 12
  fall asleep
The vomiting is violent and often accompanied
  by diarrhoea
The child becomes very upset and cries a great
  deal

The child may have a large, sweaty head and — CALC CARB 12
  tend to be fat
The teeth are slow to erupt
The stool appears chalky
The child either hates or loves milk but either
  way, milk makes him worse

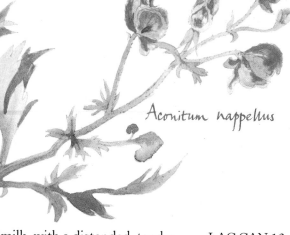

Aconitum nappellus

Intolerance of milk, with a distended, tender — LAC CAN 12
  abdomen after taking it

The child fails to thrive and is constipated, — MAG CARB 12
  with pale, dry and crumbly stools

Aversion to milk, which causes diarrhoea — NAT CARB 12
The abdomen is distended
Loud rumblings are heard and the wind moves
  around, causing pain

The child refuses the breast and vomits after each feed

The head sweats during sleep and the sweat may be offensive

SILICA 12

DOSAGE

The selected remedy should be taken three times a day until an improvement occurs.

HEADACHE

Most headaches in children come on from eye strain, tiredness, or emotional problems, but migraine can occur in children, although not usually under the age of five. A condition called abdominal migraine, in which there are repeated attacks of abdominal pain followed by sickness and headache, can also develop in children. A headache often occurs with head colds and infectious diseases like chicken-pox. Sinusitis-induced headaches usually occur in older children.

A child with recurrent headaches, a severe headache which does not quickly settle, or a severe headache with a raised temperature should be seen by a doctor.

KEY FEATURES	TREATMENT
After a blow to the head	ARNICA 30
Flushed face with shiny bright eyes Comes on suddenly and is a throbbing pain, usually worse on the right side	BELLADONNA 30

Severe and throbbing
The face is flushed, the feet are cold
The pain is worse after midnight

FERRUM MET 30

Starts in the neck and spreads over the head to one eye
Worse in the morning and better after urinating
The patient feels listless

GELSEMIUM 30

The head feels heavy after being in the sun
The face is pale

GLONOINE 30

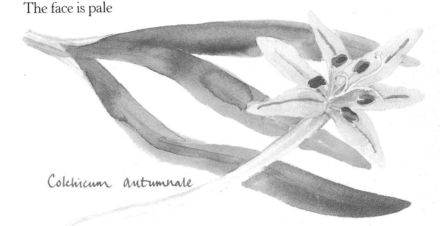

Colchicum autumnale

After mental exertion
Usually one-sided, with blurring of vision on the affected side
Accompanied by vomiting

IRIS 30

The child gets tired easily
The ache occurs more often in girls and comes on after a lot of school work

PHOS ACID 30

DOSAGE

The selected remedy should be taken every thirty minutes until an improvement occurs and is maintained.

INFLUENZA

(see Colds, p. 29)

NAUSEA

(see Digestive Upsets, p. 35)

NIGHTMARES

These tend to occur soon after the child falls asleep and cease on waking. However the child may appear to be awake when he is not. He does not remember the attack when fully awake. Children may have bad or frightening dreams more frequently than adults. These often follow some upsetting event, emotional trauma, or after watching a frightening television programme.

KEY FEATURES	TREATMENT
Restless sleep with worrying dreams	ACONITE 30
Fears the dark and going to bed May shout out while still asleep	BELLADONNA 30
Twitches and screams while asleep Very weird dreams	HYOSCYAMUS 30
Restless sleep with troubled dreams	PULSATILLA 30

DOSAGE

The selected remedy should be taken at bedtime. It may be repeated during the night if necessary.

NAPPY (DIAPER) RASH

Two main causes are responsible for this condition: detergents or soap not adequately rinsed out of the nappy (diaper) cause an irritation of the skin and a fine red rash with a few small, raised pimples; infrequent nappy (diaper) changes allow the ammonia in the urine to irritate and burn the skin.

KEY FEATURES	TREATMENT
The urine smells like ammonia	BENZOIC ACID 6
Diffuse redness all over the nappy (diaper) area	MEDORRHINUM 6
Worse after bathing, better if left exposed to the air	SULPHUR 6

DOSAGE

The selected remedy should be taken three times a day until an improvement occurs and is maintained.
Calendula cream may be used sparingly on the rash at each nappy (diaper) change.

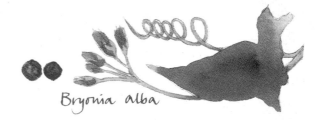

Bryonia alba

NOSEBLEEDS

Epistaxis

Children are notorious nose-pickers and this may be the cause of the bleed. However, most nosebleeds in children start spontaneously and, in spite of seeming very heavy, are usually of minor significance.

If the bleeding has not stopped within about half an hour, or if it seems especially heavy, the child should be taken to the nearest accident and emergency department.

KEY FEATURES	TREATMENT
After any injury to the nose	ARNICA 30
After excitement Accompanied by fear	ACONITE 30
Bright red blood Profuse flow	FERRUM PHOS 30
Darker blood Drips rather than pours	HAMAMELIS 30

DOSAGE

A dose of the selected remedy should be taken every fifteen minutes until the bleeding ceases.

SLEEP PROBLEMS

It is important to discover the cause of the sleeplessness and not to allow the child to become dependent on medication in order to sleep. However, for a short-term problem homeopathic treatment is ideal as it produces no actual sedation but allows the child to relax into a normal satisfying sleep.

KEY FEATURES	TREATMENT
Fear, agitation, excitement, or anxiety At the start of a feverish illness	ACONITE 30
Anxiety about the next day's happenings	ARG NIT 30
Fear of going to bed Flushed face, dilated pupils May 'see' frightening things	BELLADONNA 30
Jerking of the arms With colic One cheek red, the other pale	CHAMOMILLA 30
Over-active mind All senses are over-acute Ready to play and quite happy	COFFEA 30
Awake and lively late at night	CYPRIPEDIUM 30
The mind is full of bewildering images	HYOSCYAMUS 30

With many fears and troublesome thoughts	PHOSPHORUS 30

DOSAGE

One dose of the selected remedy should be taken about one hour before the child goes to bed and another dose at bedtime. A third dose may be taken during the night, if necessary.

THROAT, Sore

This is a very common condition in children, indicated by redness at the back of the throat. A raised temperature occurs in only about one third of cases. It sometimes precedes an attack of acute tonsillitis.

KEY FEATURES	TREATMENT
Sensation of a splinter in the throat when swallowing	ARG NIT 30
The throat is dark red, rough and sore	
The tonsils are inflamed and sore	BARYTA CARB 30
Smarting pain on swallowing	
Comes and goes suddenly	BELLADONNA 30
Hot, red skin	
Dry mouth and throat	
Pain extends to the ear	CAPSICUM 30
A rough, scraping sensation in the throat	DULCAMARA 30
After catching cold in damp weather	
Sensation of a splinter in the throat	HEPAR SULPH 30
The throat feels raw, as if scraped	
The tonsils are inflamed and swollen	

Tearing pain in the throat	LACHESIS 30
Chronic sore throat	
Mucus sticks in the throat	
White patches on the throat	NITRIC ACID 30
Sharp, sore, stinging pain makes swallowing difficult	
Pain in the throat, worse on coughing	PHOSPHORUS 30
Ulcerated sore throat	
The throat feels hot	PHYTOLACCA 30
Pain at the root of the tongue extends to the ear	

DOSAGE

The selected remedy should be taken three times a day for four days.

TOOTHACHE
and Teething Problems

Teething babies tend to be restless, tearful and generally irritable. Some pull at their ears and show excessive hand chewing. The best evidence that a baby is teething is, of course, the appearance of an erupting tooth in the gums. Teething symptoms without evidence of any other illness, such as a raised temperature, cough or diarrhoea, points to teething being the correct diagnosis.

KEY FEATURES	TREATMENT
Pain after exposure to cold, dry air or cold foods or drinks	ACONITE 30
Hot and/or cold food causes pain	BRYONIA 30

		KEY FEATURES	TREATMENT
Terrible pain; the child is inconsolable Worse at night Teething in babies	CHAMOMILLA 30	Large lumps of curd-like vomit are brought up Followed by great exhaustion With yellow-green diarrhoea preceded by stomach cramps	AETHUSA 12
Pain from tooth decay The teeth look yellow	KREOSOTE 30	From an overloaded stomach or after too much rich food The tongue is coated white No appetite	ANT CRUD 12
The teeth are very sensitive to the touch Excessive salivation	PLANTAGO 30		
Pain from bad teeth or gum boil Much worse at night With increased salivation The teeth feel loose or too long	MERC SOL 30	With diarrhoea The patient is very anxious and chilly	ARS ALB 12

DOSAGE

The selected remedy should be taken at thirty-minute intervals until there is lasting relief.

Ruta graveolens

VOMITING

The nausea which often precedes it, and the vomiting itself, may be caused by overeating or drinking, by infection, by travel sickness or as part of other illnesses such as whooping cough.

If the vomiting is associated with severe abdominal pain, if it does not settle soon after starting treatment, if dehydration is suspected or if the vomiting becomes worse or more frequent, immediate medical attention must be sought.

Intense nausea and sweating Straight after eating Profuse salivation	IPECAC 12
After overeating Much belching and distension Worse in the morning	NUX VOM 12
Vomits food and drink as soon as they are warmed in the stomach	PHOSPHORUS 12

DOSAGE

A dose of the selected remedy should be taken every thirty minutes until an improvement is maintained.

43

INFECTIOUS DISEASES

Measles

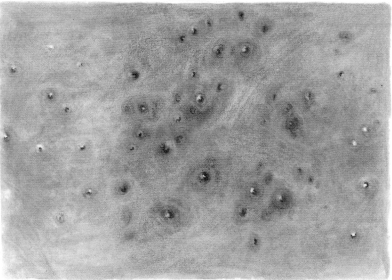

Chicken pox

CONTENTS

Chicken-pox	45
German Measles	45
Glandular Fever	45
Measles	46
Mumps	47
Scarlet Fever	48
Shingles	48
Whooping Cough	49

*T*hese illnesses are also known by the collective title of 'communicable diseases' as they are capable of being passed from one person to another. Their spread is brought about in one of several different ways: by physical contact, by breathing in infected air droplets from an ill person's sneezes or coughs, by handling an already infected object such as a cup or spoon, and by coming into contact with a 'carrier', a person who can spread the disease without showing signs of suffering from it.

Although the infectious diseases are most commonly found in children, adults are not immune. In fact, if they contract one, they are usually quite ill with it.

While infectious diseases are self-limiting (that is, they last for only a certain number of days), homeopathic treatment can be used to shorten the duration of the illness, prevent it becoming too severe, and in some cases, if given early enough, prevent the disease from becoming established in the patient. However, if the patient's condition deteriorates, expert medical advice should be obtained.

CHICKEN-POX

The incubation period for this illness is 12–14 days. The eruption starts as a small, flat, red patch which goes on to form the typical, slightly raised, blister-like spots of chicken-pox. These take 2–4 days to form, then they start to break down and crust over. The temperature will be slightly raised and a cough is often present.

KEY FEATURES	TREATMENT
In the early stages when the child is hot and thirsty, restless and anxious	ACONITE 30
For an irritable, whining child The remedy helps to bring out the eruption With a cough	ANT TART 12
Headache, which makes sleeping difficult The eyes are bright, the face flushed	BELLADONNA 12
Intense itching in a restless child The most commonly used remedy	RHUS TOX 12

DOSAGE

Aconite 30 should be taken every two hours for four doses as early as possible in the illness. Otherwise the selected remedy should be taken three times a day for three or four days.

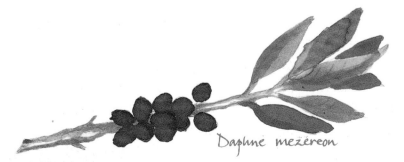

Daphne mezereon

GERMAN MEASLES
Rubella

This is a short-lasting infectious illness with an incubation period of 11–21 days (usually 18). The rash is often over within a few hours and in most cases the glands at the back of the neck are slightly enlarged, and sometimes tender and painful.
No specific treatment is necessary.

GLANDULAR FEVER
Infectious mononucleosis

This debilitating condition, which tends to occur in adolescents and young adults, is caused by the Epstein-Barr virus. Although it is infectious, it is mainly spread through close contact via the oral-respiratory route and consequently has become known as the 'kissing disease'. However, most cases occur without any known contact.
The illness is usually slow to start, 1–6 weeks being common, and during this time the patient may complain of feeling listless and have vague muscle aches and headaches. The lymph nodes (glands), especially those in the neck, the groin and the armpits, then become tender and begin to enlarge. The spleen may also become enlarged. A slightly raised temperature, sore throat, jaundice and a skin rash, like that of German measles, can develop at this time and the tiredness may increase. Convalescence is often prolonged and the illness can last for 2–3 months.

It is essential to have this condition correctly diagnosed as rest is important during its course, so medical help should be sought. However, conventional medicine has nothing to offer other than rest in the treatment of this condition.

KEY FEATURES	TREATMENT
For contacts of proven cases, or during an outbreak at a college or school, prevention may be aided by taking	GLANDULAR FEVER NOSODE 30
Mental fatigue Enlarged glands in all areas, with a sore throat which makes swallowing difficult The glands may feel quite tender	BARYTA CARB 30
During the sore throat phase, when there are also painful swollen glands in the neck, groin and armpits	BELLADONNA 30
Feeling of great weakness and coldness, with enlarged glands in the neck and armpits	GRAPHITES 30
Sweaty, bad breath, feeling hot and cold	MERC SOL 30

DOSAGE

Three doses of Glandular Fever Nosode should be taken on one day as soon as possible after contact. If the epidemic continues, the nosode may be taken in a similar manner once a week until the epidemic is over.

For treatment of diagnosed cases, the selected remedy should be taken three times a day for five days.

MEASLES

This illness, which has an incubation period of 10–15 days, usually starts with the child showing symptoms similar to those of flu for 7–10 days. A dry, irritable cough is often present, and for a few days before the rash appears the temperature is raised, becoming quite high a day or two before the rash comes out.

The rash is characteristic and starts as separate, dull red areas (often first behind the ears), which rapidly join up to form the typical blotchy measles rash all over the body. The patient often has swollen eyelids and red eyes, frequently disliking bright light. The cough usually continues throughout, and often after, the illness.

KEY FEATURES	TREATMENT
In the early stages with fever, hot, dry skin, thirst and restlessness	ACONITE 30
With a dry or croupy cough	

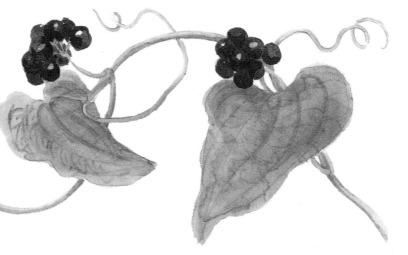

If the rash is slow to appear Dry, hard, painful cough The child dislikes being moved and develops a mild delirium	BRYONIA 30
Streaming, burning tears and a running nose with a bland discharge Light hurts the eyes	EUPHRASIA 30
The patient shows stupor, lack of thirst and an itchy, dark red skin Sneezing and a sore throat	GELSEMIUM 30
After using Pulsatilla, if swollen glands remain and the eyes and ears are affected With diarrhoea	KALI BICH 30

A dry cough at night, which is loose by day
Profuse tears and a thick, yellow, bland nasal
  discharge
Dry mouth but no thirst. Use *after* the rash
  has appeared
	PULSATILLA 30

DOSAGE

The selected remedy should be taken three times a day for 3–4 days.

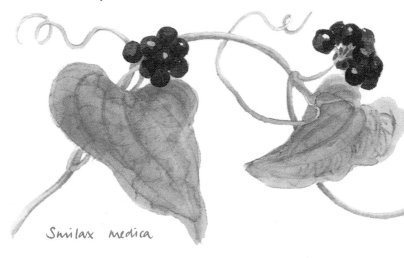

Smilax medica

MUMPS

Incubation in this disorder is 14–21 days. The characteristic feature is swelling of the salivary gland(s), mainly the parotid, which is found below and in front of the lobe of the ear. Other glands cause swelling under the jaw, producing the typical moon-faced appearance. There may be pain on eating (chewing) and often some earache. The swelling lasts 3–5 days but the illness may be prolonged if it then goes over to the other parotid gland.

Abdominal pain with severe vomiting or painful testicles all require urgent medical help.

KEY FEATURES	TREATMENT
Bright red face with swelling on the right side	BELLADONNA 30
Stiff jaw, offensive salivation and a foul, dirty tongue	MERCURIUS 30
The most commonly used remedy	PILOCARPUS 30
If the illness is prolonged	PULSATILLA 30
The swelling is on the left side and sticking pains occur on swallowing	RHUS TOX 30

DOSAGE

The selected remedy should be taken three times a day for three days. It should be continued, or another remedy selected, if the swelling then comes up on the opposite side of the face.

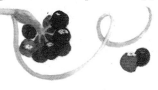

47

SCARLET FEVER
Scarletina

This is a very contagious disease which occurs mainly in children and is due to infection with the bacteria known as streptococcus. Symptoms include a raised temperature with a sore throat and swollen neck glands. The rash is scarlet in colour, starts in the armpits and groins and spreads to the rest of the body, other than around the mouth. Even the tongue becomes red and it looks a bit like a strawberry.

The possibility of the illness affecting the heart and/or kidneys is ever present, so medical advice and treatment is essential.

KEY FEATURES	TREATMENT
The skin feels rough and is rose-coloured The throat is sore, swollen and stinging The patient feels worse from warmth, requires a cool room and wants to be uncovered	APIS 30
A smooth, bright red rash with a sore throat, 'strawberry' tongue and swollen neck glands The lips, mouth, throat and skin are hot, red and dry	BELLADONNA 30
For use after Belladonna when the mouth becomes sore and ulcerated, with profuse saliva and foul breath	MERCURIUS 30
If the patient becomes restless but drowsy	RHUS TOX 30

DOSAGE

The selected remedy should be taken four times a day for three days in conjunction with any orthodox therapy prescribed by your doctor.

SHINGLES
Herpes zoster

This condition arises from the chicken-pox virus and can occur in any age group. The symptoms are those of a painful eruption, the pain often occurring 2–14 days before the rash. The rash appears on one side of the body only and the initial blotchy red patch, which is rather like a hot-water bottle burn, changes into a collection of small blisters. These eventually crust over to heal in 10–20 days.

Medical attention is needed if the eye and/or the area around the eye is involved, or if the condition is very painful or extensive.

KEY FEATURES	TREATMENT
Large blisters with burning and stinging pain Cold dressings relieve the pain	APIS 12
The blisters join together Intense burning pain, relieved by warm dressings The patient is restless, worse after midnight	ARS ALB 12
Small, very itchy blisters which dry quickly, producing thick scabs For pain which continues after the blisters have healed	MEZEREUM 12
With severe neuralgic pain, usually in the chest wall Clusters of burning-itching blisters which are very tender to the touch and worse with any movement	RANUNC BULB 12

Small blisters with itching and tingling, and the   RHUS TOX 12
surrounding skin appears swollen
Local warmth helps the pain

DOSAGE

The selected remedy should be taken four times a day until the blisters begin to dry and crust over.

In the case of Mezereum for pain that continues after the blisters have healed, take four doses a day until an improvement is maintained.

WHOOPING COUGH

This illness which can be dangerous under the age of about one year, starts with flu-like symptoms, including a hard, dry, mainly nocturnal cough which lasts for 7–14 days before the typical whooping cough spasm occurs. This makes the child red or blue in the face and vomiting frequently follows each coughing spasm.

The whoop is a hoarse intaking of breath that starts as the child recovers his breath after a bout of coughing. It occurs in only about 40 per cent of cases.

Whooping cough is a potentially serious disease which carries a greater risk of long-term ill-effects than the vaccine which is administered against it. Therefore, if there are no contra-indications in the family medical history, it is recommended that all children be given immunization. If there are good reasons for not administering the vaccine, the homeopathic remedy Pertussin may be used instead, but this should always be done under medical supervision.

KEY FEATURES	TREATMENT
Cough after eating or if the patient gets angry Much catarrh with 'rattling' sounds in the chest The patient is thirstless	ANT TART 30
Painful cough which makes the child cry	ARNICA 30
Stomach pain and tears before the cough, which is dry, violent and spasmodic Very little mucus, the cough is worse at night and after exposure to cold	BELLADONNA 30
Gagging and vomiting, with a red face and violent spasms of coughing A useful remedy early in the illness	CARBO VEG 30
The cough is worse at night when warm in bed, better in a cool room and after cold drinks With ropy, clear strings of mucus	COCCUS CACTI 30
Typical paroxysms of coughing one after the other Crawling sensation in the throat Vomiting after coughing The patient holds on to his chest when coughing because it is painful Worse at night	DROSERA 30

DOSAGE

The selected remedy should be taken every two or three hours until relief is obtained. It can then be taken three times a day for a further four or five days.

EMOTIONAL AND NERVOUS DISORDERS

The nervous system consists of two main parts: the *central nervous system*, which is made up of the brain, the spinal cord and nerves; and the *autonomic nervous system*, which consists of nerve centres called ganglia, two nerve cords and nerves.

The brain is the command centre and receives messages from nerve endings throughout the body. It then transmits messages back to them, telling them what actions to initiate.

The brain is made up of nerve cells and nerve fibres and is enclosed in three separate membranes called the meninges. Between the inner and middle membranes is a space which contains the cerebro-spinal fluid.

The cerebrum is the largest part of the brain and consists of right and left halves. The cerebellum lies behind the back end of the cerebrum and is also divided into right and left halves. The brain stem connects the cerebrum and cerebellum to the spinal cord. Most of the nerve fibres connecting the brain with the rest of the body pass down through the spinal cord, but some also come from the base of the brain itself and do not enter the spinal cord. These are the cranial nerves, which control smell, sight, hearing, taste and movements of the eye, the tongue, the jaw and the face.

The spinal cord is a tube of nervous tissue continuous with the brain stem. About 18 inches (45 cm) long, it is covered by the same membranes as those which cover the brain and enclose the cerebro-spinal fluid. It runs through the spinal canal, which is within the vertebrae (bones making up the spine) and which protects it from damage. The spinal cord connects the nerve fibres from the brain with rest of the body and has two sorts of fibres: sensory fibres, which run up and carry messages *to* the brain, and motor fibres which carry messages *from* the brain to the muscles.

On either side of the spinal cord and at the level of the gap between each vertebrae a bunch of motor nerve fibres run out of the cord and a bunch of sensory fibres run in. Each of these collections is known as a nerve root and together they are called a spinal nerve. Nerve fibres from this go to nerve endings throughout the body.

What does the nervous system have to do with emotional problems? The answer is far less complicated than the preceding description might suggest. When a person is subjected to mental, physical or emotional strain, there is an increase in tension, which makes the muscles tight and contracted. This in turn increases pressure on the nerves and possibly on the blood vessels, which can lead to a variety of physical symptoms. Anxiety, for example, can manifest itself with headaches, stomach upsets, back pain or broken sleep. Treating the whole person (emotional and physical symptoms) is the hallmark of homeopathy, and it is particularly successful in remedying emotional and nervous disorders.

THE ROLE OF THE CENTRAL NERVOUS SYSTEM

The cerebrum is the part of the brain concerned with thought, will, sensation and emotions.

The cerebellum coordinates the action of the various muscle groups which work together in a complicated combination of movements such as walking. It is also concerned with balance.

The lower part of the brain-stem contains the centres of nerve fibres which are concerned with regulation of the heart, breathing and swallowing.

The spinal cord carries sensory impulses (messages) to and motor impulses (orders) from the brain. It also contains secondary centres which control reflex actions. These are automatic actions which do not need the attention of the brain.

The autonomic nervous system consists of two chains of nerve collections called ganglia which, in the main, lie on either side of the spinal column and intermingle with the spinal nerves. It controls the automatic functions of the body, such as movements of the intestines, the beat of the heart and contraction and dilation of the blood vessels.

CONTENTS

Absent-mindedness	51
Anger and its Effects	52
Anxiety	53
Arrogance	54
Clumsiness	54
Concentration, Lack of	55
Confidence, Lack of	55
Confusion of Mind	56
Depression, Clinical	56
Eating Disorders	58
Emotional States	59
Fears and Phobias	59
Hallucinations	60
Hyperactivity	61
Hysteria	61
Indifference	62
Indolence	63
Insomnia	63
Irritability	64
Memory Loss	65
Moodiness	66
Quarrelsomeness	66
Restlessness	67
Senility	69
Sensitivity, Excessive	69
Shyness and Timidity	70

ABSENT-MINDEDNESS

It is common to forget some details of day-to-day activities, but if this forgetfulness becomes excessive and a burden, or if the patient finds it difficult to pay attention to instructions or seems preoccupied with his/her own thoughts, treatment will help. All these symptoms tend to increase with advancing years.
The features given below are additional to the absent-mindedness.

KEY FEATURES	TREATMENT
Nervous indigestion	ANACARDIUM
The patient is depressed and irritable	12
Decreased senses of smell, sight and hearing	

Poor memory	ARG NIT 12
The patient is apathetic and lifeless	AURUM 12
Debility and hypochondria Poor memory accompanied by disorders of the urinary tract and sexual weakness	CONIUM 12
Incoherent conversation with silly and nonsensical behaviour	DUBOISIA 12
Impaired coordination Numbness and tingling in the limbs	KALI BROM 12
Weak memory Confused thoughts Writes and spells words incorrectly	LYCOPODIUM 12
Loss of will-power Weak memory	MERCURIUS 12
Confusion and an impaired memory	NUX MOSCHATA 12
Slow perception Weak memory	OLEANDER 12
Vertigo and a hazy feeling The patient talks continuously	PHYSALIS 12

DOSAGE

The selected remedy should be taken twice a day for an indefinite period of time, or until an improvement is maintained.

Ranunculus bulbosus

ANGER *and its effects*

People vary in the way that they react to annoying events or individuals, but some are in a perpetual state of anger due to real or imagined grievances. Additionally, there are people who become ill from anger. These features can be used to select an appropriate homeopathic remedy.

KEY FEATURES	TREATMENT
Cannot bear to be touched or looked at Angry at every little attention Over-excitable and intense	ANT CRUD 30
Anger following a fright	ARNICA 30
Anxiety with the anger	CALC ARS 30
Wild anger Low morals Tendency to swear	CEREUS SERP 30
Complaints from anger With colic One red cheek, one pale Perspires with the anger In the very young or the very old	CHAMOMILLA 30
Abdominal pain after anger Great indignation	COLOCYNTH 30
Laughs a lot May be violent with anger and sorry afterwards	CROCUS 30
Unreasonable anger Headache following anger	IGNATIA 30
Sudden anger with an impulse to do violence	MERCURIUS 30

Ill-effects from anger with fear	NAT MUR 30
Violent temper, can't bear contradiction Generally irritable and angry Anger from loud noises which are painful The anger may lead to indigestion	NUX VOM 30
Ill-effects of anger and insults Colic after anger Suppressed anger and indignation	STAPHYSAGRIA 30

DOSAGE

The selected remedy should be taken three times a day for four days. Repeat it after this whenever necessary.

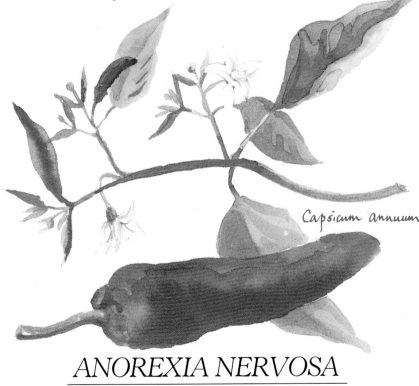

Capsicum annuum

ANOREXIA NERVOSA

(*see Eating Disorders, p. 58*)

ANXIETY

Anxiety has been defined as an exaggerated or unreasonable fear in a normal person. It is perfectly normal to worry about aspects of everyday life, but when the anxiety becomes so great that it prevents normal behaviour, the condition has become an illness and needs treatment.

KEY FEATURES	TREATMENT
Acute anxiety with agonizing terrors and fear of death Frequent palpitations The patient is inconsolable and restless	ACONITE 30
Anticipatory anxiety, with diarrhoea Hurried, irritable, nervous and lacking in self-confidence For pre-exam nerves	ARG NIT 30
Intense anxiety with great restlessness Fears something terrible will happen Worse during the night, after midnight Very chilly, exacting and fault-finding	ARS ALB 30
Anxiety leading to nausea With fear of downward motion Worsens until 11 p.m.	BORAX 30
The patient thinks he has done something wrong Uneasy and anxious with palpitations Fears loss of reason Despairs of life	CALCAREA 30
Nightly attacks of anxiety Cramps in the legs from fear	LACHESIS 30

Anxious about everything and even has anxious dreams	NAT MUR 30
The patient is certain something terrible will happen	
Very sensitive patients who are restless and fidgety	PHOSPHORUS 30
They need security and constant reassurance	
Anxiety after bad news or an emotional upset	PULSATILLA 30
The patient is weepy, touchy and needs company	

DOSAGE

The selected remedy should be taken four times a day for four days and repeated when necessary.

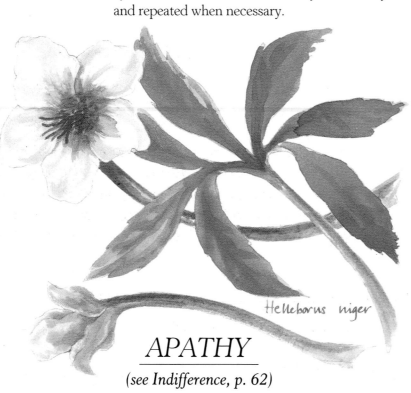

Helleborus niger

APATHY

(see Indifference, p. 62)

ARROGANCE

This feature of some patients may be used in the search for the correct homeopathic remedy for them. They have an exaggerated opinion of their own importance and ability, and show great conceit.

KEY FEATURES	TREATMENT
Headstrong and haughty when ill	LYCOPODIUM 30
Proud but with contempt for others	PLATINA 30

DOSAGE

The chosen remedy should be taken three times a day for five days and repeated when necessary.

BULIMIA NERVOSA

(see Eating Disorders, p. 58)

CLUMSINESS

Patients who show this symptom are ungainly in their movements; as they move about, they often bump into objects not really in their way. They lack manipulative skills and are very prone to dropping things.

KEY FEATURES / TREATMENT

KEY FEATURES	TREATMENT
Numbness in the hands and fingertips, so the patient drops things easily Generally clumsy	APIS 12
Great weakness in all the joints and clumsiness with the hands, so drops things easily	BOVISTA 12

DOSAGE

The remedy should be taken three times a day until an improvement is maintained.

	TREATMENT
The patient finds it impossible to study and becomes despondent because of this Desire to be with other people	SKATOL 12
The patient feels very tired and unable to think properly	TEREBINTH 12

DOSAGE

The remedy selected should be taken three times a day for five days and repeated after that when necessary.

CONCENTRATION, *Lack of*

Patients who are not able to concentrate find that they cannot put their mind totally to any problems that they have. This condition also applies to people who are incapable of giving their full attention to whatever they are doing.

KEY FEATURES	TREATMENT
Forgetful, irritable and depressed	ICHTHYOLUM 12
The patient cannot concentrate his thoughts	IRIDIUM 12
Loses the thread of a conversation	MEDORRHINUM 12
The patient feels that he lacks the power to concentrate Coordination is poor	ONOSMODIUM 12
Lack of self-control and concentration ability	OPIUM 12 *(prescription required in US)*

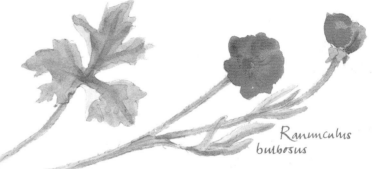

Ranunculus bulbosus

CONFIDENCE, *Lack of*

Patients who lack self-confidence doubt their own ability to carry out normal day-to-day activities and are especially diffident about undertaking any task out of the ordinary. In fact, such people are often extremely capable individuals and homeopathic treatment will help them overcome their diffidence.

KEY FEATURES	TREATMENT
Aversion to work and an irresistible desire to swear and curse The patient lacks confidence in himself and others	ANACARDIUM 30

Loss of self-confidence	BARYTA CARB 30
Absent-minded, irritable and irresolute	CALC SIL 30
Loss of self-confidence Melancholic and afraid to be alone	LYCOPODIUM 30

DOSAGE

The chosen remedy should be taken three times a day for four days. After this it should be used when necessary – three doses daily until an improvement is maintained.

CONFUSION OF MIND

This condition shows as a difficulty in understanding what is being said or what is required. Patients often have jumbled thoughts and find it hard to follow a normal conversation or perform simple tasks in the correct manner.

KEY FEATURES	TREATMENT
Vertigo with dullness of the mind	ANT TART 12
Apathy Inability to concentrate Depression	ANAGALLIS 12
Mental confusion Falls asleep while being spoken to	BAPTISIA 12
Vertigo and nausea Faintness on rising	BRYONIA 12
Confusion and delusions	CALC ARS 12

Confusion with dizziness	GLONOINE 12
Confusion with a dull headache	NAT SAL 12
Confusion in the head on rising suddenly	SALICYLIC ACID 12
Confusion of ideas The patient needs to talk a lot	STICTA 12
Mental confusion and dimness of vision	TILIA 12
Confusion and headache on waking	TRIFOLIUM 12

DOSAGE

The chosen remedy should be taken four times a day until an improvement is maintained.

DEPRESSION, Clinical

Although we all get depressed about certain day-to-day happenings, it does not last long, nor is it very severe. Patients who suffer from clinical depression can be ill for many weeks or months, during which time they become increasingly apathetic and suffer from an almost total lack of confidence. Their depression may cause considerable interference with their life, affecting concentration and relationships with other people. They are generally worse in the morning, their mood lightening as the day goes on, they may experience sleep problems, such as waking up in the early hours and not being able to get off again, there is often a loss of libido (sex drive), constipation and a total lack of appetite (sometimes the reverse occurs).

A depressed patient may also develop symptoms of illness in other parts of the body. While very real and worrying to the patient, these are imagined and no illness is actually present. Although most depression develops for no apparent reason, it can come on after events such as bereavement or severe shock, and in women as part of the menopause.

This can be a very serious illness which requires skilled professional help from a psychiatrist. The homeopathic remedies suggested should be used only in mild cases of depression and very careful and frequent checks made for deterioration.

KEY FEATURES	TREATMENT
Much worse after listening to music Great fear and anxiety	ACONITE 6
Profound melancholy and hypochondria Tendency to swear Impaired memory Very easily offended	ANACARDIUM 6
Very restless with great anguish and fear May be suicidal Thinks it useless to take treatment *All these symptoms require urgent medical help.*	ARS ALB 6
Disgusted with life and talks of committing suicide Oversensitive to noise Peevish at the least contradiction *All these symptoms require urgent medical help.*	AURUM 6
Desires to be alone Sad and reflective Avoids conversation	CARBO AN 6

Sad and hopeless	CAUSTICUM 6
Melancholic Full of contradictions Tearful	IGNATIA 6
Sad in the morning No desire to mix with others	LACHESIS 6

Crataegus oxyacantha

Profound depression The patient fears he has some incurable disease and has an aimless, hurried manner	LILIUM TIG 6
Extreme sadness in the morning on waking Loss of self-confidence Afraid to be alone Extreme apprehension	LYCOPODIUM 6
Great sadness Very anxious and full of dread for the future	MUREX 6
Depression because of a chronic illness Consolation makes the patient worse	NAT MUR 6
Saddened by lively music Worse in damp weather	NAT SULPH 6
Sad and cries easily Changeable, contradictory moods Much better out of doors	PULSATILLA 6
Very listless and apathetic	RHUS TOX 6

Indifference to the family Cries while talking of symptoms Easily offended	SEPIA 6
Irritable and apathetic Thin and weak, even though the appetite is good and he eats well	SULPHUR 6

DOSAGE

The chosen remedy should be taken three times a day. When an improvement occurs it may be stopped, but the patient will need constant reassessment as relapses are common.

EATING DISORDERS
Anorexia and Bulimia nervosa

These disorders usually, but not always, occur in adolescent girls who develop a fear of becoming fat and have distorted impressions of their own body image. Anorexia is characterized by rapid weight loss and may be preceded or followed by a cessation of the menstrual periods.
Bouts of excessive eating (bulimia) may occur in some anorectics and such binges are followed by self-induced vomiting to prevent the food being absorbed and forming fat.

These are potentially dangerous disorders and should be treated only under constant medical supervision.

KEY FEATURES	TREATMENT
The patient has a complete loathing for food and drink Sentimental and peevish	ANT CRUD 6

A complete loss of appetite The patient cannot bear any disturbance and wants to be alone	BRYONIA 6

The stomach feels full after the smallest
  amount of food or drink and can become very
  distended with wind
	CARBO VEG 6

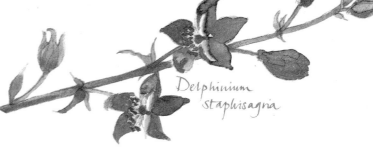

Delphinium staphisagria

Total aversion to the sight or smell of food	COLCHICUM 6
Persistent nausea, not relieved by vomiting The patient is sulky and despises everything	IPECAC 6
The appetite disappears on eating the first mouthful of food Worse with cold food The patient becomes very apprehensive	LYCOPODIUM 6
The patient vomits food as soon as it is swallowed In tall, thin, artistic types	PHOSPHORUS 6
Nausea from the smell of food cooking Wants to be alone Hates fuss and sympathy	SEPIA 6

DOSAGE

The chosen remedy should be taken three times a day until an improvement is maintained.

EMOTIONAL STATES

Strong feelings brought on by emotional events can affect people in different ways. The key features below are all related to emotional events, or are illnesses induced by emotional changes.

KEY FEATURES	TREATMENT
Illness due to emotional and physical tension	ACONITE 30
Sad and weepy, unreasonable	AMMON CARB 30
Tearful Awkward and drops things	APIS 30
Migraine due to emotional disturbances	ARG NIT 30
Ill after emotional disturbances	COCCULUS 30
Diarrhoea from emotional excitement	GELSEMIUM 30
Melancholic, sad and tearful	IGNATIA 30
Highly emotional, very weepy Changeable contradictory moods Better out of doors	PULSATILLA 30
Emotional sensitivity Music causes weeping and trembling	THUJA 30

DOSAGE

The selected remedy should be used three times a day until an improvement is maintained.

FEARS AND PHOBIAS

Most people have minor fears, such as a fear of flying, but these do not interfere with their normal lives. Indeed, if necessary, they would overcome their fear in order to, say, go on holiday abroad. Some people, however, have perpetual and/or multiple fears which disturb their everyday existence and bring on acute physical symptoms.
Whatever the fear, it can be helped by homeopathic medicine. The following list contains some of the more general remedies for fear. For more specific treatment of particular fears, professional help should be sought.

KEY FEATURES	TREATMENT
Sudden panic Great fear and anxiety Fears death but also fears the future Physical and mental restlessness	ACONITE 30
Apprehension before an event Fearful, nervous and melancholic Lacks self-confidence Impulsive, wants to do things in a hurry Great desire for sweet things Diarrhoea from fear	ARG NIT 30
Fears loss of reason and misfortune Apprehensive Forgetful	CALC CARB 30
Emotional excitement and fear leading to bodily illness Dull and listless Stage and examination fear	GELSEMIUM 30

Full of fear and imaginations Hates being left alone	KALI CARB 30
Consumed with all sorts of fears, but especially of thunder Very sensitive Restless and fidgety	PHOSPHORUS 30
Fears being alone, the dark and ghosts Worse in the evening Likes sympathy, weeps easily and is timid and irresolute	PULSATILLA 30

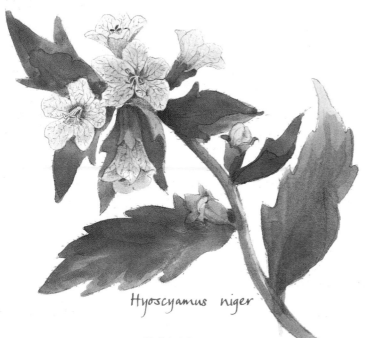

Hyoscyamus niger

DOSAGE

A dose of the selected remedy should be taken every fifteen minutes until an improvement is maintained.

If the remedy is being taken for a special event, such as an examination, it should be taken in the 30 potency three doses on the day before the event and a further dose on the morning of the event.

HALLUCINATIONS

To hallucinate means to see, hear, smell or feel something that is not there. Hallucination may occur because of some mental disorder such as schizophrenia, a brain disorder such as a tumour, after the use of certain drugs or alcohol, or with a raised temperature (especially in children).

All patients who hallucinate should be treated under medical supervision.

KEY FEATURES	TREATMENT
Sudden and severe giddiness Delirium with hallucinations	ABSINTHIUM 30
The patient thinks he is possessed by two persons or wills	ANACARDIUM 30
Hallucinations of smell and sight	ARS ALB 30
Visual hallucinations; sees monsters and hideous faces Acuteness of all the senses The body is hot, the face red	BELLADONNA 30
Mental depression; hallucinates and fears he will be killed Intellectual apathy	PLUMBUM 30
Auditory hallucinations (hears things)	STRAMONIUM 30
At night the patient is irritable and oversensitive	VALERIANA 30

DOSAGE

The selected remedy should be taken every hour for four doses.
Repeat only if the symptoms return.

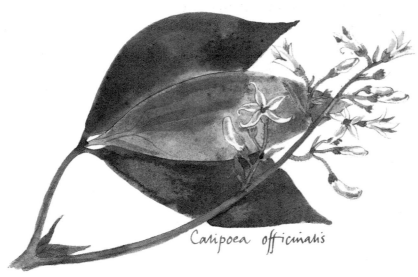

Caripoea officinalis

HYPERACTIVITY

Hyperkinesis

This is a condition, usually in a child, in which there is extreme restlessness with mental and physical overactivity.

KEY FEATURES	TREATMENT
Unusually active mind and body	COFFEA 12
Great nervous excitability	
Full of ideas	
Insomnia because of activity of the mind	

DOSAGE

The remedy should be taken twice a day until an improvement is
maintained. It should then be repeated if necessary.

HYSTERIA

*Hysteria is a nervous condition often characterized by a multitude of symptoms for which no physical cause can be found. The patient is very emotionally unstable.
The features below are some additional symptoms frequently shown in hysteria.*

KEY FEATURES	TREATMENT
Sensation of a ball in the throat	ASAFOETIDA 30
Flatulence	
Offensive diarrhoea	
Sudden changes of moods	CROCUS 30
Spasmodic twitching of muscles	
Nervous temperament	IGNATIA 30
Effects of grief and worry	
Very changeable moods	
Nervous anxiety and great irritability	KALI PHOS 30
Night terrors	
Any work seems an effort	
Fainting fits	MOSCHUS 30
Uncontrollable laughter	
Extreme coldness	
Hysterical flatulence	VALERIANA 30
Irritable and oversensitive	
Sensation of a thread in the throat	
Difficulty with breathing, anxiety and palpitations of hysterical causation	VIOLA ODORATA 30

DOSAGE

The selected remedy should be taken three times a day for one week. It may need repeating at regular intervals after this.

INDIFFERENCE

Homeopathic treatment will help people who are apathetic, caring for no one and showing no concern for themselves. The remedies given below consider not only the indifference, but also other associated symptoms. Both should be taken into account when choosing a remedy.

KEY FEATURES	TREATMENT
The patient is clumsy and drops things Tearful, jealous, fidgety and hard to please Even the brain feels tired	APIS 12
In sluggish, fat, lazy people who faint easily Need for fresh air The patient may not have recovered from a previous illness	CARBO VEG 12
Associated with debility from the loss of body fluids through diarrhoea, vomiting or bleeding The patient is apathetic, disobedient, taciturn and despondent Unable to sleep because of an overactive mind Sudden crying and restlessness	CHINA 12
Very depressed; the patient fears he is suffering from an incurable disease Aimless manner	LILIUM TIG 12
Difficult, slow comprehension with mental weakness and depression The patient becomes very anxious and restless during thunderstorms Headache from the slightest mental exertion, worse from being in the sun	NAT CARB 12
The patient feels weak and weary Consolation aggravates and leads to irritability Blinding headaches	NAT MUR 12
Listless, impaired memory, cannot collect thoughts or find the right word Effects of grief and mental shock	PHOS ACID 12
Indifferent to the family, the patient is irritable and easily offended Very sad, weeps while relating symptoms Feels cold, even in a warm room Hot flushes, weakness and excessive perspiration at the menopause	SEPIA 12

DOSAGE

The selected remedy should be taken three times a day for an indefinite time until an improvement is maintained.

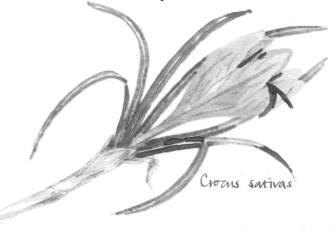

Crocus sativas

INDOLENCE
Aversion to Work

This condition applies to lazy, idle people who seem actually to dislike work and are not prepared to make any effort to help themselves or others. In choosing the correct homeopathic remedy, other features about the person involved must also be taken into account.

KEY FEATURES	TREATMENT
Due to alcoholism	CARB SULPH 6
General lethargy The head feels heavy with neuralgia over the right eye Jaundice, either now or in the past Better for eating hot food	CHELIDONIUM 6
Fat and chilly, fidgety and unable to make up his mind Music makes the patient cry Apprehensive and despondent	GRAPHITES 6
Great loquacity In jealous, suspicious people Restless, uneasy, wants to be off somewhere all the time Worse after sleep	LACHESIS 6
Aversion to his or her occupation	SEPIA 6
Lazy, irritable and depressed, very selfish, no regard for others Hates standing and has a dislike of water and washing	SULPHUR 6

DOSAGE

The selected remedy should be taken three times a day until an improvement is maintained. It will need to be restarted if there is a subsequent deterioration.

INSOMNIA

People who suffer from insomnia can be placed in one or both of two categories: those who have difficulty in falling asleep and those who have difficulty remaining asleep. Although most insomnia of the first type is stress related, early waking, often around 4–5 a.m., followed by catnapping can be an early symptom of a depressive disorder.
Homeopathic remedies can be used to correct these sleep disorders without fear of addiction to sleeping pills. They help by relaxing the mind and aiding the patient to fall into a good and refreshing natural sleep.

KEY FEATURES	TREATMENT
Anxiety caused by fear or over-excitement during the evening For insomnia associated with the start of a fever	ACONITE 30
From worry about an event the next day, such as an examination or interview	ARG NIT 30
Inability to fall asleep, or waking up at about 2 a.m. Great restlessness and a need to get up and walk around the room	ARS ALB 30

The problems of the day seem to go around and around in the mind	COFFEA 30
Inability to fall asleep because of exciting thoughts of recent events	
Great sensitivity to noise	
Sleeplessness associated with an unhappy event such as a death	IGNATIA 30
Waking at about 4 a.m. and inability to get back to sleep due to an overactive mind	LYCOPODIUM 30
Mental overactivity, going over the day's work again and again in the mind	NUX VOM 30
Anger at inability to fall asleep	
In very light sleepers who are easily disturbed by the slightest noise	SULPHUR 30

DOSAGE

The selected remedy should be taken during the evening if possible and repeated at bedtime. Another dose may be taken during the night, if necessary.

IRRITABILITY

The symptoms covered in this ailment are those associated with the main features of irritability, which may show the patient to be peevish, easily angered, grumpy and somewhat aggressive. Irritability is usually a 'built-in' feature of the patient, but certain physical conditions, such as constant pain, can lead an otherwise pleasant and calm person to become irritable. (See also Quarrelsomeness)

KEY FEATURES	TREATMENT
Weakness and restlessness with exhaustion after the slightest exertion	ARS ALB 30
Nightly aggravations	
Fear, fright and worry	
Headache and dizziness from sitting up	BRYONIA 30
Dry parched lips and mouth	
Everything irritates the patient	
Absent-minded, irresolute, lacking in self-confidence	CALC SIL 30
Anxious and intolerant	CARB SULPH 30
Sensitive, thirsty and hot	CHAMOMILLA 30
Unbearable pain	
Restlessness	
Nervous children who do not want to be touched or carried	CINA 30
The patient gets very angry	
Worse at night	
Cannot bear the slightest contradiction	HELONIAS 30
Much better if kept busy	
Very nervous, easily startled	KALI PHOS 30
In pale, sensitive, weepy females	
Hateful, vindictive, headstrong but with hopeless despair	NITRIC ACID 30
Sensitive to noise, pain and touch	
Very irritable; cannot bear noise, smells or light	NUX VOM 30
Fault-finding and sullen	

Easily offended, the patient shows an indifference to his family — SEPIA 30

Very sad and weepy, becoming anxious towards the evening

Depressed — SULPHUR 30
Thin and weak
Very selfish

DOSAGE

The selected remedy should be taken three times a day as necessary.

MEMORY LOSS
Amnesia

Total or partial loss of memory may follow physical or psychological injury, disease or drugs. Very often the amnesia applies to events immediately preceding the injury; for example, details of a car accident may be totally forgotten after the event.

Loss of memory for the recent past, but good recollection of events which occurred many years previously is frequently found in the elderly and is a normal symptom of ageing.

KEY FEATURES	TREATMENT
For recent events	ABSINTH 12
Diminished ability to concentrate, comprehend and reason	BARYTA CARB 12
Sudden loss of memory	CARBO VEG 12

Senility — CARB SULPH 12
Impotence
Dementia alternating with excitement

Marked loss of memory for names — CHLORUM 12

Confused, despondent and irritable — EUONYMUS 12
Unable to recall familiar names

General failure of mental power — KALI BROM 12
Melancholia
Loss of sexual desire

Loss of will-power — MERCURIUS 12

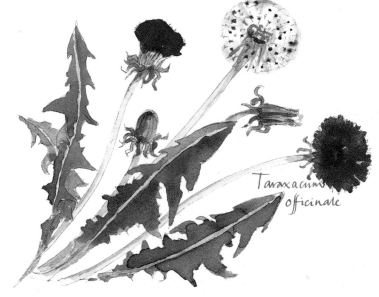

Taraxacum officinale

Slow perception — PLUMBUM 12
Speech disorders (aphasia)

Remembers everything prior to the illness — SYPHILINUM 12

DOSAGE

The selected remedy may need to be taken twice a day indefinitely.

MOODINESS

Although moodiness implies a sullen, sulky and gloomy disposition, most of the symptoms looked at in this section relate to patients whose mood changes easily and frequently.

KEY FEATURES	TREATMENT
Sentimental and moody	ANT CRUD 30
Marked alteration of moods With vivid dreams Forgetful and absent-minded	CENCHRIS 30
Weepy Clouded perception and memory Impatient	CROTALUS 30

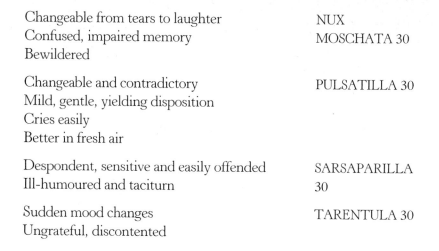

Coffea arabica

Introspective Silent brooding Sighing and sobbing after shock, grief and disappointment Very changeable moods	IGNATIA 30

Changeable from tears to laughter Confused, impaired memory Bewildered	NUX MOSCHATA 30
Changeable and contradictory Mild, gentle, yielding disposition Cries easily Better in fresh air	PULSATILLA 30
Despondent, sensitive and easily offended Ill-humoured and taciturn	SARSAPARILLA 30
Sudden mood changes Ungrateful, discontented	TARENTULA 30

DOSAGE

The selected remedy should be taken three times a day for four days.

PHOBIAS

(see Fears, p. 59)

QUARRELSOMENESS

People are quarrelsome for different reasons. Some may feel they have a definite grievance to air, but there are others of whom it might be said that their ability to argue over everything is part of their personality. It is to the latter that this section really applies. To help you pick the correct remedy, the symptoms associated with quarrelsomeness are listed. (See also Irritability)

KEY FEATURES	TREATMENT
Peevish at the least contradiction	AURUM 30
Profound depression	
Talks of suicide	
Oversensitive	
All these symptoms need urgent medical attention.	
Forever sighing and sobbing, with changeable moods	IGNATIA 30
Melancholic and uncommunicative, the symptoms follow shocks, grief and disappointment	
Irritable, cannot bear noise or smells	NUX VOM 30
The patient is sullen, fault-finding and has a fiery temperament	
Feels that death is near	PETROLEUM 30
Irritable, easily offended	
Vexed at everything	
Lazy, irritable and depressed	SULPHUR 30
Very selfish, with no regard for others	
Hates standing and dislikes water and washing	
Sudden mood changes	TARENTULA 30
Ungrateful, discontented	

DOSAGE

The selected remedy should be taken four times a day for three days.

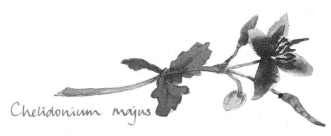

Chelidonium majus

RESTLESSNESS

Restlessness can be physical and mental and this section looks at both. The person involved will be unable to stay still, and will be worried, anxious and uneasy. By combining these symptoms with other features of the condition, the correct homeopathic remedy may be chosen.

KEY FEATURES	TREATMENT
Physical and mental restlessness	ACONITE 12
Tossing about, even when asleep	
Frequent nightmares	
Severe neuralgia with tingling and numbness	
Thirst always present and comes with fevers	
Violent palpitations	AETHUSA 12
Headache and vertigo	
Anxious and weeping	
Severe itching	AGARICUS 12
The skin feels as if burning	
Anxious and confused dreams	ALUMINA 12
Excited and very talkative	AMBRA 12
Unable to sleep	APOCYNUM 12
Cross and irritable	ARAGALLUS 12
Wanders aimlessly	
Bewildered and confused	
Wakes with arms and legs feeling swollen and heavy	ARANEA 12
Extreme coldness day and night	
Poor sleeper	

Sleepless and restless when overtired	ARNICA 12	Anxious and restless during thunderstorms	NAT CARB
Weakness and exhaustion, worse each night	ARS ALB 12	Restless and wakeful resulting from exhaustion	PASSIFLORA 12
Periodical burning pains with cold skin and extreme anxiety		Restless and fidgety	PHOSPHORUS 12
		Wakes up frequently during the night	
Hot, red skin with a flushed face and a dry mouth and throat	BELLADONNA 12	Depressed and oversensitive	
Excited mentally		Aching and soreness, weakness and restlessness	PHYTOLACCA 12
Restless sleep			
Acuteness of all senses		The first sleep is restless	PULSATILLA 12
Restless sleep at time of a period	CALCAREA 12	Tired in the afternoon, wide awake in the evening	
Anxious restlessness ending in rage	CANTHARIS 12	Thirstless, peevish and chilly	
At night with tearing pains in the bones and joints	CAUSTICUM 12	Extreme restlessness	RHUS TOX 12
		Constant changing of position	
Loss of energy		Joints and tendons ache	
Restless legs at night		Great apprehension at night	
Peevish and restless with colic	CHAMOMILLA 12	Insomnia with restlessness, fever and anxious dreams	SECALE 12
Especially useful with children			
Nervousness and nightly restlessness during teething	COCA 12	Depression, restlessness, coldness, spinal tenderness and restless feet associated with a period and the menopause	ZINC MET 12
Great nervous agitation	COFFEA 12		
Sleeplessness			
Fever with flushed cheeks	IODUM 12		
Apathetic			
Restless sleep with nightmares	KALI BROM 12		
Grinds teeth in sleep			
Sleeps during the day but restless at night because of heat	MAG MUR 12		
Bad nightmares			

DOSAGE

The selected remedy should be taken four times a day until an improvement is maintained. Repeat if and when necessary.

Ruta graveolens

SENILITY

This condition of mental and physical deterioration is associated with ageing.

KEY FEATURES	TREATMENT
Impairment of all functions due to old age Coldness and numbness Music causes weeping Nervous hypersensitivity	AMBRA 12
Senile dementia, the patient feels as if he is two people Very easily offended The memory is poor and the patient becomes very absent-minded	ANACARDIUM 12
Senile dementia, with confusion and loss of confidence, loss of memory and childish behaviour	BARYTA CARB 12
The patient feels sad and hopeless but is intensely sympathetic General health is very poor	CAUSTICUM 12
In thin, scrawny women who are run down and anxious With cataracts	SECALE 12

DOSAGE

The selected remedy should be taken three times a day for an indefinite period or until an improvement occurs which is maintained.

SENSITIVITY, *Excessive*

Although it is possible to be sensitive and react to virtually any stimulus, mental or physical, this section applies to mental oversensitivity only. People who are oversensitive are usually easily offended and consequently often quite irritable.

KEY FEATURES	TREATMENT
In light-haired females who are sensitive and romantic	COCCULUS 6
In nervous, sensitive and often anaemic individuals who show easy flushing Susceptibility to chest complaints	FERRUM PHOS 6
In easily excitable patients with a dark complexion Mild disposition Quick to perceive, rapid to act Weeps very easily	IGNATIA 6
In pale, irritable, lachrymose females with menstrual irregularities The slightest work seems impossible Nervous fears	KALI PHOS 6
Melancholic and afraid to be alone, individuals are apprehensive and the slightest thing may annoy them	LYCOPODIUM 6
Very irritable and hypersensitive to all stimuli, sullen and fault-finding	NUX VOM 6
Oversensitive, restless and fidgety	PHOSPHORUS 6
Despondent, easily offended, ill-humoured and taciturn	SARSAPARILLA 6

Emotional sensitivity	THUJA 6
Music causes weeping and trembling	
Easily tired	

DOSAGE

The selected remedy should be taken twice a day until an improvement is maintained.

SHYNESS AND TIMIDITY

Shy people are generally not at ease in the company of others, especially strangers. They are often timid, easily frightened, reluctant to initiate conversation and may blush easily. Shy children will cling to their parents and may cry if they feel out of their depth.

KEY FEATURES	TREATMENT
Intensely shy and blushes very easily	AMBRA 30
Often depressed, dislikes company but afraid to be alone	CONIUM 30

Fat and chilly individuals in whom music causes tears	GRAPHITES 30
Apprehensive, despondent and unable to make decisions	
Disinclined to converse	KALI PHOS 30
Absent-minded, anxious and indolent	KALI SIL 30
Irresolute with a mild, gentle, yielding disposition, weeps easily	PULSATILLA 30
Nervous, easily startled and hypochondriacal	SABADILLA 30

DOSAGE

The selected remedy should be taken three times a day for four days. It may need repeating after approximately six weeks.

WEEPINESS

(See Emotional States, p. 59)

WORK, AVERSION TO

(See Indolence, p. 63)

Delphinium staphisagria

THE HEAD, SCALP AND FACE

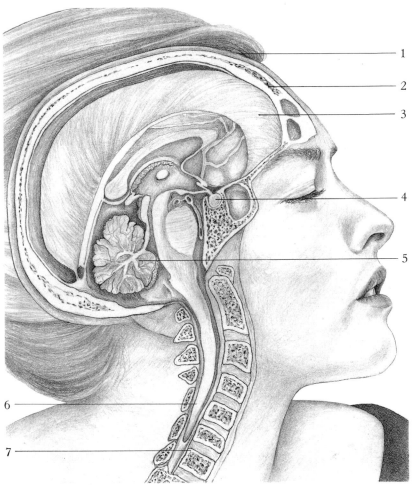

1
2
3
4
5
6
7

1	Scalp	5	Cerebellum
2	Cranium (*Skull*)	6	Spinal cord
3	Cerebrum (*Brain*)	7	Spine
4	Pituitary gland		

CONTENTS

Bell's Palsy	72
Dandruff and Eczema of the Scalp	72
Face, Burning Sensations in	73
Face, Discoloration of	73
Face, Pain in	74
Hair Loss/Baldness	75
Headache	76
Migraine	78

The skull, which sits on top of the spinal column, consists of two parts: the brain case, which is called the cranium and is formed from eight bones, and the face which is made up from fourteen bones. After infancy twenty-one of these twenty-two bones become so closely joined together that they become, in effect, a single bone. The exception is the lower jaw bone, the mandible, which is attached by a joint resembling a hinge to the cranium in front of the ear.

It is the cranium that forms the protective case which contains the brain and its upper part is covered by the scalp. The lower part of the skull, which is concealed beneath the muscles of the neck, is known as the base of the skull and it is through this that the spinal cord passes down into the spinal canal.

Underlying the skin of the face are many small muscles which control the movement of the eyelids, the nose and the mouth, thereby altering facial expression. In addition, there are larger muscles concerned with the process of mastication (chewing).

BELL'S PALSY

This is a condition of sudden onset which produces a weakness in the facial muscles on one side of the face. There are no other muscles or parts of the body involved. The eyelid on the affected side cannot be totally closed or opened, the side of the mouth droops, making eating a little difficult, and saliva may dribble.

Medical advice should be obtained.

KEY FEATURES	TREATMENT
After exposure to cold, dry air Tends to be left-sided	ACONITE 30
Marked distortion of the mouth Tends to be left-sided Trembling of the jaw Improves with rest	CADMIUM SULPH 12
Usually right-sided Some pain may be present The mouth weakness may be marked	CAUSTICUM 12
Hot, heavy, flushed face The eye symptoms are marked with vertigo	GELSEMIUM 12
Left-sided facial paralysis The face feels hot	SENEGA 12

DOSAGE

The selected remedy should be taken three times a day until an improvement occurs and then stopped. Repeat if a deterioration develops.

DANDRUFF AND ECZEMA OF THE SCALP

Although dandruff can occur at any age, it is most commonly found in young adults and is often at its worst soon after puberty. A form can be found in babies.
The scalp becomes covered with small white or yellowish flakes of dead skin which come away when the hair is brushed.
Eczema of the scalp and dandruff are frequently found at the same time.

KEY FEATURES	TREATMENT
The scalp itches and there is some hair loss	AMMON MUR 6
The scalp itches intolerably Circular bare patches develop The scalp is rough, appears dirty, is sensitive and covered with dry scale Worse during the night	ARS ALB 6
The scalp feels sore and is very dry	BADIAGIA 6
Dandruff often associated with eczema elsewhere on the body	KALI MUR 6
Dandruff often associated with ringworm of the scalp	KALI SULPH 6
The hair is very dry Intense itching, worse at night	MEDORRHINUM 6
Itching of the scalp Hair falls out in large bunches	PHOSPHORUS 6
Profuse, scaly dandruff	SANICULA 6

White, scaly dandruff	THUJA 6
Dry hair which easily falls out	
Greasy facial skin	
Eczema of the scalp with swollen glands in the neck	VIOLA TRICOLOR 6

DOSAGE

The selected remedy should be taken three times a day until an improvement is maintained.

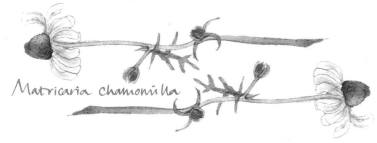

Matricaria chamomilla

FACE, Burning Sensations in

A sensation of heat in the face is usually an indication of abnormality, particularly if it persists for more than a few minutes. Conditions which may cause this sensation are shingles, neuralgia (nerve pain) and erysipelas. It may also accompany a feverish illness and is sometimes a feature in hay fever. Flushing from being overheated, after exercise, from too much alcohol or the menopause are other causes, but in these circumstances the burning soon goes. (See also Face, Pain in)

KEY FEATURES	TREATMENT
The facial muscles feel stiff and may twitch Itching and burning	AGARICUS 30
Itching vesicles which burn when touched	CANTHARIS 30

The body and face feel hot; any movement, or uncovering, makes the patient feel icy cold	NUX VOM 30
The face is red, burns and itches	STRONTIA 30

DOSAGE

The selected remedy should be taken four times a day for three days.

FACE, Discoloration of

Although the normal colour of the face in Caucasians varies from quite pale to very red, alteration to the colour of the face may be an indication of illness elsewhere in the body. The face becomes hot and flushed with many illnesses that cause a temperature rise, such as tonsillitis or flu. In liver disease the patient may become jaundiced and the face then appears yellow. A pale face can indicate anaemia, a blue, cold, sweaty face develops in shock and after severe conditions such as a heart attack, while a purple-red face can be found with raised blood pressure.

All other aspects of the patient should be considered in conjunction with this symptom in order to select the correct remedy.

KEY FEATURES	TREATMENT
Red and hot	ACONITE 12
On rising after lying down the face becomes deathly pale	
Palpitations accompanied by a red face	AGARICUS 12

73

Red after a stroke	ARNICA 12	Red and flushes easily	SULPHUR 12
Hot, red and flushed, with dilated pupils and a dry mouth	BELLADONNA 12	The lips are red and dry The nose is red and scabby	
Red with a sudden loss of consciousness	CANTHARIS 30	Pale, blue and icy cold, and the patient collapsed	VERATRUM ALB 30
Red, but the patient feels cold Severe bursting headache	CAPSICUM 12		

DOSAGE

Remedies in the 12 potency should be taken twice a day until an improvement is maintained.
Remedies in the 30 potency should be taken every fifteen minutes *while waiting for medical assistance.*

Blue and covered in a cold sweat	CARBO VEG 30
Yellow, especially on the cheeks and nose, with jaundice	CHELIDONIUM 12
Bloated and red, whereas the complexion is normally sallow	CHINA 12
Fiery-red and becomes flushed after the least pain or exertion	FERRUM MET 12
Red, even though the patient is anaemic	GRAPHITES 12
Greyish-yellow complexion with blue circles around the eye	LYCOPODIUM 12
Swollen, red and puffy The lips may appear black Deep-seated facial neuralgia	MERC CORR 12
Pale, blue and florid	NAT PHOS 12
Yellow blotches and pale or sallow	SEPIA 12
Red with facial neuralgia, worse in cold, damp weather	SILICA 12
Red and the patient looks anxious and sweaty With a fever	SPONGIA 12

FACE, Pain in
Facial Neuralgia

Facial pain often stems from the trigeminal nerve and is confined to one side or the other. Although the cause is not usually apparent, being in a draught may bring it on, especially after driving with the window open on a cold day. Other causes can be local skin infections, shingles, toothache, dental abscess, sinusitis and injury.

This condition requires expert medical help.

KEY FEATURES	**TREATMENT**
Pain on the left side Tingling and numbness The patient feels restless Jaw pain	ACONITE 30

The facial muscles feel stiff and may twitch Sensation of the face being pricked with ice-cold needles	AGARICUS 30
The facial muscles twitch The face is flushed, red and hot	BELLADONNA 30
The face is hot, heavy and flushed The facial muscles feel tight and the chin quivers Vertigo may be present	GELSEMIUM 30
The pain comes on after breakfast, starts below one eye and soon involves the whole face	IRIS 30
Left-sided pain with the face purple, mottled and puffy	LACHESIS 30
The face is red The teeth become painful and the pain may extend to the ear Extreme sensitivity to cold air The pain is relieved by local warmth	MEZEREUM 30
Coldness and numbness on the right side of the face The pain comes and goes gradually	PLATINA 30
Redness and burning of the cheeks The pain extends in all directions from the upper jaw	SANGUINARIA 30
The eye, cheek, teeth and temple all hurt, they are very sensitive to touch and seem ice-cold to the patient Symptoms improve in the evening	SPIGELIA 30
Left-sided pain The eye and nose discharge clear fluid The pain is as if the parts had been crushed Talking, sneezing, clenching the teeth and temperature changes aggravate the pain, which occurs at the same time each day, usually in the morning and afternoon	VERBASCUM 30

DOSAGE

The selected remedy should be taken every half hour until an improvement occurs and is maintained.

HAIR LOSS/BALDNESS
Alopecia

The commonest form of hair loss is the slowly progressive baldness that affects men and, occasionally, elderly women. It involves the gradual loss of hair from the crown and temples. Another form of hair loss called Alopecia areata may develop in older children and adults. In this condition small bald patches suddenly appear and may slowly enlarge over the next week or so. After about 6–10 weeks, fine hair starts to grow again and the whole condition clears within approximately two more months. Other types of baldness do occur but are far less common.
Symptoms associated with hair loss are listed below.

KEY FEATURES	TREATMENT
Recurrent headaches	ANT CARB 6
Scrotal eczema	ALUMEN 6

The scalp itches and is numb	ALUMINA 6
Chronic nasal catarrh and itching of orifices	FLUORIC ACID 6
Premature baldness with greying of the hair at an early age	LYCOPODIUM 6
Oily sweating of the scalp	MERCURIUS 6
Baldness following acute, exhausting illnesses	THALLIUM 6
Moist eczema of the head and face with extreme itching Bald spots occur	VINCA MINOR 6

DOSAGE

The selected remedy should be taken twice a day until an improvement occurs.

HEADACHE

Headaches may be due to many different causes. Some of the main ones are: stress and tension, periods, eye strain (from watching too much television, for example), sinusitis and raised blood pressure.

In treating a headache with a homeopathic remedy the features of the pain itself are of the utmost importance. Its site, route of progression and any associated symptoms elsewhere in the body must also be noted.

Sudden and severe, frequent or constant, and unresponsive headaches may need investigation. A doctor should be consulted.

KEY FEATURES	TREATMENT
Tearing headache from mental exertion Pain in the forehead and back part of the head The patient is quite irritable	ANACARDIUM 30
Sensation of the head being enlarged With vertigo The pain is better for pressure	ARG NIT 30
The pain is worse on the right side and in the frontal region Throbbing pain, sharp at times and greatly aggravated by light, noise, jarring and lying down The face is flushed and red	BELLADONNA 30
Pain starts in the front, then goes over the head to the neck, and even to the shoulders and back Worse in the morning and from any movement; even movement of the eyes makes the pain worse	BRYONIA 30
Sharp, lancing pains in and over the eyes, shooting up to the top of the head, which feels as if it will lift off Sharp pain from the neck to the frontal region, which appears to go through the head, not over it	CIMICIFUGA 30
Violent throbbing of the neck arteries, feeling as if the skull will burst With anaemia	CHINA 30
Vertigo is a marked symptom Pain in the back of the head and neck	COCCULUS 30

A dull heavy ache and the eyelids feel heavy   GELSEMIUM 30

Pain starts in the back of the head, then goes over the head to settle in one eye.

Feeling of a band around the head

Worse in the morning, relieved by passing urine

The patient is listless and dull

The pain is throbbing and may be in any part of the head   GLONOINE 30

Relieved in the open air and worse if the head is bent back

The head feels heavy, as if congested   IGNATIA 30

Sensation of a nail being driven into the back of the head

Stooping helps the pain

The attack often ends by vomiting and passing a large amount of urine

The headache comes from arthritis in the neck (spondylosis).   IPECAC 30

The bones feel crushed or bruised, and even the tongue feels bruised

Nausea and vomiting

Intense, throbbing pain over the eyes with a disturbance of vision   IRIS 30

Pain usually on one side of the head or the other, but not both

Bitter, sour vomiting may occur when the headache is at its worst

From close academic work

Throbbing, hammering pain accompanied by visual effects such as zigzags   NAT MUR 30

Worse sunrise to sunset, and from heat and noise

In the morning, following a stomach upset   NUX VOM 30

Pain either in the back of the head or over one eye

Vomiting and violent retching may accompany pain

A 'hangover' headache

The pain is either in the forehead or over the eyes and tends to change its position   PULSATILLA 30

Worse from warmth and mental exertion, and in the evening

Associated with a period, a gastric upset, or rheumatism

The pain starts in the morning and begins in the back of the head, goes over the top and settles in the right eye   SANGUINARIA 30

Sleep brings relief

Noise and light cannot be tolerated

Vomiting of food and bile when the headache is at its worst

The pain is sharp and seems to shoot upwards through the brain   SEPIA 30

The patient can bear neither light nor noise

Pain relieved by sleep and violent exercising

Related to a period

With nausea and vomiting

Nervous headache from excessive mental exertion   SILICA 30

Starts in the back of the head and travels over the top to become established over the right eye

Noise, motion and jarring are intolerable

Relieved by wrapping the head up warmly

Headache as described under Silica, except it settles in the left eye — SPIGELIA 30
Starts in the morning, worst at midday and goes in the early evening

DOSAGE

The selected remedy should be taken two-hourly until an improvement is maintained.

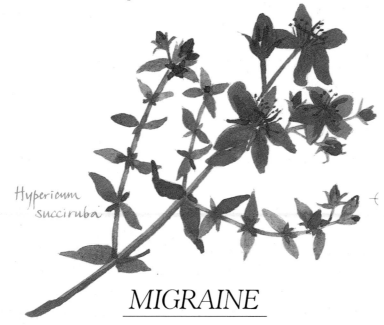

Hypericum succiruba

MIGRAINE

There are several features that distinguish migraine from a simple headache. There is usually a preceding aura, which may be seen as blurred vision, zigzags, or flashes of light. Less commonly there is abdominal pain or numbness of the tongue, face or even a limb. A severe headache, usually involving only one half of the head, comes on as the aura goes. Vomiting and nausea are frequently present, and there is often a dislike of light. Attacks tend to recur.

Migraine can start at any age, from about five onwards. It tends to subside after the age of fifty-five. Note that any of the remedies for headache (pp 76–8) may also be useful in treating migraine.

This type of headache should be diagnosed by a doctor.

KEY FEATURES	TREATMENT
After worry or prolonged studying Pressing-outward pain The ears are sensitive to the least noise and tinnitus develops	CIMICIFUGA 30
Frontal pain with a sore scalp The pain starts over the right eye and extends backwards through the head With vertigo, visual disturbance and stomach-ache	EUONYMUS 30
Left-sided pain with a feeling of pressure on top of the head The neck cracks when moving the head Worse in the morning until noon	NICCOLUM 30
Sensation of a band around the head Violent dizziness Better in the open air	PRIMULA VERIS 30
Dull frontal pain, worse over the right eye The eyeballs 'ache' and the face is flushed The patient is restless	SCUTELLARIA 30

DOSAGE

The selected remedy should be taken every two hours until an improvement is maintained.

THE EYE

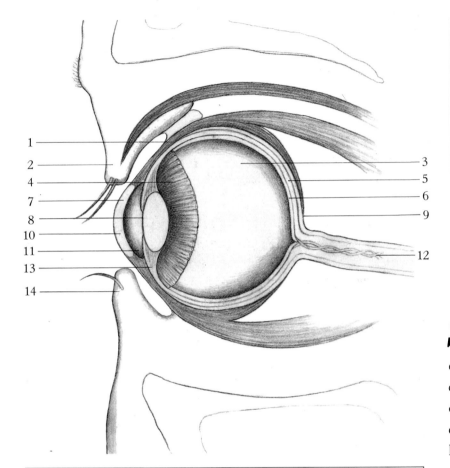

1	Conjunctiva	8	Lens
2	Upper eyelid	9	Sclera
3	Vitreous humour	10	Cornea
4	Iris	11	Aqueous humour
5	Choroid	12	Optic nerve
6	Retina	13	Ciliary muscle
7	Pupil	14	Lower eyelid

CONTENTS

Black Eye	80
Conjunctivitis	80
Discharge from the Eye	81
Eyelids, Inflammation of	82
Eyelids, Turning In or Out	83
Eye Strain	83
Itching of the Eyes	84
Styes	84
Swelling of the Eye and Eyelids	85

Shaped like a globe, the eye is set in the orbit, a bony socket in the skull bone. It is partially covered by the eyelid. The visible part of the eye is covered by a thin, transparent membrane called the conjunctiva which, if it becomes inflamed, makes the blood vessels dilate and the white part of the eye appear red. The tear glands continuously secrete a watery fluid which protects the conjunctiva by keeping it moist.

The eye is composed of several parts. The cornea is the transparent front part of the otherwise opaque, firm, fibrous covering of the eyeball called the sclera. It is the sclera which maintains the shape of the eye.

The iris is the coloured part of the eye. In its centre is the pupil, which is black and acts as a diaphragm, controlling the amount of light entering the eye. Behind the pupil is the lens, which is elastic and can alter its shape rapidly. Acting with the cornea, it reduces the size of objects seen, focusing them on to the sensitive inner surface of the eye, the retina.

The lens divides the eye into a clear, fluid-containing front portion called the anterior chamber, while the posterior chamber at the back contains a jelly-like substance called the vitreous humour. The retina contains many nerve endings and nerve fibres which go to the optic nerve. This in turn passes through an aperture in the bone at the back of the orbit on its way to the brain.

BLACK EYE

An injury to the area around the eye may lead to pain and discoloration with some swelling. The bruised tissues will then go through the normal colour changes of bruising.

Unless there has been a separate blow to both eyes, a patient with two black eyes following an accident needs immediate hospital attention as this may indicate a fracture of the base of the skull.

KEY FEATURES	TREATMENT
Bruising, swelling and pain	ARNICA 30
Better after a cold application to the eye	LEDUM 30
The eyeball itself feels tender	SYMPHYTUM 30

DOSAGE
The selected remedy should be taken once every hour for five doses.

CONJUNCTIVITIS

Inflammation of the conjunctival membrane makes the white of the eye look red due to the dilatation of small blood vessels within it. The symptoms often start with irritation, which is followed by a painful feeling of grit in the eye. At first the eye waters more than usual, but soon this turns to a pus-like discharge which causes the lids to stick together when the eyes are closed for prolonged periods. The condition is very infectious and may spread to the other eye. Recurrent attacks of conjunctivitis may be of an allergic origin.

If the pain is severe, the vision affected in any way, or a foreign body or eye ulcer suspected, a doctor should be consulted.

KEY FEATURES	TREATMENT
The eyelids are dry, burning and smarting, especially in the morning In chronic cases	ALUMINA 6
The lids are swollen, red and puffy The tears burn and sting Dislike of light The conjunctiva is bright red With sudden piercing pains	APIS 30
Pus is invariably present The conjunctiva may be scarlet red, puffy and swollen	ARG NIT 30
Pustular conjunctivitis The eye is very sensitive to cold and feels better if closed	CLEMATIS 30

Extreme sensitivity to light and excessive tears | CONIUM 30
The eyes are worse in dim light

Diffuse redness with marked dislike of light | EUPHRASIA 30
The eyes water continuously with acrid and
  burning tears
The lids may burn and swell
With a catarrhal cold and headache

The eyes and lids are red and inflamed, and the | HEPAR SULPH 30
  eyeballs sore to the touch
With a profuse pus-like discharge
The eye is very sensitive to touch and air
Corneal ulceration may follow
If corneal ulceration is suspected, seek medical advice.

The eyelids are affected, the eyes themselves | NAT ARS 30
  feel weak and heavy, and water in the wind
The lids stick overnight

Chronic conjunctivitis with copious, thick | PICRIC ACID 6
  yellow discharge

The discharge is profuse, bland and white/ | PULSATILLA 30
  yellow in colour, and the lids are inflamed and
  sticky
Worse in the warmth

DOSAGE

Remedies in the 30 potency should be taken four times a day for
three days.
Remedies in the 6 potency should be taken twice a day until there is
a sustained improvement.

DISCHARGE FROM THE EYE

The usual cause is an infection of the conjunctiva (conjunctivitis). The discharge is watery at first and there is a sensation of grit in the eye. The discharge soon becomes thicker and pus-like and the lids may stick together overnight.
In hay fever and other allergic conditions a clear, watery eye discharge may develop. This can be bland or acrid. A foreign body in the eye may produce the same symptoms, but can usually be seen for removal.

An eye discharge with pain, or one that does not quickly respond to treatment, should be referred to a doctor.

KEY FEATURES	TREATMENT
Pus-like discharge with swollen conjunctiva and a red eye	ARG NIT 30

Hyoscyamus niger

Inflammation of the eye with a thick yellow discharge	CALC SULPH 30
Visual field defect; the patient sees only half of an object	
A thick yellow discharge with a granular rash on the lids	DULCAMARA 30
Colds always affect the eyes	
The discharge is acrid, thick and burns the lids	EUPHRASIA 30
The eyes constantly water	

A profuse, burning, acrid discharge makes the lids red and swollen	MERCURIUS 30
A thick, profuse, yellow, bland discharge makes the eyes itch and burn and the lids are inflamed and stick together	PULSATILLA 30

DOSAGE

The selected remedy should be taken three times a day for five days.

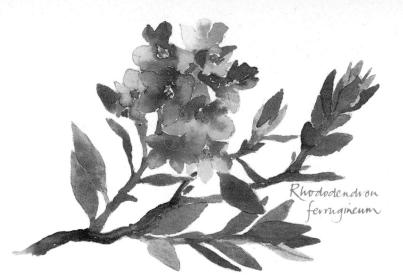

Rhododendron ferrugineum

EYELIDS, Inflammation of
Blepheritis

Redness of the eyelids is often associated with eczema elsewhere in the body, but especially on the scalp. Scaling of the lids is also present and irritation is common.

KEY FEATURES	TREATMENT
The lids appear red and thick	ARG MET 12
The lids are itchy, swollen and scaly, and worse in the morning Sensitivity to bright light	CALC CARB 12
The lids become swollen and may ulcerate Sensation of a film in front of the eyes, worse after exposure to cold	CAUSTICUM 12
The lids feel heavy and difficult to open Vision is blurred and smoky Extreme pain around the eye	GELSEMIUM 12
The lids are red, swollen and feel dry A honey-like exudate forms on the lids	GRAPHITES 12
Extreme pain around the eye with excessive tears, sensitivity to light and smarting lids	IPECAC 12
The lids burn and are swollen and puffy from fluid Small granules on the lids	KALI BICH 12
Ulceration and redness of the lids Styes are frequent	LYCOPODIUM 12
The lids are red and feel hot with excessive tears, spasmodic sneezing and runny nose	SABADILLA 12
The lids burn and may ulcerate With eczema elsewhere	SULPHUR 12
The lids stick at night and are dry and scaly by day Styes are frequent	THUJA 12

DOSAGE

The selected remedy should be taken three times a day until an improvement is maintained.

EYELIDS, Turning Out or In
Ectropion or Entropion

These conditions tend to occur in the elderly. When the lid turns inward, damage to the eye can be caused by the eyelashes pricking the eyeball. When the lid turns outward, the flow of tears is interfered with and the eye appears to be constantly watering. Surgical correction may be necessary.

KEY FEATURES	TREATMENT
The lids are swollen, red, inflamed and turn out	APIS 12
The lashes turn inward and cut against the eyeball	BORAX 12
Loss of eyelashes The skin around the eye is dry and scurfy	PETROLEUM 12

DOSAGE

The selected remedy should be taken twice a day until an improvement occurs and then stopped. Repeat the treatment as and when necessary.

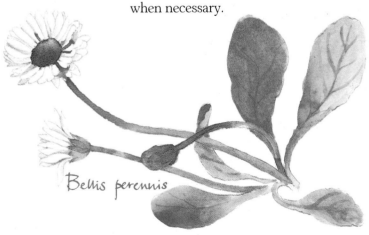

Bellis perennis

EYE STRAIN

People whose work involves a lot of reading, such as students or those working for long periods of time at a visual display unit (VDU), may suffer from eye strain. This manifests itself as eye ache, difficulty in focusing and possibly headaches.

It is advisable to have a sight test if this condition is recurrent.

KEY FEATURES	TREATMENT
Reading is difficult as the letters seem to move The lids twitch and are red, itchy and burning	AGARICUS 12
Eye strain from close work Worse in the warmth The eyes ache, feel tired and are better for closing or pressure	ARG NIT 30
A film seems to be in front of the eye The lids are inflamed	CAUSTICUM 30
Eye strain with long sight	CINA 12
The eyes feel hot and tired, and vision may become blurred The lids may twitch	MAG PHOS 30
Tired eyes from reading or writing, the letters start to run together and a headache occurs (especially in children)	NAT MUR 30
The vision becomes blurred The eyes feel heavy and pain extends to the left temple May be associated with migraine	ONOSMODIUM 30

The eyes tire, even without much use	PHOSPHORUS 12
It is easier to see things by shading the eyes with the hand	
Sensation of a mist before the eyes and letters may appear	
Eye strain from any cause	PILOCARPUS 12
The eyes tire easily and smart	
Vision becomes hazy	

DOSAGE

Remedies in the 12 potency should be used twice a day or until glasses are prescribed.
Remedies in the 30 potency should be taken every two hours for three doses.

ITCHING OF THE EYES

Irritation of the eye (itching and watering) is usually caused through allergy, as in hay fever. If the cause is known, it is obviously wise to avoid the irritant whenever possible.

KEY FEATURES	TREATMENT
Excessive tears and intolerable itching of the eyelids	AMBROSIA 6
The eyes smart and burn	
The pupil is large and bright, with a dislike of light	AGNUS 6
The eye itself itches	
Itching and smarting, with swelling, heat and soreness	FAGOPYRUM 6

Itching and soreness of the lids with red and inflamed conjunctiva	ZINC MET 6
Symptoms worse in the inner part of the eye (nose side)	

DOSAGE

The selected remedy should be taken every hour until an improvement is maintained.

STYES

These are small boils that occur in the eyelid. Irritation of the lid is often the first sign and is soon followed by redness, pain and swelling of the affected lid.

KEY FEATURES	TREATMENT
For recurrent styes	APIS 30
The whole lid becomes swollen, and sharp, piercing pains develop	
The conjunctiva becomes red	
The lids are dry, red and scaly and there is intolerance of artificial light	GRAPHITES 30
In the inner angle of the eye (the nose side)	LYCOPODIUM 30
The lids become red and ulcerate	
With thick, profuse, yellow discharge	PULSATILLA 30
The lids become inflamed and stick	
The eyes itch and burn	
The eye feels tender to the touch	SILICA 30
Aversion to light as it causes sharp pains which run through the eye	

The margins of the eye itch	STAPHYSAGRIA 30
The eyes appear sunken	
Recurrent styes	
The lids stick overnight and are dry and scaly	THUJA 30

DOSAGE

The selected remedy should be taken four times a day for three days.

SWELLING OF THE EYE AND EYELIDS

The most likely cause of this condition is an allergy such as hay fever. The white of the eye can swell considerably and in these circumstances medical help should be sought. Other causes of swelling are conjunctivitis, infection of the eyelid, eczema of the lids, inflamed cysts in the lids and injury.

Any unexplained swelling in or around the eye requires medical diagnosis.

KEY FEATURES	TREATMENT
The lids are swollen, red and puffy, burning and stinging	APIS 30
The conjunctiva is red, the tears hot and sudden piercing pains occur	
The conjunctiva swells and there is an abundant pus-like discharge	ARG NIT 30
The lids are sore, thickened and swollen	
The eyes ache and feel tired	

Swelling around the eye	ARS ALB 30
The tears feel hot and cause soreness of the lids	
Intense dislike of light	
The eyes continually water	EUPHRASIA 30
The lids swell and burn	
Frequent inclination to blink	
The tears are acrid	
The lids are red and swollen and may crack	GRAPHITES 12
Eczema of the lids	
Swelling over the upper lids and across the bridge of the nose	KALI CARB 12
The lids stick together overnight	
The lids become red, puffy and sore, and the eyes feel sore and hot	MERC CORR 30
The tears are acrid	
Worse at night	
The eyes appear almost closed because of great swelling	RHUS VEN 30

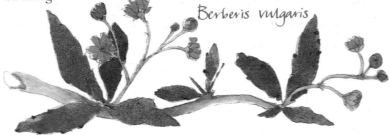

Berberis vulgaris

DOSAGE

Remedies in the 30 potency should be taken every two hours for four doses, then three times a day for a further two days. Remedies in the 12 potency should be taken twice a day until an improvement occurs, then stopped. Repeat the treatment as and when necessary.

THE EAR

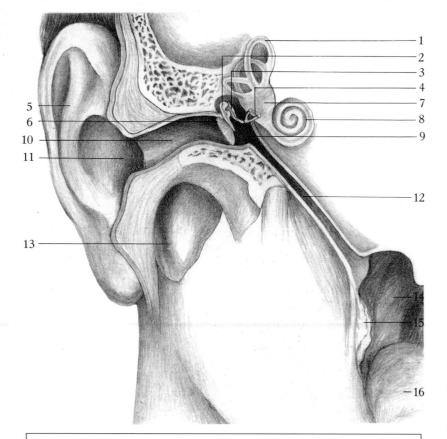

1 —
2 —
3 —
4 —
7 —
8 —
9 —
5
6
10
11
12 —
13 —
14
15
16

CONTENTS

Catarrh and Obstruction of the Eustachian Tube	87
Deafness	88
Earache with Discharge	88
Earache without Discharge	89
Ear, Noises in	90
Eczema of the Ear	91
Injuries to the Ear	91
Menière's Disease	92
Travel Sickness	92

*T*he ear is normally described as being in three parts: the external, middle and inner ear. The first two are purely concerned with collecting and transmitting sound from the outside to the inner ear, which, apart from hearing, also controls balance.

The external ear comprises the pinna, which is both protective and functional as it collects and directs sound waves down the external auditory canal and on to the ear drum.

The middle ear is a tympanic cavity deep in the skull bone. The ear drum (tympanic membrane) is its external wall and the middle ear bones (auditory ossicles) are located just inside it. These are called the hammer (malleus), the anvil (incus) and the stirrup (stapes) because of their shape. When sound-waves hit the drum they cause it to vibrate and these vibrations are transmitted via the three ossicles to the cochlea to produce the sensation of hearing.

1 Semicircular canal	9 Tympanic cavity
2 Hammer (*Malleus*)	10 External auditory canal
3 Anvil (*Incus*)	11 Concha
4 Stirrup (*Stapes*)	12 Eustachian tube
5 Pinna	13 Mastoid process
6 Tympanic membrane (*Ear drum*)	14 Mouth
	15 Tonsil
7 Vestibule	16 Tongue
8 Cochlea	

From the cavity of each middle ear the narrow eustachian tube runs down to the back of the nose just where it joins the throat. In this way the middle ear is open to outside air and the ear drum then has equal air pressure on either side of it which allows it to move freely. If one or both of the eustachian tubes are blocked with catarrh, the drum cannot vibrate freely and partial but temporary deafness ensues.

Unfortunately these tubes can also allow infection into the middle ear which may lead to a condition called otitis media. If left untreated, this may lead to a hole forming in the ear drum which bursts outwards to let the infection out of the middle ear. Infection of the middle ear can also (rarely) spread inwards into the bony mass found just below the ear (the mastoid process) to produce the condition known as mastoiditis.

The inner ear is a complex structure and consists of a vestibule, semicircular canals and the cochlea. The vestibular apparatus is concerned with balance. In it are the semicircular canals which contain fluid and have many nerve endings in their walls. When the head is moved the fluid presses on different parts of the walls and the nerve endings then send a message to the brain to let it know what position the head is in. Excessive movements can produce confused messages getting through and cause motion sickness.

The cochlea is the essential organ of hearing. It looks rather like the shell of a snail, and its cavity lying in fluid contains numerous tiny strands, rather like hairs. If stimulated by a particular sound, each of these hairs passes on information about that sound via the auditory nerve to the brain.

CATARRH
and Obstruction of the Eustachian Tube

The symptoms produced when the eustachian tube is blocked are temporary deafness and, very often, pain. Pressure changes experienced when ascending or descending suddenly (as in a plane) can produce both symptoms, as can catarrh, which is a common cause of obstruction.

KEY FEATURES	TREATMENT
Roaring and buzzing in the ears, words and sounds echo unpleasantly	CAUSTICUM 30
Naso-pharyngeal catarrh with deafness	GRAPHITES 30
Naso-pharyngeal catarrh with tinnitus	HYDRASTIS 30
Sharp, stitching pains The middle ear becomes inflamed and produces a tenacious, stringy, pus-like discharge	KALI BICH 30
Deteriorating hearing Stuffy sensation in the naso-pharynx Snapping noises in the ear with a middle-ear catarrhal inflammation	KALI MUR 30

DOSAGE

The selected remedy should be taken three times a day for five days.

DEAFNESS

Deafness may be congenital or can be a complication of an infectious disease such as measles. It may be partial or complete, permanent or temporary. There are many possible causes, the commonest being wax in the ear, infection in the external or middle ear, catarrh in the eustachian tube, disease of the middle-ear bones, noise and advancing years. The key features below occur in conjunction with deafness.

KEY FEATURES	TREATMENT
Catarrh	ALLIUM SAT 30
Calcium deposits on the drum Hardening of the middle-ear bones Roaring noises in the ears	CALC FLUOR 12
Eczema of the external ear, worse in damp weather or surroundings	CALENDULA 12
Chronic middle-ear catarrh Accumulation of wax Ringing or roaring noises in the ear	CAUSTICUM 12
Chronic middle-ear infection Progressive deafness Buzzing noises in the ear High-pitched sounds heard best	CHENOPODIUM 12
Roaring noises in the ear Pus-like discharge with eustachian catarrh	HYDRASTIS 30
Eczema of the external ear, worse after using steroid ear drops	LOBELIA 12
Vertigo with noises in the ear Menière's disease	NAT SAL 12
Following measles	PULSATILLA 30
Infected discharge	VIOLA ODORATA 30

DOSAGE

Remedies in the 12 potency should be taken twice a day until an improvement is maintained.
Remedies in the 30 potency should be taken three times a day for four days.

EARACHE with Discharge

The pressure of hardened wax or a foreign body in the canal may cause earache. It may also be caused by a chemical irritant such as hair lacquer or shampoo getting into the canal, and sometimes from the chlorine in swimming pools. However, most earache is caused through infection, which may be in the external auditory canal (otitis externa) or in the middle ear (otitis media).

If earache fails to clear quickly, medical help should be sought.

KEY FEATURES	TREATMENT
The skin around ear is raw and burning Thin, offensive, acrid discharge and a roaring noise with each bout of pain	ARS ALB 30
Sudden onset with violent burning and throbbing pain The patient is very hot and red Thin, burning discharge with delirium	BELLADONNA 30

Violent, unbearable pain and restlessness	CHAMOMILLA 30
The patient (usually a child) is very fretful	
Throbbing, pulsating pain with cracking noises and a discharge of mucus and pus	CALC CARB 30
Hearing is affected	

Calendula officinalis

Paroxysms of throbbing pain	FERRUM PHOS 30
Noises in the ear	
Discharge of mucus and pus which may be blood-stained	
Smelly discharge with throbbing noises in the ear and diminished hearing	HEPAR SULPH 30
Boils in the canal	
Thick, yellow, stringy discharge	KALI BICH 30
Swelling, usually of the left ear, and tearing pain	
The discharge has an offensive odour like rotten meat	PSORINUM 30
The ear is hot, red and swollen	PULSATILLA 30
Darting pains, worse at night, a profuse, thick, yellow-green discharge and ringing noises in the ears	

Smelly discharge	SILICA 30
Great sensitivity to noise	
Roaring sounds in the ears	
For chronic inflammation with a thin, acrid, offensive discharge	TELLURIUM 12
The ear canal is very sensitive to touch	

DOSAGE

Remedies in the 12 potency should be taken twice a day until an improvement is maintained.
Remedies in the 30 potency should be taken three times a day for four days.

EARACHE *without Discharge*

Pain in the ear most commonly occurs in the early stages of infection, either in the outer ear, middle ear or eustachian tube, which, if untreated, may eventually lead to a discharge developing. Excessive wax in the outer canal of the ear can occasionally cause some discomfort, especially if water gets behind it after bathing or swimming.
Any of the following, if not treated, may lead to a discharge. The remedy will then need to be changed.

KEY FEATURES	TREATMENT
The external ear is hot and red	ACONITE 30
Stinging, cutting or throbbing pains are worse after exposure to cold, dry wind and at night	
Pain shoots up from the throat	ALLIUM CEPA 30

89

The external ear is red and sore Stinging pain	APIS 30
Shooting pain from the throat The tonsils are swollen	GELSEMIUM 30
Severe neuralgic pain, worse behind the right ear and in cold air	MAG PHOS 30
Shooting pain radiates from the throat and is worse on swallowing	PHYTOLACCA 30
Toothache may also be present The hearing becomes very acute Pain appears to go from ear to ear	PLANTAGO 30

DOSAGE

Remedies in the 12 potency should be taken twice a day until an improvement is maintained.
Remedies in the 30 potency should be taken three times a day for four days.

Ringing, roaring, pulsating ear noises Deafness or words re-echo Chronic middle-ear catarrh	CAUSTICUM 12
Deafness and vertigo	CHIN SAL 12
Violent ringing, buzzing and roaring in the ears Hearing is defective	CHIN SULPH 12
Throbbing in the ear with an infection	FERRUM PHOS 30
Roaring and singing sounds develop Excessive ear wax	LACHESIS 12
Roaring and ringing, deafness and vertigo	SALICYL ACID 12
Humming and roaring accompanied by a headache The ears feel hot internally	SANGUINARIA 30
Whizzing noise in the ear Catarrhal deafness preceded by ultra-sensitive hearing	SULPHUR 12

DOSAGE

Remedies in the 12 potency should be taken twice a day until an improvement is maintained.
Remedies in the 30 potency should be taken three times a day for four days.

EAR, Noises in
Tinnitus

Hearing tends to deteriorate with age and in some people noises, heard only by them, may develop in their ears. The commonest sounds heard are those of ringing and roaring, but virtually any other sound may be present.

KEY FEATURES | **TREATMENT**

Buzzing and singing noises in the ear and head Hearing is impaired Menière's disease may also occur	CARB SULPH 12

ECZEMA OF THE EAR

Eczema around the ear or in the outer canal will usually lead to irritation and scratching. Cracks, especially behind the ear, tend to occur and these occasionally discharge or become infected.

KEY FEATURES	TREATMENT
Moist, scabby eruption with cracks behind the ear and a gluey, honey-like, thick discharge	GRAPHITES 12
Sore, crusty eruption behind the ear	OLEANDER 12
Hard, dry, cracked skin behind the ear easily becomes infected	PETROLEUM 12
The skin may bleed from scratching	

DOSAGE

The selected remedy should be taken twice a day until an improvement occurs, then stopped. Repeat the treatment as and when necessary.

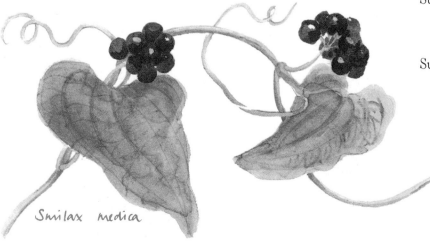

Smilax medica

INJURIES TO THE EAR

The external ear canal is very easily damaged, so attempts to remove wax from within the ear by using cotton-wool buds and the like should never be attempted. Blows to the ear may cause internal as well as external damage, and sudden, very loud noises can also cause injury. The use of personal stereos to listen to loud music may also lead to internal injury and possibly eventual hearing loss in some ranges.

All but superficial injuries need prompt medical attention. Injuries or bleeding within the ear canal, particularly after a head injury, and those caused by exposure to sudden loud noises must be treated in a hospital urgently.

KEY FEATURES	TREATMENT
Bruising, external pain and superficial bleeding	ARNICA 10M take every hour for 4–6 doses.
Superficial puncture wound or an insect bite	LEDUM 200 take three times a day for two days.
Superficial wound which becomes infected	HEPAR SULPH 30 take four times a day for three days.

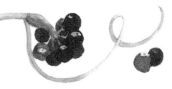

MENIÈRE'S DISEASE

This is a disorder of the inner ear. It normally occurs in adults and consists of recurring bouts of extreme dizziness with some loss of hearing and tinnitus (noises in the ear). An attack may last from several hours to several days.

Medical diagnosis is needed for this condition.

KEY FEATURES	TREATMENT
Dull headache and vertigo In younger people	AMMON IOD 30
Deaf to the human voice, but great sensitivity to other sounds and better for high-pitched sounds Buzzing in the ear	CHENOPODIUM 30
Deafness and tinnitus	CHIN SAL 30
Vertigo and deafness with noises in the ear	NAT SAL 200

DOSAGE
The selected remedy should be taken four times a day for two days.

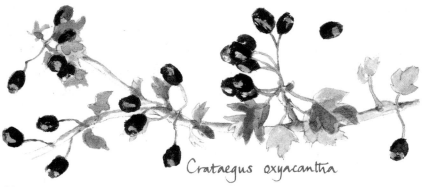

Crataegus oxyacantha

TRAVEL SICKNESS

This is due to a disturbance of the balance mechanism in the inner ear. It can take many different forms, from simple nausea to severe vomiting, and can occur in both children and adults. It may be produced by any form of transport on air, sea or land.

KEY FEATURES	TREATMENT
The most frequently indicated remedy Headache in the back of the head and neck which is worse for lying on the painful area Metallic taste in the mouth An aversion to the sight or smell of food, accompanied by a dry throat and distended abdomen	COCCULUS 30
Increased salivation The patient feels better for eating and in the warmth, and better lying down, but with head raised	PETROLEUM 30
Better with eyes closed Tight feeling around the head The face is pale with a cold sweat Worse from tobacco fumes and much better in open air	TABACUM 30

DOSAGE
The treatment should commence the night before the journey and the following regime with the selected remedy is recommended: one dose at bedtime; one dose on waking; one dose about an hour before travelling; one or two doses during the journey, depending on its duration.

THE NOSE AND SINUSES

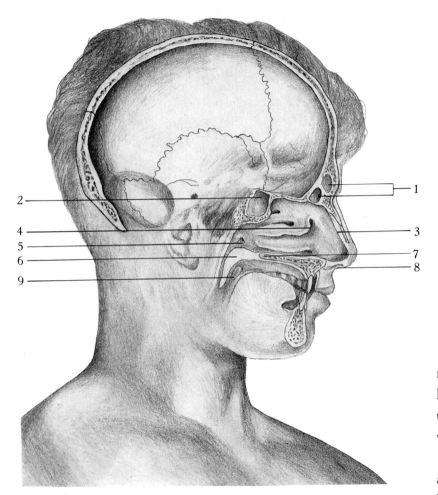

CONTENTS

Catarrh, Chronic	94
Colds	95
Hay Fever	96
Nasal Blockage/Snuffles	98
Nasal Discharge	99
Nasal Irritation/Itching	100
Nasal Polyps	100
Nosebleeds	101
Sense of Smell Disorders	101
Sinusitis	102

*T*he nose is the start of the respiratory tract and its shape is maintained by a frame of bone and cartilage. The front of the nasal cavity consists of cartilage which, unlike bone, can withstand hard knocks without being damaged. The base is formed from the upper surface of the hard palate in the front and the soft palate, which is behind.

The nasal cavity itself is divided into two separate areas, right and left, by a vertical septum made of cartilage at the front and bone behind. Jutting out from both side walls are three curved turbinates made of bone which divide each cavity roughly into three separate horizontal areas.

1	Frontal sinuses	6	Soft palate
2	Sphenoidal sinuses	7	Hard palate
3	Septum	8	Nostril
4	Turbinates	9	Tonsils
5	Eustachian tube		

The two nostrils open downwards and at their opening have a hairy lining which stops large dust particles from entering the respiratory tract. The lining mucous membrane secretes a fluid which keeps it moist, and a network of blood vessels within keeps it warm so that air going into the lungs is filtered, warmed and moistened.

As the blood vessels are thin-walled and near the surface of the mucous membrane, bleeding from burst blood vessels is quite common in the area at the front of the nasal cavity. (The medical name for a nosebleed is epistaxis.)

In the area at the side of and above the nose are several air-filled cavities within the bones of the face called sinuses and these each have an opening into the nasal cavity. The main ones are at either side of the nose below the eyes (the maxillary sinuses) and at either side of the forehead above the eyes (the frontal sinuses).

Other openings into the nasal cavity are for the tear ducts, which run from the inner corner of each eye. At the back of the nose, where it becomes the upper throat or nasopharynx, there are openings for the eustachian tubes. Also at this junction are the adenoids. These are formed of spongy tissue which, if infected, may swell and make breathing through the nose difficult.

The nerves responsible for the recognition of smells sit in the roof of the nose and run for a short distance within the mucous membrane covering the septum and outer walls of the nasal cavity. When a cold causes the mucous membrane to become swollen, air is prevented from reaching the upper part of the nose and this leads to a loss of the sense of smell.

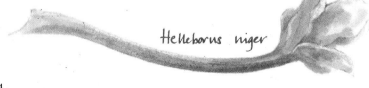

Helleborus niger

CATARRH, *Chronic*

Recurrent or chronic nasal catarrh may be produced in several different ways, each one influencing the symptoms. If the cause is allergic, the discharge is watery and sneezing frequent. If associated with chronic or recurrent sinusitis, the discharge contains mucus and pus and is profuse. In small children catarrh in the form of snuffles may persist for weeks because the nasal passages are narrow and the child is unable to blow its nose to clear the discharge of mucus and pus which has formed. Chronic catarrh may also be caused by the prolonged use of nasal decongestants and sprays.

KEY FEATURES	TREATMENT
The nose is swollen and there is a profuse, thick, yellow discharge The nasal membrane is sore	ARS IOD 6
Dull frontal headache and a yellow-coated tongue Food tastes bitter	COLLINSONIA 6
Chronic nasal catarrh with formation of green crusts in the nose The catarrh has an offensive smell	ELAPS 6
Dull frontal headache Ulcers may form on the nasal septum	FLUORIC ACID 6
Snuffles in fat babies Pressure and pain at the root of the nose The discharge is thick, ropy and green-yellow in colour The frontal sinuses become inflamed	KALI BICH 6

		KEY FEATURES	TREATMENT
The catarrh affects the nose and the pharynx Intense itching of the nose	MEDORRHINUM 6	Used within a few hours of the symptoms appearing, it may stop the cold from developing For colds caught in frosty, cold and dry, windy weather The patient is hot, thirsty, shivery and restless, and worse in a stuffy atmosphere	ACONITE 30
The discharge is yellow, offensive and corrosive Worse in both hot and cold weather	NITRIC ACID 6		
The nasal membrane is dry and congested Nasal polyps may be present	SANGUINARIA 6	The eyes and nose stream and the watery discharge makes the nose and upper lip sore Frequent bouts of sneezing Worse in a warm room and better in the fresh air	ALLIUM CEPA 30
Heavy, lumpy post-nasal discharge which is coughed up through the mouth Thick green plugs and crusts	SEPIA 6		
Chronic catarrh with foul breath and a crawling sensation in the nostrils Nasal polyps Loss of the sense of smell	TEUCRIUM 6	In changeable weather Painful, frequent sneezing bouts All discharges are burning and the upper lip becomes sore The nose feels blocked at night, with intense irritation in the nostrils The patient is very chilly but wants frequent small, cold drinks	ARS ALB 30

DOSAGE

The selected remedy should be taken twice a day until an improvement occurs, then stopped. Repeat the treatment as and when necessary.

COLDS

A cold is an acute infection caused by a virus and is highly infectious. A sore throat is an early symptom and at this stage there is a clear, watery, nasal discharge with a tendency to sneeze. After a day or two this goes on to become a thick discharge of mucus and pus which may block the nose. A dry cough also occurs after a few days. The temperature may or may not be raised in adults, but it usually is in babies and small children.

KEY FEATURES	TREATMENT
After getting cold and wet, or becoming chilled when overheated Much sneezing, made worse in a cold room The eyes and nose both stream and the eyes become sore and red Pains in the neck, back and limbs	DULCAMARA 30
The eyes are red and watery, and the tears irritating A bland nasal discharge The cold is worse at night but the cough is worse during the daytime	EUPHRASIA 30

Slow onset in warm, moist weather Headache and the arms and legs feel heavy and ache Chills seem to run up and down the spine Sore nostrils and sensation of a lump in the throat	GELSEMIUM 30
In cold, dry weather Much sneezing and the nasal discharge, which starts as thin and watery, becomes thick, yellow and offensive The patient is exceptionally cold and hates even the slightest draught	HEPAR SULPH 30
Violent sneezing and extreme thirst The eyes and nose become sore and red from the acrid, watery tears and nasal discharge, and there is a frontal headache The patient feels hot and cold alternately	KALI IOD 30
Creeping chilliness at first, which leads on to a sore throat, foul breath, green-yellow catarrh and a dry, tickly cough Profuse sweats	MERCURIUS 30
After being in the cold or exposed to cold, dry winds The nose alternates between being blocked at night and runny during the day The patient becomes very chilly and irritable	NUX VOM 30
The cold is persistent and the patient produces bland, thick, green-yellow catarrh The nose becomes blocked (especially on the right) in the evening and at night, and also in a warm room	PULSATILLA 30

Pain in the face and nose
The sense of smell is affected
Lack of thirst

DOSAGE

Aconite may be taken every hour in the first few hours of the illness until an improvement occurs. Otherwise the selected remedy should be taken four times a day until an improvement occurs, then stopped.

HAY FEVER

This sometimes distressing condition is caused by an allergy to one or more pollens and mostly occurs in the spring and summer. The main symptoms, which are due to irritation of the membranes of the nose and eye, are bouts of violent sneezing with streaming eyes. The nose may also stream, but this may alternate with a stuffed-up nose. Other symptoms which may develop are itching of the roof of the mouth, itching in the ears, and in some patients a mild form of asthma with a sensation of tightness in the chest.

KEY FEATURES	TREATMENT
The eyes may swell and sting, but the tears are bland Acrid nasal discharge makes the nose and upper lip become sore Frequent sneezing Headache, felt at the back of the head, often accompanies the hay fever Symptoms worse indoors and in the evening	ALLIUM CEPA 12

The eyes feel burning hot, while the tears are acrid and sting the cheek   ARS ALB 12

Thin, burning nasal discharge irritates the upper lip

Nose frequently blocked

Tickling sensation in one spot in the nose, not helped by the violent sneezing which may occur

The patient feels worn out and is better indoors and for warmth

Pain over the root of the nose   ARUM TRIPH 12

Frequent sneezing with a burning nasal discharge but at times the nose feels blocked

The sneezing is worse at night

Itching in the eyes, nose and roof of the mouth   ARUNDO 12

Thin, watery nasal discharge which later becomes thicker and yellow-green

The condition comes on in late summer, or even in the autumn   DULCAMARA 12

The eyes swell and stream tears

Constant sneezing, and although the nose streams, it feels blocked

The skin feels hot and dry

Patient better at rest and indoors, much worse after rain

The eyes burn, itch and stream with burning tears   EUPHRASIA 12

Profuse, watery, but bland nasal discharge

Frequent sneezing is worse in the evening and at night, but a cough may develop, which is worse during the day and often goes away at night

The eyes feel hot, heavy and look bloodshot   GELSEMIUM 12

The nose streams a burning discharge, mainly in the morning

The nose tingles and there is violent sneezing

Dry, burning throat, hot face and aching limbs

Swallowing produces pain in the ears

Excessive sweating and all the symptoms are worse in the morning

Cyclamen europaeum

The eyes smart and swell with burning, profuse tears   KALI IOD 12

With pain in the sinuses

Profuse nasal discharge, at first thin, watery and burning, becomes thick, yellow and offensive

Violent sneezing

Nose becomes red, tender and sore

The patient feels altenately hot and chilly and is worse in the mornings and evenings

Eyelids swollen and itchy   NAT MUR 12

Profuse tears sting the eyes

Frequent violent sneezing with a burning, profuse, watery nasal discharge

Symptoms much worse around 10 a.m.

97

Eyes and nose itch terribly, and the irritation goes to the throat	NUX VOM 12
Frequent sneezing in distressing prolonged bouts	
Watery nasal discharge, much worse indoors, but the nose becomes blocked when outdoors and at night	
Hot face, but the patient feels chilly and becomes bad-tempered	
Eyelids hot and red, but the profuse tears are bland	SABADILLA 12
Thin nasal discharge becomes thicker and then the nose feels sore and blocked	
Prolonged attacks of violent sneezing may cause a severe headache and nosebleeds	
Symptoms worse from odour of apples, garlic, onions and flowers	

DOSAGE

The selected remedy should be taken every half hour until an improvement occurs, and then stopped. Repeat as and when necessary.

If the cause of the allergy is known, it is useful to take a potency of it during the winter months to desensitize. The commoner triggers of hay fever are all available for this purpose and may be obtained from homeopathic pharmacies. In most cases Mixed Pollen 30 and House Dust Mite 30 are the remedies required. For densensitization take the selected remedy three times a day on one day each week from one month before the start of the hay fever season.

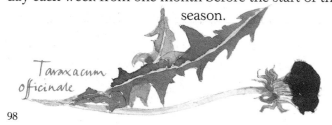

Taraxacum officinale

NASAL BLOCKAGE/SNUFFLES

The nose may become blocked from catarrh, from polyps, from injury or from a foreign body in the nose. Catarrh usually follows any irritation of the lining of the nose, such as a cold or inhalation of an irritant. Hay fever and other allergies cause blocking with a considerable amount of (usually watery) discharge and sneezing. The discharge is thicker when associated with sinusitis, as is the discharge in babies which causes snuffles and a nasal drip, often for weeks. (See also Chronic Catarrh, p. 94)

KEY FEATURES	TREATMENT
The nose feels dry but there may be a scanty, watery discharge	ACONITE 12
The blockage is mainly at night, making breathing through the nose difficult For children who get 'snuffles'	AMMON CARB 12
Sneezing does not clear the nose Thin, watery, burning discharge	ARS ALB 12
Acrid, burning discharge The nose is so obstructed that breathing through the mouth is necessary Boring pain in the nose	ARUM TRIPH 12
The nose is completely blocked up Usually occurs in cold, wet weather	DULCAMARA 12
Chronic catarrh with a stuffed-up sensation	EUCALYPTUS 12
Snuffles, especially in fat babies Pressure and pain at the root of the nose and a thick, ropy, greenish-yellow discharge	KALI BICH 12

The nose feels very dry and blocked with much crusting	LYCOPODIUM 12
Children wake during the night rubbing their nose because of the snuffles	
Blockage comes on after two or three days of a thin, watery discharge from the nose	NAT MUR 12
Loss of smell and taste	
The blockage is mainly in the right nostril and worse in the evening	PULSATILLA 12
Abundant yellow mucus in the morning	
The sense of smell is diminished	

DOSAGE

The selected remedy should be taken four times a day for four days.

NASAL DISCHARGE

This entry deals with the types of nasal discharge the patient may experience and should be used in conjunction with Chronic Catarrh (see p. 94)

KEY FEATURES	TREATMENT
Copious watery, very acrid discharge	ALLIUM CEPA 12
Thin, watery, irritating, acrid discharge, or a profuse, thick, yellow discharge	ARS IOD 12
Acrid, burning discharge	ARUM TRIPH 12
Profuse, thick, foul discharge which runs down the throat at night	COPAIVA 12

Profuse, fluent discharge with a cough	EUPHRASIA 12
Thick, offensive discharge	HEPAR SULPH 12
Profuse watery discharge, or thick, ropy, greenish-yellow discharge	KALI BICH 12
Profuse, acrid, hot, watery, thin discharge	KALI IOD 12
Thick, yellow discharge and salty mucus	NAT SULPH 12
Chronic catarrh with yellow, offensive, corrosive discharge	NITRIC ACID 12
Copious mucus discharge	RUMEX 12
Copious, watery, nasal discharge	SABADILLA 12
Chronic, thick, greenish discharge	SEPIA 12
Post-nasal bland mucus discharge	SPIGELIA 12

DOSAGE

The selected remedy should be taken twice a day until an improvement occurs, then stopped. Repeat the treatment as and when necessary.

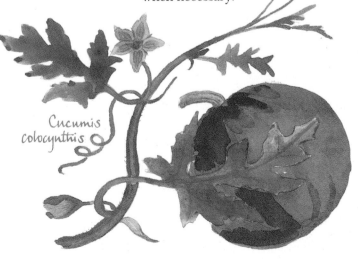

Cucumis colocynthis

NASAL IRRITATION/ITCHING

When internal, this symptom is invariably due to something inhaled to which the patient is allergic. It is common in hay fever. External irritation may be due to the same cause, but can also occur in eczema and with some nasal discharges.

KEY FEATURES	TREATMENT
Irritation and tingling of the nose with a constant desire to sneeze	ARS IOD 12
The tip of the nose is red and scabby with itching around the nostrils	CARBO VEG 12
The nose itches all the time and the patient wants to rub and pick at it until it bleeds	CINA 12
Itching and tickling in the soft palate and naso-pharynx	GELSEMIUM 12
The nose feels dry but there may be a slight watery, burning discharge	
Intense irritation of the nose, throat and larynx	KALI PERM 12
Itching at the end of the nose with sneezing, worse in the morning	SILICA 12
Itching and redness with a burning sensation	STRONTIA 12

DOSAGE

The selected remedy should be taken every two hours until an improvement is maintained.

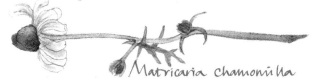

Matricaria chamomilla

NASAL POLYPS

These are soft, elongated, shiny, greyish growths which develop from the nasal lining and may obstruct the nostril. They are not malignant but often recur after surgical removal. They are associated with chronic sinusitis, hay fever and other allergies which affect the nose. They are a cause of mouth-breathing and snoring.

KEY FEATURES	TREATMENT
When the nose is obstructed with several polyps	CADMIUM SULPH 6
The nose feels dry and the nostrils become sore Smelly yellow discharge from the nose	CALC CARB 6
For the treatment of existing polyps and to prevent them recurring	FORMICA 6
With frequent nosebleeds and chronic catarrh	PHOSPHORUS 6
The nose feels dry and congested With diarrhoea after a cold Many nasal polyps	SANGUINARIA 6
With enlargement of the adenoids Chronic dry catarrh with dry scabs and easily occurring nosebleeds	SULPHUR 6
Chronic catarrh with foul breath and many polyps	TEUCRIUM 6

DOSAGE

The selected remedy should be taken twice a day until an improvement occurs, then stopped. Repeat the treatment as and when necessary.

NOSEBLEEDS
Epistaxis

These usually occur for no apparent reason, but may develop when there is a cold or other infectious illness, after injury or picking the nose, with raised blood pressure or in certain blood diseases. The lining of the nose just before the nasal opening is very prone to damage and most bleeding occurs from this area.

If the bleeding has not stopped within about half an hour, or if it seems especially heavy, the patient should be taken to the nearest accident and emergency department. Repeated nosebleeds require medical investigation.

KEY FEATURES	TREATMENT
After any injury to the nose	ARNICA 30
After excitement and for a nosebleed accompanied by fear	ACONITE 30
Bright red blood which flows profusely	FERRUM PHOS 30
Darker blood which drips rather than pours	HAMAMELIS 30

DOSAGE

A dose of the selected remedy should be taken every fifteen minutes until the bleeding stops.

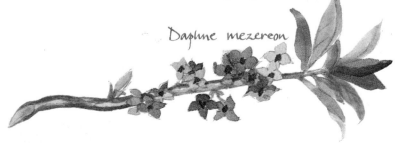

Daphne mezereon

SENSE OF SMELL DISORDERS

Loss of the sense of smell commonly occurs with nasal conditions such as colds and catarrh. It normally returns soon after the illness is over. Occasionally in the elderly there is a diminution of the sense of smell and this may be progressive.

KEY FEATURES	TREATMENT
Diminished sense of smell, with a runny nose and sore, cracked, red nostrils	ALUMINA 6
Frequent sneezing Sense of smell affected	ANACARDIUM 6
Sense of smell very acute	CARB ACID 6
Loss of sense of smell, with a thick, ropy, green-yellow nasal discharge and violent sneezing	KALI BICH 6
Sense of smell very acute	LYCOPODIUM 6
Loss of sense of smell The nose becomes blocked, especially on the right side Yellow mucus, worse in the morning	PULSATILLA 6
Chronic catarrh with loss of sense of smell The breath is foul	TEUCRIUM 6

DOSAGE

The selected remedy should be taken twice a day until an improvement occurs, then stopped. Repeat the treatment as and when necessary.

SINUSITIS

Sinus infection usually follows a nasal cold, but the symptoms vary, depending on which sinus is affected.

In frontal sinusitis there is always a severe headache with tenderness over the affected sinus. There is usually a fever and a blood-stained nasal discharge occasionally occurs.

In maxillary sinusitis a nasal discharge of mucus and pus always occurs and a headache is common but not invariably present. There is tenderness over the affected sinus and a low-grade fever is sometimes present.

KEY FEATURES	TREATMENT
Maxillary sinusitis with bad breath and a hot head but cold body The patient has a taste of bad eggs	ARNICA 30
Severe pain in the face and a violent headache, worse at night	AURUM MET 30
Frontal sinusitis, with a bursting, splitting headache, much worse on any movement Nosebleed in the morning which relieves the headache	BRYONIA 30
Chronic catarrh, with the nose feeling blocked Dull headache and tenderness over the frontal sinuses	EUCALYPTUS 6
Sinusitis after a cold Dull, pressing pain in the forehead on the affected side The scalp and neck muscles are painful Thick, tenacious discharge in back of throat	HYDRASTIS 30
Pain at the root of the nose extends to the frontal sinuses The nasal discharge is thick and ropy Loss of sense of smell Especially useful for chronic frontal sinusitis	KALI BICH 6
Profuse, hot, watery, acrid nasal discharge Pain in the affected frontal sinus and often facial pain on the same side	KALI IOD 30
Frontal sinusitis, with a blinding headache from sunrise to sunset Either a thin, watery nasal discharge or the nose is blocked and breathing through the nose is difficult	NAT MUR 30
Frontal sinusitis, often right-sided, with pain at the root of the nose and a blocked nostril on the affected side Pain and thick yellow catarrh, worse in the evening	PULSATILLA 30
Maxillary sinusitis The face is red and the pain throbbing and tearing, worse in cold, damp conditions Dry, hard crusts form in the nose and bleed when attempts are made to clear the nose	SILICA 30
Frontal sinusitis with burning pain in the forehead The eyelids feel heavy	VIOLA ODORATA 30

DOSAGE

Remedies in the 30 potency should be taken three times a day for three days.

Remedies in the 6 potency should be taken twice a day until an improvement is maintained.

THE MOUTH, TONGUE AND LIPS

CONTENTS

Bad Breath	104
Cold Sores	104
Lips and Mouth, Cracked	104
Mouth, Irritation in	105
Mouth Ulcers	106
Salivation Problems	107
Tongue, Coating/Discoloration of	107

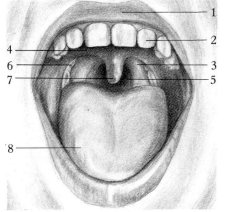

1	Lips
2	Teeth
3	Fauces
4	Soft palate
5	Pharynx
6	Tonsils
7	Uvula
8	Tongue

The mouth is lined with mucous membrance, and its roof, which separates it from the nasal cavity, is formed by the hard palate in front and the soft palate behind. The uvula can be seen hanging down from the back of the soft palate.

The tongue is a muscular organ covered on top by a tough mucous membrane which has the nerves of taste within it. The sensations of sweet, acid, salt and bitter are detected by the tongue and the palate. The tongue is very mobile and can move in most directions. It is involved in speech, in chewing food and helps in swallowing.

There are three pairs of salivary glands which have ducts opening into the mouth. These are the right and left parotid glands, found below the ear, the sublingual glands which lie under the tongue, and the submaxillary glands below the angular corner of the lower jaw. All these glands produce saliva which is essential to food digestion.

BAD BREATH
Halitosis

Bad breath may occur for a short while after eating heavily flavoured food such as curry or garlic. Chronic bad breath may be a sign of dental diseases, mouth ulcers, infection in the nose, throat or lungs, and mouth-breathing.

KEY FEATURES	TREATMENT
Bitter or putrid taste in the mouth Affecting girls at puberty Ulcers on the gums	AURUM MET 6
The breath smells mouldy Mouth and tongue ulcers, and the mouth feels hot and tender	BORAX 6
The breath has an offensive, sickly smell Sensation that the uvula has enlarged	CROCUS 6

Thick, offensive, dry, green-yellow crusts form on the back of the mouth, producing very foul breath	ELAPS 6
The breath smells like urine, with sour belching and burning blisters on the tongue	GRAPHITES 6
Great increase in saliva The gums become spongy, sore and bleed easily The tongue is yellow, flabby, thick and teeth-indented The breath has an offensive smell	MERCURIUS 6
Dry mouth with no thirst The tongue is yellow or white and covered by a tenacious mucus The breath is offensive	PULSATILLA 6
Bad breath from infected gums	SILICA 6
The breath is offensive and smells of onions	SINAPSIS NIG 6
The tongue is fissured and painful Foul odour from the mouth with an offensive taste	SPIGELIA 6
The tongue is dry, red, sore and shiny, with burning at its tip The breath feels cold and smells foul	TEREBINTH 6
Chronic nasal catarrh produces bad breath	TEUCRIUM 6

DOSAGE

The selected remedy should be taken four times a day until an improvement occurs, then stopped. Repeat the treatment as and when necessary.

COLD SORES

These fluid-filled blisters develop on and around the lips as a result of infection by the herpes simplex virus. Often recurring, they may be brought on by mild trauma such as dental treatment, sunlight and physical or emotional strain.

KEY FEATURES	TREATMENT
Foul-smelling breath and mouth ulcers The patient is very thirsty	CAPSICUM 12
The tongue is dry and rough, the throat sore and the saliva tenacious and soapy All symptoms are much worse for cold	DULCAMARA 12
The mouth feels dry and the tongue and lips feel numb, dry and may tingle With a deep crack in the centre of the lower lip	NAT MUR 12
Blisters around the mouth, and sometimes chin The corners of the mouth ulcerate; the tongue is sore, red at the tip, coated and cracked	RHUS TOX 12

DOSAGE

The remedy should be taken four times a day for three days.

LIPS AND MOUTH, *Cracked*

The commonest cause of cracking is the simple drying that occurs with cold weather. However, it also occurs with upper respiratory tract infections, cold sores and is said to be related to vitamin B2 (riboflavin) deficiency.

KEY FEATURES	TREATMENT
Marked redness of the lips, which are cracked and dry Food tends to taste bitter and sour	ALOE 12
The tongue is coated thick white The saliva tastes salty	ANT CRUD 12
The corners of the mouth are sore and cracked, and the roof of the mouth feels sore The saliva is profuse and acrid	ARUM TRIPH 12
The lips are parched, dry and cracked The mouth is dry and the patient has a great thirst	BRYONIA 12
The lips are dry and cracked, the breath is foul and the tongue red Much slimy mucus in the mouth and the gums bleed easily	HELLEBORUS 12
Cracks also at the side of the nostrils	LAC CAN 12
Scaly, itching herpes on the face and at the corners of the mouth	LYCOPODIUM 12
Numbness and tingling of the tongue, lips and nose Eruptions around the mouth, with small blisters on the lips The lips and corners of the mouth are dry, ulcerated and cracked Deep crack in the middle of the lower lip	NAT MUR 12
The lips are cracked and dry, the gums bleed and the tongue feels swollen	PHOS ACID 12
The lips are pale and the corners of the mouth cracked The lips are pale, with a red and itchy eruption on the chin	ZINC MET 12

DOSAGE

The selected remedy should be taken three times a day until an improvement occurs, then stopped. Repeat the treatment as and when necessary.

MOUTH, Irritation in

This is mainly found in hay fever and other allergic conditions, but can also be present with mouth and throat infections.

KEY FEATURES	TREATMENT
Irritation in the nose and the roof of the mouth Hay fever preceded by burning and itching of the roof of the mouth	ARUNDO 12
Scaly, itching herpes on the face and at the corners of the mouth	LYCOPODIUM 12
Violent itching in the roof of the mouth with a dry, contracted throat and difficulties in swallowing	STRYCHNINUM 12
The mouth feels scalded and there is a sensation of heat down the oesophagus The palate itches and the uvula feels elongated	WYETHIA 12

DOSAGE

The selected remedy should be taken every two hours until relief is maintained.

MOUTH ULCERS

Mouth ulcers can occur as a result of infection, either in the mouth or elsewhere in the body, from such conditions as throat infections, thrush, measles, glandular fever and the herpes simplex virus which produces cold sores. They may also develop through a shortage of vitamins B or C, with some anaemias, mechanical trauma from ill-fitting dentures or jagged teeth, excessive alcohol, tobacco and hot, spicy foods. Some drugs cause mouth ulcers and an individual sensitivity to toothpaste or mouthwash may occasionally be a cause.

KEY FEATURES	TREATMENT
Ulcers on the roof of the mouth	AGARICUS 30
With dryness and a burning sensation The gums are unhealthy and bleed easily	ARS ALB 30
The mouth feels hot and tender, the ulcers bleed on touch and when eating	BORAX 30
Small white ulcers in the mouth and throat Burning sensation in the mouth, pharynx and throat, with difficulty in swallowing liquids	CANTHARIS 30
The tongue becomes covered in small white ulcers	CARBO VEG 30
The gums and the mouth are painful and bleed easily on contact Ulcers in the corners of the mouth	HEPAR SULPH 30
The ulcers are white, the tongue coated grey-white and the neck glands enlarged	KALI MUR 30
White, raw, burning ulcers leading to foul breath The gums become swollen, spongy and bleed The tongue is dry and cracked at the tip and catches on the teeth	LACHESIS 30
Ulcers in the mouth and throat, increased salivation and the gums become spongy and recede	MERCURIUS 30
Small white ulcers, the gums appear white and swollen, and bleed easily, producing blood in the saliva	NUX VOM 30
The gums are sore, the tongue red and cracked, and ulcers form at the corners of the mouth Blisters around the mouth and chin	RHUS TOX 30
The tongue is white, with small white ulcers on the tongue and in the mouth The saliva has a metallic taste and the breath is foul	SARSAPARILLA 30
Ulceration in the mouth and at the back of the throat, with a dry, burning sensation The tongue is white and feels scalded	SANGUINARIA 30

DOSAGE

The selected remedy should be taken four times a day until an improvement occurs, then stopped. Repeat the treatment as and when necessary.

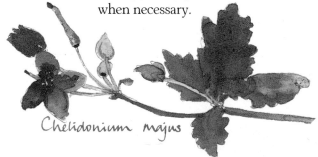

Chelidonium majus

SALIVATION PROBLEMS

Stones may develop in the duct (tube) leading from the salivary gland to the mouth and in these circumstances insufficient saliva gets through to the mouth. Starvation may also lead to a decreased secretion, while increased secretion may develop with certain tumours. Salivation increases normally as a response to chewing and the smell, sight, taste and thought of food.

KEY FEATURES	TREATMENT
Diminished salivation The saliva is sticky and frothy, and the tongue feels scalded	BERBERIS 12
Increased salivation The throat burns, with a constant feeling of phlegm in it With mouth ulcers	EUCALYPTUS 12
Salivation is greatly increased, tasting foul and coppery, and making the breath foul too The mouth and tongue feel sore	MERCURIUS 12
Excessive saliva which has a dry, bitter taste The tongue feels rough and swollen	PTELEA 12
Excessive saliva that runs out of the mouth when the patient sleeps Mouth ulcers and the tongue develops cracks along its length	SYPHILINUM 12

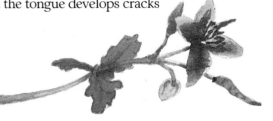

Sore throat and hoarseness with excessive saliva The salivary glands feel full	TRIFOLIUM 12
Increase in saliva and the mouth feels scalded	VERATRUM VIR 12

DOSAGE

The selected remedy should be taken four times a day until an improvement occurs, then stopped. Repeat the treatment as and when necessary.

TONGUE, *Coating/Discoloration of*

The tongue can be affected in many disorders and this list can be used to select the correct remedy if its appearance is abnormal. However, it is always wise to take note of any other symptoms that the patient may have before making a final choice of remedy.

KEY FEATURES	TREATMENT
The tongue is coated white The tip tingles and the gums get inflamed and feel hot	ACONITE 6
The tongue is thickly coated and feels as though scalded	AESCULUS 6
The tongue is coated thick white Cracks are present in the corners of the mouth	ANT CRUD 6

The tongue is fiery red, swollen and raw, feeling as though scalded	APIS 6	The tongue is coated white with bright red edges and there is profuse salivation	LAC CAN 6
The tip of the tongue is red and painful	ARG NIT 6	The tongue is dry, black, cracked and swollen	LYCOPODIUM 6
The tongue feels burnt and is dry and brown	BAPTISIA 6	The tongue is coated brown, feels thick and is blistered	MEDORRHINUM 6
The tongue is red at the edges and coloured like a strawberry	BELLADONNA 6	The tongue is yellow, flabby, thick and teeth-indented	MERCURIUS 6
The tongue is coated yellowish or dark brown, and the tongue, throat and mouth are very dry Excessive thirst	BRYONIA 6	The back of the tongue is coated white-yellow and has cracked edges	NUX VOM 6
The tongue is coated white or yellow-brown and covered in small, painful, red or white ulcers	CARBO VEG 6	The tongue is dry, smooth red or white, but not thickly coated	PHOSPHORUS 6
		The tongue has a red tip and feels rough and scalded	PHYTOLACCA 6
The tongue is coated yellow and everything eaten tastes bitter	CHAMOMILLA 6	The tongue is yellow or white and covered with a tenacious mucus	PULSATILLA 6
The tongue is yellow and has teeth imprints on its sides	CHELIDONIUM 6	The tongue is red, cracked and coated all over, except for the tip	RHUS TOX 6
Cracks in the corners of the mouth, the tongue is coated yellow and there is great thirst	EUPATORIUM 6	The tongue is dry and red at the edges	
The tongue feels numb, is coated yellow and trembles Bad taste in the mouth and bad breath	GELSEMIUM 6	The tongue is dry and cracked, and there is tingling at the tip, which feels stiff	SECALE 6
The tongue is mapped, red, shiny, smooth and dry Sensation of a hair on the tongue	KALI BICH 6	The tongue is white but with a red tip and red borders	SULPHUR 6
		The tongue is white or yellow and has a red streak down the middle	VERATRUM VIR 6
The tongue appears coated with brownish mustard The mouth is excessively dry, especially in the morning	KALI PHOS 6		

DOSAGE

The selected remedy should be taken four times a day for three days.

THE TEETH AND GUMS

CONTENTS

Abscess	110
Gums, Bleeding	110
Toothache	111
Tooth Decay	112

*T*he teeth are hard, bony structures set in the jaw. Each tooth consists of two main parts: the crown, which is the enamelled portion of the tooth projecting above the gum, and the root, which is the part embedded in the jaw.

Inside each tooth is a central cavity which contains the tooth-pulp. This is a very sensitive and soft tissue containing blood vessels, lymph vessels and nerves, which enter the tooth through a small opening at the base of the root. Covering the pulp is a hard substance, the dentine, which forms the greater part of the tooth.

The teeth erupt through the gums in two main stages. The temporary milk teeth, twenty in number, start to appear around the seventh month. Normally they have all erupted by the end of about two and a half years and are eventually replaced by permanent teeth. The permanent teeth, of which there are thirty-two, normally start to appear between the ages of six and eight.

The gums consist of firm, fleshy tissue which covers the part of the jaw from which the teeth grow, and the neck of the tooth (the junction between the crown and the root).

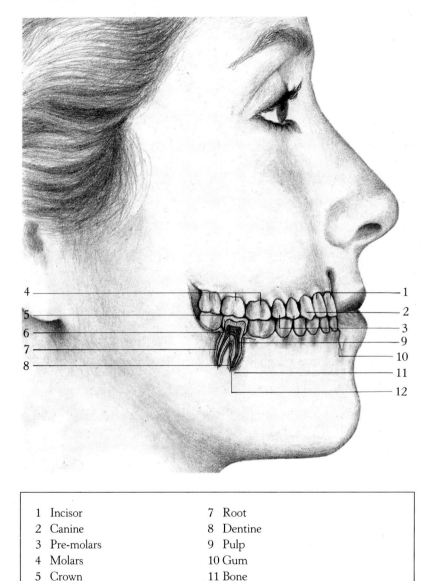

1	Incisor	7	Root
2	Canine	8	Dentine
3	Pre-molars	9	Pulp
4	Molars	10	Gum
5	Crown	11	Bone
6	Enamel	12	Nerve and blood supply

ABSCESS or Gumboil

This is the equivalent of a boil and it develops in relation to a tooth. The symptoms are pain in the jaw, which is always present in adults but not necessarily in children, tenderness of the affected tooth, and swelling and redness of the surrounding gum and possibly that part of the face overlying the area involved.

Dental and/or medical treatment may be necessary.

KEY FEATURES	TREATMENT
Very painful and throbbing The mouth feels dry The face overlying the abscess is red and hot	BELLADONNA 30
The patient complains of, and appears to be in, great pain The face is pale	BORAX 30
The abscess forms a hard swelling on the jaw The teeth are loose and hurt if food comes into contact with them	CALC FLUOR 30
Mainly in the gum With swelling and toothache, which may cause facial neuralgia	HEKLA LAVA 30

DOSAGE

The selected remedy should be taken every two hours until relief is found or until expert advice has been obtained.

GUMS, BLEEDING

Gingivitis and Pyorrhoea

The gums may bleed for several reasons, which can vary from over-enthusiastic brushing to a variety of diseases, of which the most common is gum infection. Gingivitis causes a red, spongy, painful swelling of the gums, which bleed easily from brushing. This condition may arise from pyorrhoea, which is a more straightforward gum infection in which small quantities of pus appear in the hollow between the tooth and the gum.

For both these conditions dental advice should be obtained.

KEY FEATURES	TREATMENT
The mouth is sore and the breath smells bad The gums are sore and bleeding The jaw hurts on opening the mouth	ALUMINA 30
The gums detach from the teeth and bleed easily	ANT CRUD 30
The gums bleed easily and the teeth hurt, although not diseased	ARG NIT 30
Sore taste in the mouth Toothache from cold or hot The gums bleed	CALC CARB 30
The teeth are very sensitive, especially when eating The gums retract and bleed easily when cleaning the teeth	CARBO VEG 30
The gums and mouth are painful to the touch and the gums bleed	HEPAR SULPH 30

Very painful and rapidly decaying teeth with spongy, bleeding gums	KREOSOTE 30
The gums are swollen, spongy and bleed Toothache radiates to the ears	LACHESIS 30
The gums are spongy, recede and bleed easily Much tooth decay, and the teeth are loose and tender	MERCURIUS 30
Putrid breath with bleeding gums, and the teeth become loose	NITRIC ACID 30
The gums are swollen, white and bleeding Toothache, worse for cold	NUX VOM 30
Bleeding gums retract from the teeth, which feel cold	PHOS ACID 30
Swollen, ulcerated gums that bleed easily Persistent bleeding after tooth extraction	PHOSPHORUS 30
Spongy gums which bleed easily and black, crumbling teeth	STAPHYSAGRIA 30
The teeth become loose and the gums bleed	ZINC MET 30

DOSAGE

The selected remedy should be taken four times a day for four days.

TOOTHACHE

Whatever the reasons for its occurrence, toothache should be treated according to the other symptoms accompanying it. The pain is usually due to dental caries (decay) and is generally worse for sweet and cold. If the pain is made worse by heat, the caries has probably reached the pulp of the tooth and an abscess may then develop.

KEY FEATURES	TREATMENT
Pressing the teeth together sends shocks through the head, eyes and ears	AMMON CARB 30
In decayed teeth, especially before a period	ANT CRUD 30
Pain in sound, good teeth	ARG NIT 30
Before a period	BARYTA CARB 30
Relieved by cold mouthwashes, but worse for eating Neuralgic pain in the face at the same time	BISMUTH 30
With vertigo and cold feet before a period	CALC CARB 30
Worse from warm drinks, especially coffee During pregnancy	CHAMOMILLA 30
Better for pressing the teeth firmly together and from warmth	CHINA 30
Eased by ice-cold water	COFFEA 30
Dry mouth with burning tongue and painful gums and teeth	COLCHICUM 30
With abdominal pain	COLOCYNTH 30
Better for ice-cold water	FERRUM MET 30
Pulsating pain	GLONOINE 30
With swelling of the jaw	HEKLA LAVA 30
Pulling, tearing pain leading to facial neuralgia and depression	HYPERICUM 30

111

Worse after drinking coffee or smoking	IGNATIA 30
With bleeding gums	KALI PHOS 30
Pain radiates to the ears	LACHESIS 30
With swollen cheeks, relieved by warm applications	LYCOPODIUM 30
The teeth are very tender and sore	
In the lower molars	LYCOPUS 30
During pregnancy, worse at night and from cold	MAG CARB 30
Pain from cutting wisdom teeth	
Better for heat and hot drinks	MAG PHOS 30
In pregnancy	NUX MOSCHATA 30
The mouth becomes very dry	
The teeth are very sensitive and sore to touch	PLANTAGO 30
Better while eating but worse in cold air	
With neuralgia of the eyelid	
Relieved by holding cold water in the mouth	PULSATILLA 30
In damp weather and before a storm	RHODODEN-DRON 30
Tearing pain, worse after eating and from the cold	SPIGELIA 30
During a period and after dental extraction	STAPHYSAGRIA 30
Pain in the teeth on blowing the nose	THUJA 30

DOSAGE

The selected remedy should be taken every two hours until relief occurs.

TOOTH DECAY
Caries

Dental caries, or tooth decay, occurs when sweet or starchy food particles get stuck between the teeth or form a film over them. These particles start to ferment and form an acid, which eventually erodes the hard enamel covering the crown and enters the dentine, which it begins to destroy.

Dental advice should be obtained.

KEY FEATURES	TREATMENT
The teeth develop slowly and decay rapidly	CALC PHOS 12
Decay from eating excessive sweet foods	COCA 12
Early decay of teeth	FLUORIC ACID 12
Facial neuralgia with and from the decaying teeth	HEKLA LAVA 12
Very rapid tooth decay in teeth which are dark and crumbly	KREOSOTE 12
The teeth are loose, tender and decay easily	MERCURIUS 12
Decay in the roots and violent pain extending to the ear	MEZEREUM 12
Worse at night	
The teeth decay and are very sensitive along the gum margin	THUJA 12
The gums retract	

DOSAGE

The selected remedy should be taken twice a day while waiting to see a dentist.

THE THROAT

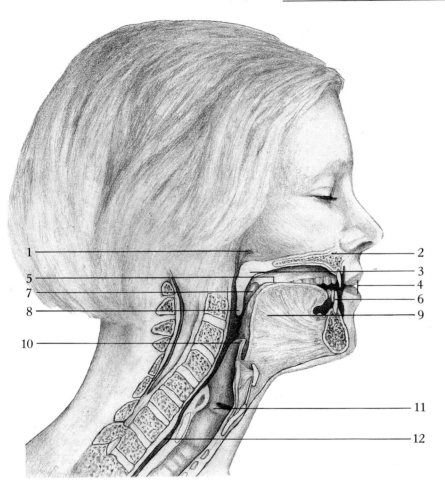

1	Adenoids	7	Tonsils
2	Hard palate	8	Uvula
3	Soft palate	9	Muscles of the tongue
4	Lips	10	Epiglottis
5	Tongue	11	Larynx
6	Teeth	12	Oesophagus

CONTENTS

Adenoids	114
Hoarseness and Voice Loss	114
Stammering	115
Throat, Sensations in	115
Throat, Sore	116
Tonsillitis	118

Another name for the throat is the pharynx. This cavity at the back of the nose and mouth connects the mouth to the gullet (oesophagus), which takes the chewed food to the stomach, and the voice-box (larynx), which allows the air breathed in to flow to the windpipe (trachea) and on to the lungs.

As it is vital that food does not go to the lungs, the entrance to the larynx is automatically closed during swallowing by the contraction of its surrounding muscles. It is sealed tight by the epiglottis. In the larynx are the vocal cords which enable us to make sounds and speak.

On either side at the back of the throat are the tonsils. These are composed of tissue which helps destroy infective organisms such as bacteria. While doing this, the tonsils become swollen and inflamed, and tiny pockets of pus show on their surface. Repeated attacks of tonsillitis can lead to chronic enlargement of the tonsils. Infection from the diseased tonsils sometimes finds its way up the eustachian tube to the middle ear.

ADENOIDS

Some enlargement of the adenoids is normal in children up to about the age of ten. After this the adenoids start to regress. Excessive enlargement can lead to nasal speech, snoring, breathing through the mouth and temporary deafness. Chronic infection of the adenoids may be associated with recurrent tonsillitis and middle-ear infection (otitis media).

KEY FEATURES	TREATMENT
With enlarged tonsils	AGRAPHIS 30
Chronic enlargement of the adenoids	CALC PHOS 30
With nasal polyps	SULPHUR 30

DOSAGE

The selected remedy should be taken four times a day for three days.

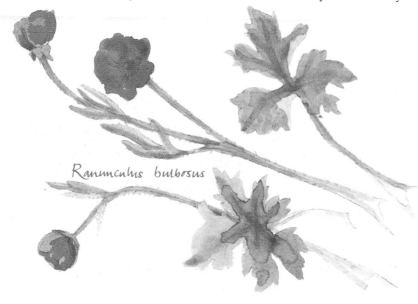

Ranunculus bulbosus

HOARSENESS AND VOICE LOSS

Laryngitis

Acute inflammation of the larynx interferes with its normal function and produces hoarseness or even complete voice loss. Overuse of the voice can lead to the same symptoms.

If the condition does not respond to treatment or lasts for more than twenty-one days, a medical opinion should be sought.

KEY FEATURES	TREATMENT
The temperature is raised, the throat feels rough and the voice becomes hoarse Thin, frothy sputum is present	ACONITE 30
Burning rawness in the throat and total voice loss	AMMON CAUST 30
Rawness and burning in the larynx Copious mucus which looks like boiled starch but is easily coughed up Chronic laryngitis in singers	ARG MET 30
The voice suddenly changes Painful, dry cough with hoarseness and rawness From overuse of the voice	ARUM TRIPH 30
Of sudden onset with a red, dry throat and an aversion to fluids	BELLADONNA 30
Worse in the evening and after exposure to cold dry wind	CAUSTICUM 30

Slight fever, slight cough, slight amount of sputum All worse in a draught	HEPAR SULPH 30
Worse in the evening, the larynx hurts when talking and the voice sounds rough and hoarse	PHOSPHORUS 30
The throat feels very dry and talking is painful The chest also feels sore, with an unproductive cough	SENEGA 30
Harsh barking cough The throat is sensitive to touch and worse in bed	SPONGIA 30

DOSAGE

The selected remedy should be taken four times a day for four days.

STAMMERING

Often exacerbated by stress, stammering is an inability to speak without involuntary stops and repetitions.

KEY FEATURES	TREATMENT
The remedies listed here should be tried, one at a time, for one month. If there is a response, continue for a further two months.	BELLADONNA 6 BOVISTA 6 CUPRUM MET 6 STRAMONIUM 6

DOSAGE

Take one dose twice a day.

THROAT, *Sensations in*

These headings are self-explanatory and may be used in conjunction with other throat symptoms or on their own.

KEY FEATURES	TREATMENT
Of a splinter, especially on swallowing	ARG NIT
Of sand in the throat	CISTUS CAN
Of a lump	GRAPHITES
Sharp, splinter-like pain	HEPAR SULPH
Of a plug, which goes on swallowing	IGNATIA
Of a fish bone	KALI CARB
Of a lump, which goes on swallowing	LACHESIS
Of a hair	NAT MUR
Of a splinter, due to ulcers	NITRIC ACID
Of a hot ball	PHYTOLACCA
Of a string hanging down the throat	VALERIANA

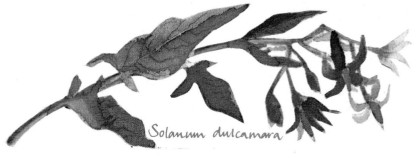

Solanum dulcamara

DOSAGE

The selected remedy should be taken in the 12 potency three times a day until an improvement occurs.

THROAT, *Sore*

Although many healthy throats are red (more so in smokers), a sore, red throat with a raised temperature is indicative of infection and may precede acute tonsillitis (see p. 118). Other illnesses in which there may be a sore, red throat are influenza, the common cold, glandular fever and adenoid infections.

If the symptoms do not clear quickly, medical help should be sought.

KEY FEATURES	TREATMENT
After being in a cold, dry atmosphere The throat is dry, burning and red	ACONITE 30
Sore throat with difficulty in swallowing	AETHUSA 30
The throat is dark red, rough and sore Sensation of a splinter in the throat when swallowing	ARG NIT 30
Sore, inflamed throat with bad breath Mouth ulcers may develop Solids cause gagging when swallowing	BAPTISIA 30
Of sudden onset The throat appears bright red, is very dry and often worse on the right Constant desire to swallow, but swallowing is difficult Aversion to drinks Sleep is restless and delirium may occur	BELLADONNA 30
Dry mouth, tongue and throat with excessive thirst	BRYONIA 30
Better for warm drinks	CALC FLUOR 30
Very inflamed throat with a burning and feeling of intense constriction Burning sensation in the mouth and pharynx Blisters may form in the mouth	CANTHARIS 30
Smokers' sore throat with a burning, smarting sensation Pain extends to the ears and is worse in the cold	CAPSICUM 30
Rough, scraping sensation after catching cold in damp weather	DULCAMARA 30

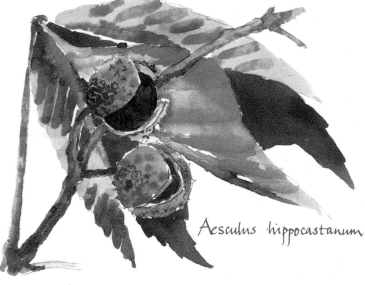

Aesculus hippocastanum

Pain extends to the ears and the throat feels rough	GELSEMIUM 30
The throat is very dry with stinging pains, mainly on the right The patient holds the neck while talking Worse in moist, warm conditions	GUAIACUM 30

Sensation of a splinter or lump in the throat, which feels raw, as if scraped
Pus may be present — HEPAR SULPH 30

Sensation of a lump in the throat, relieved by swallowing — IGNATIA 30

The tongue is yellow at its base
Sticky tenacious mucus with a sensation of dryness and burning — KALI BICH 30

Ulcerated throat with an upset stomach — KALI MUR 30

Sensation of a lump in the throat goes on swallowing, but returns afterwards
Swallowing is painful and mucus seems to stick in the throat
Worse after sleep
For irritable, nervous sore throats — LACHESIS 30

Thirstless but with a dry throat — LYCOPODIUM 30

Dryness and soreness with a constant desire to swallow, which is painful
Intense inflammation, rawness and smarting
The breath is offensive — MERCURIUS 30

The uvula is swollen and there is intense burning in the throat, worse for pressure — MERC CORR 30

Sensation of a splinter or fishbone, with sharp, sore, stinging pain
The throat ulcerates, swallowing is difficult, white patches appear and there is an offensive discharge — NITRIC ACID 30

In a smoker and/or drinker
For people who use their voice a lot
Rawness and a scraping sensation — NUX VOM 30

The throat may ulcerate and the pain is worse on coughing — PHOSPHORUS 30

A dark red, hot-feeling throat with pain on swallowing which may radiate to the ear — PHYTOLACCA 30

The throat feels swollen and the epiglottis dry and burning
Tendency to hoarseness — WYETHIA 30

DOSAGE

The selected remedy should be taken three times a day for four days.

Datura stramonium

117

TONSILLITIS

The tonsils, which are on either side at the back of the mouth, can become acutely inflamed, often quite suddenly. The symptoms include a sore throat and fever, and all cases have a pus-like discharge. Offensive breath and a coated tongue are also usually present.

If there is no response to treatment within twelve hours, a doctor should be consulted.

KEY FEATURES	TREATMENT
Smarting pain on swallowing Colds always go on to tonsillitis The glands of the neck and behind the ears are enlarged For chronic tonsil enlargement	BARYTA CARB 30
The throat is bright red with much pus and exudate The tonsils are swollen, especially on the right side Swallowing is difficult and produces sharp pains which are felt in the tonsils	BELLADONNA 30
Useful if taken early in the attack Violent, burning headache The limbs ache The throat feels hot	GUAIACUM 30
Rigors and chills Sharp, sticking pain in the tonsils and a throbbing throat Pus forms on the tonsils	HEPAR SULPH 30
The throat has a grey look with white spots and enlarged tonsils	KALI MUR 30
Dark red or purple tonsils Much external swelling and tenderness Starts on the left side Pain shoots to the ear on swallowing Aggravation from hot drinks	LACHESIS 30
Rarely needed at the onset Use when pus is present with thick, tenacious saliva and foul breath Very swollen, dark red tonsils	MERCURIUS 30
Pain at the root of the tongue which extends to the ears on swallowing The tonsils are large and dark blue Intense dryness, smarting and burning in the throat	PHYTOLACCA 30

DOSAGE

The selected remedy should be taken four times a day for four days.

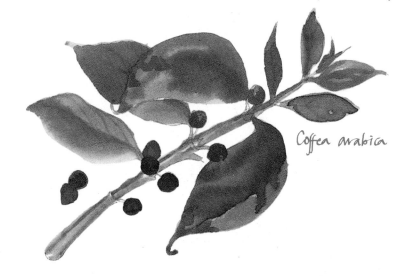

Coffea arabica

118

THE CIRCULATORY SYSTEM

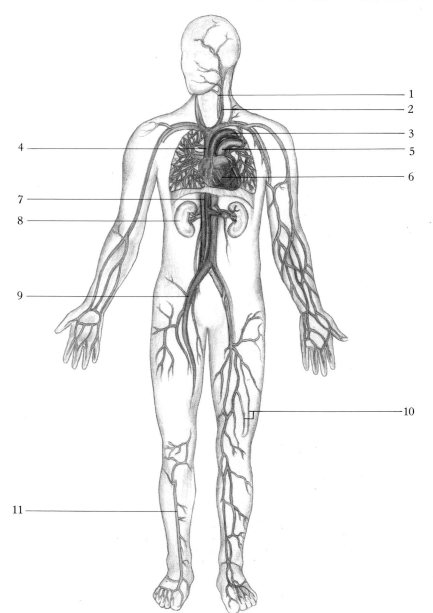

CONTENTS

Angina	121
Blood Pressure, Raised	122
Hardening of the Arteries	123
Heart Attack	124
Heart-rate, Rapid	125
Palpitations	125

1 Carotid artery
2 Jugular vein
3 Aorta
4 Superior vena cava
5 Pulmonary vein
6 Heart
7 Inferior vena cava
8 Kidney
9 Femoral artery
10 Superficial veins
11 Tibial artery
12 Pulmonary artery
13 Right atrium
14 Left atrium
15 Right coronary artery
16 Left coronary artery
17 Left ventricle
18 Right ventricle

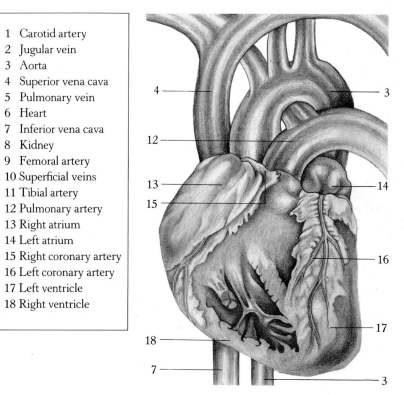

The system consists of the heart, the blood vessels and the circulation.

The heart is a hollow, muscular organ about the size of a closed fist and is to be found in the chest between the two lungs. It has four chambers, the two on the right being the right atrium and ventricle, which have the tricuspid valve between them, and the two on the left being the left atrium and ventricle, which have the bicuspid or mitral valve between them. These valves ensure that the blood circulates through the heart in the correct direction. Between the left ventricle and the aorta is the aortic valve and between the right ventricle and the pulmonary artery is the pulmonary valve.

The heart pumps blood around the body in three types of blood vessel. The arteries have thick, elastic walls and their own pumping action which helps the heart to transport blood to all parts of the body. They gradually narrow, becoming arterioles, then capillaries, which lead to venules that widen to become veins.

The veins have thinner walls and are less elastic than arteries. A series of valves in them allows the blood to be returned to the heart.

Capillaries are minute vessels that connect the smallest arteries to the smallest veins, their very thin walls allowing the exchange of substances through them. In this way oxygen and nutrients enter the tissue cells and waste matter is removed from them.

The blood returning to the heart after circulating around the body enters it at the right atrium. It then goes via the right ventricle and pulmonary artery to the lungs, where it is re-oxygenated. It is then returned to the heart via the pulmonary vein, which takes the blood to the left atrium. From here it enters the left ventricle and passes into the aorta, where it starts its circulation through the body once again.

While passing through the lungs, the blood is in the pulmonary circulation. While going around the rest of the body it is in the systemic circulation. Both are inter-related in forming a complete and closed route around the body. The regular contraction and relaxation of the heart propels blood around the circulatory route. On average the heart beats about seventy times a minute at rest, but in practice this may vary from about sixty to ninety beats per minute in some people.

During contraction (systole) of the heart, the pressure generated forces the blood through the arteries to move it onwards. During relaxation (diastole) of the heart, the onward motion of the blood continues because of the elasticity of the arterial wall. This is shown as the regular beating action called the pulse. When the systolic and diastolic pressures are higher than normal, the blood pressure is said to be raised, a condition called hypertension.

Although the blood goes round the body in a closed circuit, some of its fluid called plasma escapes through the walls of the capillaries, bathes the tissues directly, giving up proteins and food materials and collecting waste products of tissue metabolism in return. It then enters into the lymph vessels, becoming known as lymph, and goes via another circulatory route called the lymphatic system back into the main blood circulation. Along the course of the lymphatic vessels are groups of glands known as lymph nodes. These act as filters, preventing the passage of bacteria and toxic material into the bloodstream. Should infection occur, the glands become enlarged and painful.

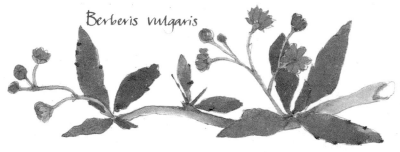
Berberis vulgaris

ANGINA
Angina pectoris

Angina (heart pain) occurs because of changes in the arteries which take blood to the heart. Put simply, they are supplying too little blood for the heart muscle to function normally, and this may lead to chest pain. The pain does not usually occur at rest; rather it comes about through increased activity by the heart, such as exercise, or in anaemia and obesity. Angina can occur in virtually any adult age group but patients over forty-five years of age are those most commonly affected.

The chest pain is described as a tightness or feeling of constriction, and in approximately half the patients involved pain will radiate down one or both arms and occasionally to the throat or jaw. The arm pain is often described as a numbness. Pain during exertion, after a heavy meal or from excitement is characteristic. The pain usually passes off after a few minutes' rest, but if it continues, the possibility of a heart attack must be considered.

In well over half the cases of angina shortage of breath occurs and raised blood pressure is present. Note that anxiety, inflammation of the oesophagus and gall bladder, as well as peptic ulceration can produce very similar pains.

Unexplained chest pain should always be referred for initial medical examination and diagnosis.

KEY FEATURES	TREATMENT
Anxiety with palpitations Intense pain around the heart, shooting down the left arm, with numbness in the fingers	ACONITE 30
The pain is worse during the night	ARG NIT 30
Pain radiates to the region of the left elbow	ARNICA 30
The chest feels as if constricted by an iron band Suffocating feeling with a cold sweat	CACTUS 30
Angina with asthma and muscle cramps	CUPRUM MET 30
Pain radiates from the back of the breastbone to the arms With much flatulence and laboured breathing	DIOSCOREA 30
The slightest exertion brings on the angina With palpitations and shortage of breath	GLONOINE 30
Violent cramping pain extends to the armpit and down the arm to the fingers, with a numb sensation in the arm	LATRODECTUS 30
Angina with pain in the right arm	LILIUM TIG 30
Constricting pains around the heart	MAG PHOS 30
Pain extends to the nape of the neck, left shoulder and arm Great anxiety and fear of death	NAJA 30
The pain is sharp and lancing, alternating with voice loss	OXALIC ACID 30
A drink of hot water relieves the pain, which is violent and greatly aggravated by motion	SPIGELIA 30
Pain, accompanied by faintness, suffocation and an anxious sweat, comes on after midnight	SPONGIA 30

Pain over the heart, radiating in all directions   TABACUM 30
Pain and shortage of breath, worse for lying on
    the left side

DOSAGE

The selected remedy should be taken immediately when the
symptoms occur and repeated every twenty minutes until there is an
improvement. It should then be taken at increasing intervals, if
necessary.

BLOOD PRESSURE, Raised

Hypertension

*There are several causes of raised blood pressure, but in the
majority of cases no cause is found. These patients are said to
have essential hypertension.*
*Apart from an increased blood-pressure reading, symptoms
may be absent, but some patients complain of dizziness,
tinnitus (noises in the ear) and headache. Nosebleeds probably
occur more often than in non-hypertensive patients.*

Initial diagnosis and investigation of this condition should be made
by a doctor. Homeopathic treatment may be possible, but should
always be administered under medical supervision.

KEY FEATURES   **TREATMENT**

Pain behind the breastbone at night   AURUM MET 6
The patient becomes very despondent and may
    feel suicidal
With hardening of the arteries

The blood pressure may be very high   BARYTA CARB 6
Palpitations, worse when lying on the left side
The pulse is full and hard

Violent, irregular palpitations   COFFEA 6
Headache, worse for noise and smell
Sleeplessness

The nose feels very blocked and swollen   IODUM 6
Palpitations from the least exertion
Anxiety and depression together

Raised blood pressure at the menopause   LACHESIS 6
Headaches, fainting and flushing
The heart feels too large and there is cramp-
    like pain in the chest wall over the heart

The heart-rate is very rapid   LYCOPUS 6
With pain over the heart area
With cardiac asthma and rheumatism
The pulse becomes weak, irregular and rapid
With nosebleeds and frontal headaches

Rapid, irregular heart-rate   SPARTIUM 6
With angina
With a profuse flow of urine
With excessive wind

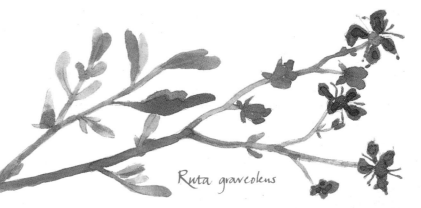

Ruta graveolens

The face becomes flushed easily Strong arterial pulse Vertigo with headache and nausea	STRONTIA 6
The pulse is slow, soft, weak and irregular Constant burning pain over the heart The face is flushed and congested, and the patient quite quarrelsome	VERATRUM VIR 6

DOSAGE

The selected remedy should be taken twice a day. Frequent blood pressure checks and patient reassessment should be made and the treatment changed or modified if necessary.

HARDENING OF THE ARTERIES

Arteriosclerosis

This condition occurs as part of the ageing process, the walls of the arteries becoming harder and less elastic. It may occur anywhere in the body, the reduced blood-flow arising from it leading to a variety of conditions. These include raised blood pressure, angina, dizziness, leg pains during exercise, vertigo, headache and mental confusion.

KEY FEATURES	**TREATMENT**

Sensation of the heart stopping for a second or two, followed by a loud rebound Raised blood pressure and despondency Pain beneath the breastbone at night	AURUM MET 12

Senile dementia, leading to confusion and
  mental weakness
Swellings in the artery wall (aneurysms),
  palpitations and raised blood pressure
	BARYTA CARB 12

Asthma, headaches, vertigo and tinnitus in the elderly Raised blood pressure	BARYTA MUR 12
Heart conditions in the elderly	CACTUS 12
Weakness of the mind and body, with vertigo, trembling and palpitations	CONIUM 12
Extreme shortage of breath, with heart pain and excessive fluid retention Pulse irregular, feeble and intermittent	CRATAEGUS 12

Early hardening of the arteries, which is rapidly
  progressive
With ice-cold extremities
The patient may be thin and scrawny with very
  shrivelled skin
	SECALE 12

With raised blood pressure producing a flushed face and pulsating arteries With vertigo and nausea	STRONTIA 12
Very rigid arteries in the elderly Rapid, irregular heart	STROPHAN-THUS 12
Hardening in the coronary arteries	TABACUM 12

DOSAGE

The selected remedy should be taken twice a day. It may be necessary to continue its use for some time, especially in the very elderly.

HEART ATTACK

Coronary thrombosis/Myocardial infarction

The symptoms are a sudden, agonizing, constricting chest pain which may radiate to the neck, jaw or arms, mainly the left. The patient is usually in shock, cold and sweaty with a grey complexion and a shallow, rapid pulse. The pain does not pass off with rest.

This condition requires urgent medical attention. Homeopathic treatment and first-aid procedures should be used while waiting for medical assistance.

KEY FEATURES	TREATMENT
Great anxiety and difficulty in breathing Numbness and tingling in the fingers Better when sitting up	ACONITE
Chest pain after exertion or fatigue The chest feels sore and bruised	ARNICA
The heart feels as if grasped and squeezed The lower part of the chest feels tied down The pain makes the patient cry out Occurs around 11 a.m. or 11 p.m.	CACTUS
Weakness and numbness in the left arm The skin is blue The patient fears the heart will stop if he moves about Slow pulse	DIGITALIS
The patient wakes from sleep feeling smothered and therefore unable to lie down	LACHESIS
Violent chest and left-arm pain Very rapid pulse and great difficulty in breathing	LATRODECTUS
Pain wakes the patient The heart feels as if in a vice The patient bends double to try to ease the pain	LILIUM TIG
Palpitations With irregular pulse Paroxysms of suffocation and tightness across the upper chest	TABACUM

DOSAGE

While waiting for the doctor, use the highest potency you have and repeat at five-minute intervals until relief is obtained.

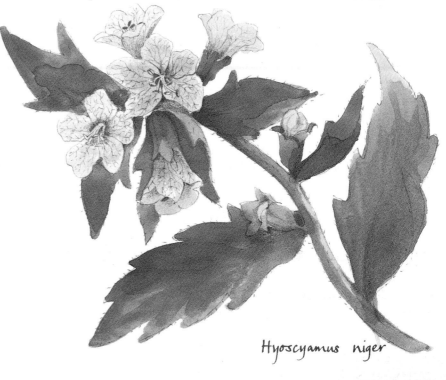

Hyoscyamus niger

HEART-RATE, Rapid
Tachycardia

In this condition the heart beats normally, but at two or three times its normal rate for short periods ranging from several minutes to a few days. It is only rarely associated with serious heart disease. In a proportion of cases the heart-rate may be over 140 per minute.

If the heart-rate does not return to normal, a medical opinion should be sought.

KEY FEATURES	TREATMENT
Rapid heart-rate alternates with a slow rate (bradycardia)	ABIES NIG 30
The patient shows fear and anxiety Pain in the left shoulder, with tingling in the fingers	ACONITE 30
From smoking in nervous young men	AGNUS 30
After excitement Wakes the patient around 2 a.m.	IBERIS 30
With a constrictive feeling about the chest	IODUM 30
With chest pain	KALMIA 30
Alternation between fast and slow heart-rate	MORPHINUM 30 (prescription required in US)
The heart and chest feel constricted, and the heart feels as if cold The body is shaken by the rapidity of the heartbeat	NAT MUR 30
Rapid or slow heart-rate Pain over the heart, radiating from the centre of the breastbone	TABACUM 30

DOSAGE

The selected remedy should be taken every three hours until relief is obtained.

PALPITATIONS

These are rapid, regular heartbeats of which the patient develops an unpleasant awareness.

KEY FEATURES	TREATMENT
With burning and distension of the stomach and abdomen	ABIES CAN 6
Palpitations, with anxiety, fainting and tingling in the fingers	ACONITE 6
Pain over the heart, palpitations and shortage of breath	ADONIS VER 6
Violent palpitations, with vertigo, headache and restlessness	AETHUSA 6
Irregular, violent palpitations after smoking	AGARICUS 6
Palpitations with the sensation of a lump in the chest, worse in the open air The patient has a pale face	AMBRA 6
Palpitations on waking, accompanied by fear, cold sweat, loud and difficult breathing and trembling hands	AMMON CARB 6

125

In the elderly	ANACARDIUM 6	Violent palpitations with anxiety, when lying on the left side	PHOSPHORUS 6
Worse when lying on the right side	ARG NIT 6	With trembling while sitting still	RHUS TOX 6
Pulse more rapid in the morning	ARS ALB 6	With contracted, intermittent pulse	SECALE 6
Violent, throbbing palpitations from exertion	BELLADONNA 6	Violent and intermittent	SEPIA 6
Violent palpitations, worse when lying on the left side	CACTUS 6	Frequent bouts accompanied by a foul mouth odour	SPIGELIA 6
Just before a period			
At night and after eating	CALC CARB 6	Just before a period	SPONGIA 6
Nervous palpitations, especially after excessive excitement	COFFEA 6	Anaemia with palpitations and breathlessness	STROPHAN-THUS 6
With a period	CROTALUS 6	When lying on the left side	TABACUM 6
From the slightest movement	DIGITALIS 6	With anxiety and noisy breathing	VERATRUM ALB 6
From the slightest exertion, laughing or coughing, and accompanied by vertigo	IBERIS 6	With difficult breathing, anxiety and hysteria	VIOLA ODORATA 6
With a burning sensation in the heart region	KALI CARB 6	During coitus	VISCUM ALB 6
Worse on bending forward	KALMIA 6		
With fainting during a period	LACHESIS 6		
During the night, lying on the left side and at about 4 a.m.	LYCOPODIUM 6		
From nervous irritation	LYCOPUS 6		
While sitting, better for moving about	MAG MUR 6		
Fluttering, palpating heart, often with heartburn	NAT MUR 6		
With shortage of breath in heart disease, worse thinking of it	OXALIC ACID 6		
In growing children	PHOS ACID 6		

DOSAGE

The selected remedy should be taken every twenty minutes until an improvement is maintained.

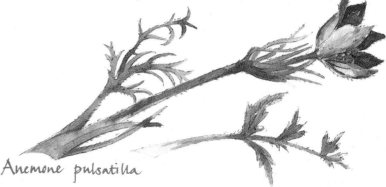

Anemone pulsatilla

THE RESPIRATORY SYSTEM

CONTENTS

Asthma	128
Bronchitis, Acute and Chronic	130
Chest Pain	132
Colds and Influenza	133
Coughs	134
Suffocation, Feeling of	136

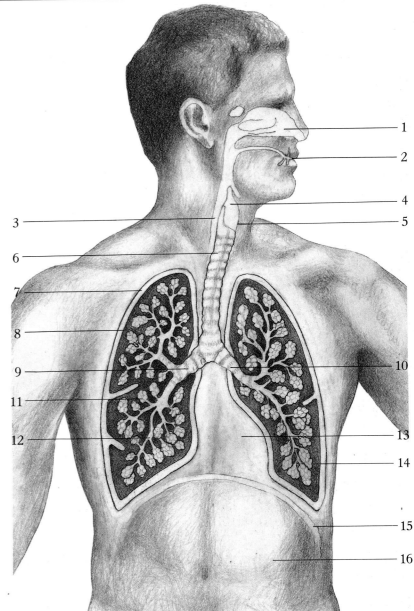

The most important function of the respiratory system is the inhalation of oxygen and the exhalation of carbon dioxide, an exchange of gases that takes place in the lungs.

In breathing, air is drawn in through the nose and/or mouth and passes through the throat (pharynx) into the larynx. The nasopharynx acts as a filter to prevent dust and foreign matter from entering the windpipe (trachea).

The trachea divides at its lower end into the right bronchus and the left bronchus (the bronchi). These go to the two lungs, where they branch out in all directions as tiny tubes (bronchioles) which

1	Nasal cavity	9	Right bronchus
2	Mouth	10	Left bronchus
3	Oesophagus	11	Alveoli
4	Larynx	12	Bronchioli
5	Vocal cords	13	Space for the heart
6	Trachea	14	Left lung
7	Pleura	15	Diaphragm
8	Right lung	16	Abdominal cavity

end in innumerable minute cavities (alveoli). These are lined with many blood vessels and it is in the alveoli that the exchange of oxygen and carbon dioxide takes place.

The trachea and bronchi are kept open by means of cartilage rings in their walls. The membrane which lines these walls secretes a mucus substance which prevents dust and bacteria from entering the lungs. When inflammation is present, this secretion is increased and becomes the sputum that is usually coughed up.

The lungs are two sponge-like organs that occupy most of the chest cavity. They lie on either side of the heart and each is covered by a very thin membrane, the pleura. This folds back on itself to be attached to the inner surface of the chest wall and thereby produces a closed space between the folds called the pleural cavity. Inflammation of the pleura gives rise to pleurisy.

Movement of the chest wall and the thick, domed-shaped muscle (the diaphragm) which forms the floor of the chest cavity and separates it from the abdominal cavity, makes the lungs expand and contract about sixteen times a minute to carry out the exchange of gases needed for the body or receive its oxygen. During physical exertion, nervous excitement and many diseases the respiratory rate is considerably increased.

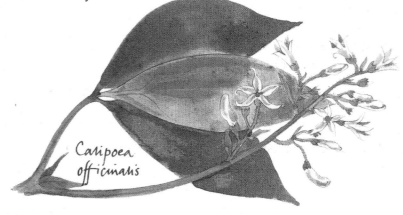

Canpoea
officinalis

ASTHMA

Asthma is an illness in which spasm in the respiratory tract produces wheezing and breathlessness. It may be associated with a chest infection, but can also be triggered by allergy, exercise or stress, and psychological factors. It tends to recur but complete cures have been effected with homeopathy.

This is a serious condition that can occur at any age and, on rare occasions, can be fatal. Expert medical help should be sought if there is not a quick and satisfactory response to homeopathic treatment at home.

KEY FEATURES	TREATMENT
Sudden violent attack after exposure to cold, dry winds	ACONITE 30
The patient is restless, very fearful and anxious	
Hoarse, dry, croupy cough and the slightest movement adds to the shortage of breath	
Much mucus formation and the chest rattles with it	ANT TART 30
Extreme shortage of breath, the patient becomes increasingly weak, drowsy and sweaty, is unable to raise any mucus and may require help to sit up to breathe	
Pale, thirstless and irritable, the tongue thickly coated	
All these symptoms require urgent medical help.	
With a cough that is aggravated on lying down	ARALIA 30
Attack after the first sleep, about the middle of the night	
Sensation of a foreign body in the throat	
With frequent sneezing	

Between midnight and 3 a.m. — **ARS ALB 30**
The patient is restless and fears death by suffocation
Better bending forward, for warmth applied to the chest wall and from warm drinks
Worse in cold air

In the very elderly and weak — **BAR MUR 30**

Alternating with an itchy skin rash — **CALADIUM 30**

In the very elderly with blue skin — **CARBO VEG 30**

Worse in damp weather — **CHINA 30**

Alternating with vomiting — **CUPRUM MET 30**
Suffocative attacks, worse around 3 a.m.
The face goes blue with coughing
All these symptoms require medical help.

When talking and with laryngitis — **DROSERA 30**

With great shortage of breath and palpitations — **EUCALYPTUS 30**
Expectoration of white, thick mucus

Worse in dry, cold air, better in damp — **HEPAR SULPH 30**

Attacks when the weather changes, or before a storm, and worse in foggy weather — **HYPERICUM 30**
Better after a profuse sweat

Sudden onset of wheezing made much worse by moving about; the patient is anxious and feels as if a weight on the chest is causing suffocation — **IPECAC 30**
Constant cough which may cause gagging and vomiting but the patient is unable to cough up phlegm

Cold perspiration, particularly on the extremities, the tongue is quite clear
All these symptoms require medical help.

Attacks between 3 and 4 a.m. — **KALI BICH 30**
The patient sits up, better for bending forward
Coughing up stringy, yellow mucus gives some relief

Worse at 3 a.m. and better for leaning forward — **KALI CARB 30**

Worse for eating — **KALI PHOS 30**

With hay fever and spasms of sneezing — **LACHESIS 30**

Attacks with a feeling of weakness and nausea — **LOBELIA INF 30**
Profuse salivation and the attack is preceded by a prickling sensation all over the body

Starts with a head cold and is worse in the evening — **NAJA 30**
Cardiac asthma

Worse in damp weather — **NAT SULPH 30**
With hay fever
Attacks usually starting around 4 to 5 a.m. with a productive cough, the sputum being copious and greenish
The patient sits up and holds his chest in order to breathe during the attack
Loose bowels after each attack

With a gastric disturbance — **NUX VOM 30**
Relieved by belching and loosening the clothing
Constricted feeling in the lower part of the chest

Attacks started or made worse from inhalation of any kind of dust	POTHOS 30
Better lying down and with the arms spread out	PSORINUM 30
In children who wake around midnight with a laryngeal cough and suffocation The nose is blocked and the patient has to breathe through his mouth With profuse sweating *All these symptoms require medical help.*	SAMBUCUS 30
Stress-induced asthma The voice becomes high-pitched and there is a great sense of suffocation with a tight feeling across the chest	STRAMONIUM 30
In bronchial and cardiac asthma Great shortage of breath, worse when walking up stairs	STROPHAN-THUS 30
In children Worse in the afternoon, at 3 a.m. and in cold, damp air	THUJA 30
Without anxiety but attack gets worse towards the morning	ZINGIBER 30

DOSAGE

In acute asthmatic attacks the selected remedy should be taken every fifteen minutes until there is an improvement. It should then be taken at increasing intervals as necessary.
Constitutional treatment should be taken between attacks to treat and cure the disorder. This should always be given under medical supervision.

BRONCHITIS, *Acute and Chronic*

Acute bronchitis is characterized by a cough which has been present for only a short time, fever and detectable infective sounds in the chest, and frequently follows a cold. It occurs mainly in the first few years of life, although it may occur at any age, and its incidence starts to rise again after the age of forty-five.
Chronic bronchitis may be defined as a habitual productive cough which recurs at intervals in response to irritation of the lungs by respiratory infections, smoking and atmospheric pollution. Apart from the cough, there is shortage of breath on exertion. Chronic bronchitis tends to be a slowly progressive disease in people over fifty years of age.

These conditions require expert medical help.

KEY FEATURES	TREATMENT
After being in a dry, cold wind With anxiety, restlessness and fear The cough is hard, dry and painful	ACONITE 30
In young infants and the very elderly Wheezing with a rattling cough, but little sputum is coughed up In children the coughing is infrequent, with drowsiness and laboured breathing With vomiting of food or mucus *All these symptoms require urgent medical help.*	ANT TART 30

Dry, hacking cough and a tickling sensation in the larynx
Worse in the evening and at night
Dry, hot, flushed skin
Tendency to drowsiness but cannot sleep

BELLADONNA 30

Very short of breath, with a dry cough that seems to start in the stomach and is worse after eating
Stitching pains in the chest, worse for any movement

BRYONIA 30

In the elderly, with a loose rattle in the chest on coughing
Hoarseness in the evening
The sputum is profuse and yellow

CARBO VEG 30

Following measles or whooping cough
The cough is loose and rattling, the sputum hard to cough up

CHELIDONIUM 30

In the elderly
Easy expectoration of greeny sputum
Worse when the weather changes to cold and wet

DULCAMARA 30

In infants
Much mucus, with a spasmodic cough which ends in choking and gagging
The face is pale and there is great shortage of breath
All these symptoms require urgent medical help.

IPECAC 30

Tough, tenacious sputum which may have a blue tinge
Croupy cough, worse towards morning and causes stomach-ache

KALI BICH 30

Intense shortage of breath with a choking cough worse at 2–3 a.m.
Stitching pains in the right side of the chest
The sputum is difficult to get up
All these symptoms require urgent medical help.

KALI CARB 30

Fever with alternations of chill and heat
Desire for cold drinks that make the cough worse
Rough, sore feeling from the throat down to the middle of the chest
Dry, raw, exhausting cough with watery, saliva-like or (more commonly) yellow sputum containing mucus and pus

MERCURIUS 30

In delicate, tall, slender patients
Dry tickling cough with a tearing pain under the breastbone and a suffocative feeling in the upper part of the chest
The cough is worse going from warm to cold air and the patient feels better after sleep
The phlegm contains mucus and pus, may be blood-streaked and has a salt-sweet taste
All these symptoms require medical help.

PHOSPHORUS 30

Long-standing chronic bronchitis

SULPHUR 30

DOSAGE

For acute attacks of bronchitis the selected remedy should be taken four times a day for three days.
For chronic bronchitis the selected remedy may be taken in the 12 potency twice a day on two days a week.

CHEST PAIN

Pain in the chest may be caused by something as simple as a pulled muscle or a blow. In these conditions the pain decreases day by day. However, pain may also be a sign of other much more serious conditions.

The main illnesses that may cause chest pain are: a heart attack; angina; a tear in the main blood vessel, the aorta (dissecting aneurysm); a blood clot in the lung (pulmonary embolus); a chest infection; a burst breathing tube in the lung (spontaneous pneumothorax); regurgitation of acid from the stomach up the gullet (relux oesophagitis); a perforated stomach ulcer.

Sudden severe chest pain for which there is no apparent cause requires urgent diagnosis by a doctor. Homeopathic treatment and first-aid procedures should be used while waiting for medical assistance.

KEY FEATURES	TREATMENT
Great anxiety and difficulty in breathing, with numbness and tingling in the fingers Better when sitting up	ACONITE
After exertion or fatigue; the chest feels sore and bruised	ARNICA
The heart feels as if grasped and squeezed The lower part of the chest feels tied down and the pain makes the patient cry out Pain often occurs around 11 a.m. or 11 p.m.	CACTUS
With weakness and numbness in the left arm and the skin is blue The patient fears the heart will stop if he moves about The pulse rate is slow	DIGITALIS
The patient wakes from sleep feeling smothered and unable to lie flat	LACHESIS
Violent chest and left-arm pain, the pulse is very rapid and the patient has great difficulty in breathing	LATRODECTUS
Pain wakes the patient, with the heart feeling as if in a vice The patient bends double to try to ease the pain	LILIUM TIG
With palpitations, the pulse may be irregular and there are paroxysms of suffocation and tightness across the upper chest	TABACUM

DOSAGE

While waiting for the doctor, use the selected remedy in the highest potency you have and repeat at five-minute intervals until relief is obtained.

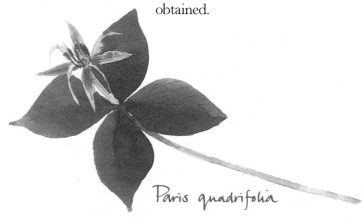

Paris quadrifolia

COLDS AND INFLUENZA

The common cold is an infection caused by a very widespread virus. Symptoms include a runny nose, which can cause problems with breathing through the nose, headache, sore throat, cough, generalized aching and malaise. The temperature is raised, but the whole illness is usually over within a few days.
Influenza produces virtually the same symptoms, but they tend to be more severe and last for a longer period.

KEY FEATURES — **TREATMENT**

After exposure to cold, dry weather or to winds and draughts — **ACONITE 30** three doses over three hours
Chilliness followed by fever; the nose is dry and feels blocked
Bouts of sneezing

The nose is sore from an acrid, burning discharge, worse in a warm room — **ALLIUM CEPA 30**
Profuse, bland watering of the eyes
Prolonged sneezing

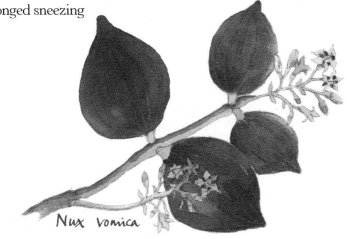

Nux vomica

A thin, watery nasal discharge makes the upper lip sore — **ARS ALB 30**
The patient is very chilly
The eyes water
Much sneezing occurs
Thirst for cold drinks

Blocked nose with yellow nasal catarrh — **ARUM TRIPH 30**
The nostrils become sore

Shivering and sneezing — **DULCAMARA 30**
Great chilliness, or the patient feels hot and cold alternately

Catarrhal snuffles in children when the nose seems blocked — **ELAPS 30**

A cold of slow onset with general malaise and body ache — **GELSEMIUM 30**
The head is hot and feels full
The patient is very chilly
Sneezing accompanied by a bland, watery nasal discharge
Colds in mild, damp weather
Sore throat

Violent sneezing — **MERCURIUS 30**
The nose drips a green-yellow, offensive discharge
Sore throat, hoarse voice, and tickly dry cough with bad breath and profuse sweating
The patient feels chilly and shaky

In cold, dry weather — **NUX VOM 30**
The nose is alternately blocked and running, blocked at night, running during the day
Much sneezing and the throat feels scraped
The patient is unable to get warm

133

Persistent cold with a thick, bland, yellow nasal discharge   PULSATILLA 30

The lips are chapped and sore

Pain in the face and nose which feels stuffed at night, but runs in the morning and out of doors

Better in fresh air

DOSAGE

With the exception of Aconite, which, if taken early enough in an attack, will prevent it becoming a full-blown cold, the selected remedy should be taken four times a day until there is an improvement. It may then be stopped.

COUGHS

Most coughs occur without any apparent cause being found. They can, however, signify many other conditions, from a simple cold to a cancer of the lung. They are usually associated with a cold or other upper respiratory infection and as such are of minor importance.

A prolonged cough, unresponsive to treatment, may indicate a serious chest condition and requires investigation.

KEY FEATURES	TREATMENT
Hard, dry, barking cough with little or no phlegm	ACONITE 12
The cough sounds loose and rattling, but no phlegm is coughed up	ANT TART 12
Spasmodic night cough after the first sleep Relieved by coughing up tough mucus	ARALIA 12
Dry, hacking cough in violent bursts that seems to come from a tickle in the larynx	BELLADONNA 12
Dry, painful cough causing the patient to hold his chest to stop the pain Pain appears to go to other parts of the body, such as the head Worse in a warm room	BRYONIA 12
Sensation of a feather in the throat brings on the cough Coughing causes a piercing pain in the chest The cough is dry at first but later there is profuse, salty phlegm	CALC CARB 12
A tickling cough relieved by drinking cold water causes rawness in the throat, hoarseness and voice loss Coughing causes urine to dribble	CAUSTICUM 12
In whooping cough Each paroxysm of coughing ends in the vomiting of clear, ropy sputum	COCCUS CACTI 12
A dry, spasmodic, hacking cough, worse at night on lying down In the elderly, where the phlegm tends to be swallowed as they become fatigued by coughing	CONIUM 12
Accompanied by vomiting and relieved by drinks of cold water In whooping cough and other cases where the coughing attacks come in quick succession	CUPRUM MET 12

A spasmodic cough which comes on in the evening and every effort to cough up phlegm ends in vomiting — DROSERA 12

Hoarse, croupy cough, where it is easy to bring up phlegm but doing so causes choking
Worse in cold air and after drinking cold water — HEPAR SULPH 12

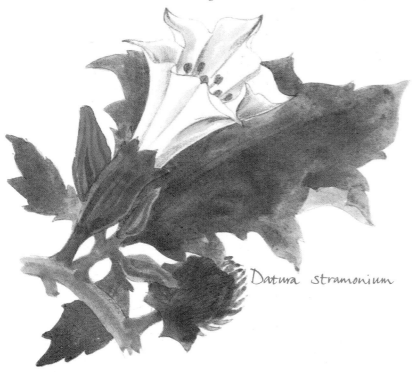

Datura stramonium

Nervous, dry, spasmodic cough
Coughing increases the desire to cough even more
Worse in the evening and on lying down — IGNATIA 12

A hard, barking cough which seems to start in the stomach
With yellow, stringy sputum which is difficult to cough up — KALI BICH 12

Spasmodic cough coming in paroxysms, with phlegm being coughed up; worse at night and on lying down — MAG PHOS 12

Dry, tickling cough, worse at night and relieved by drinks of water — OPIUM 12 *(prescription required in US)*

Worse on going from a warm room into the cold
The larynx feels raw and is worse from talking
Pain under the breastbone — PHOSPHORUS 12

A persistent cough, worse in cold air and when lying down at night
Much better in warm air and the patient will put his head under the bedclothes to achieve this — RUMEX 12

With stitching pain in the stomach
Salty phlegm is coughed up, mainly in the morning
With vomiting and soreness of the chest relieved by pressure — SEPIA 12

Violent bursts of coughing cause urine leakage, a flow of tears and sneezing, but little phlegm is coughed up
Sharp, sticking pains, worse for coughing — SQUILLA 12

Dry, croupy cough which wakes the patient
Better for a warm drink but worse in a hot room or lying with the head low — SPONGIA 12

DOSAGE

The selected remedy should be taken every thirty minutes until an improvement occurs. It may be repeated as necessary.

SUFFOCATION, *Feeling of*

Total suffocation implies a cessation of breathing as a result of drowning, smothering or some other cause that cuts off the air supply to the lungs. In practice, a feeling of suffocation simply means that not enough air is getting into the lungs. This occurs with asthma, pneumonia and lung disease such as chronic bronchitis.

All cases require expert medical help.

KEY FEATURES	TREATMENT
Between midnight and 3 a.m. The patient is restless and fears death by suffocation Better for bending forward, for warmth applied to the chest wall and from warm drinks Worse in cold air	ARS ALB 30
Asthma alternating with vomiting Worse around 3 a.m. The face goes blue with coughing	CUPRUM MET 30
Sudden onset of wheezing made much worse by moving about; the patient is anxious and feels as if there is a weight on the chest causing suffocation With a constant cough which may cause gagging and vomiting, but the patient is unable to cough up phlegm With cold perspiration, particularly on the extremities	IPECAC 30
In delicate, tall, slender patients With a dry, tickling cough, a tearing pain under the breastbone and a suffocative feeling in the upper part of the chest The cough is worse going from warm air into cold and the patient feels better after sleep The phlegm contains mucus and pus, may be blood-streaked and has a salt-sweet taste	PHOSPHORUS 30
In children who wake around midnight with a laryngeal cough and feeling of suffocation The nose is blocked and the patient has to breathe through his mouth With profuse sweating	SAMBUCUS 30
In stress-induced asthma The voice becomes high-pitched and there is a great sense of suffocation with a tight feeling across the upper chest	STRAMONIUM 30
With palpitations, an irregular pulse and paroxysms of suffocation and tightness across the upper chest	TABACUM 30

DOSAGE

The selected remedy should be taken every ten minutes while waiting for medical help.

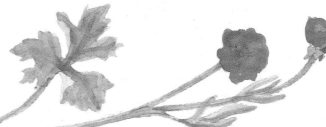

Ranunculus bulbosus

THE DIGESTIVE SYSTEM

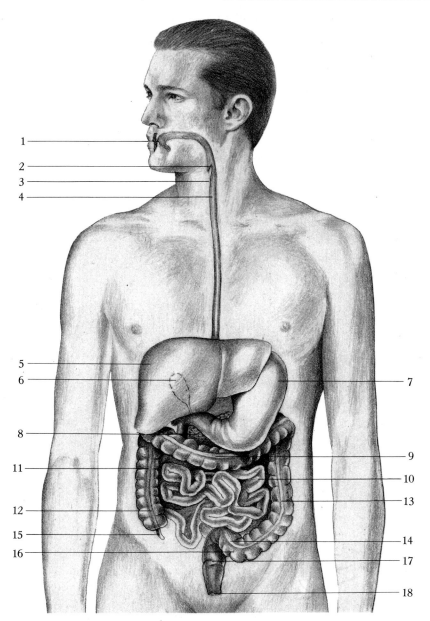

CONTENTS

Appetite, Loss of	139
Belching/Flatulence	139
Colic	140
Colitis	141
Gallstones and Gall-bladder Disease	143
Heartburn	143
Indigestion	144
Jaundice	145
Ulcers, Gastric and Duodenal	146

After being swallowed, most foods need to be digested so that they can be changed into a form that can be absorbed into the bloodstream. This process takes place in the alimentary canal, where chemical secretions from glands in its walls alter the ingested food and drink into a form that can be absorbed and utilized by the body.

1	Mouth	10	Small intestine
2	Epiglottis	11	Ascending colon
3	Throat	12	Caecum
4	Oesophagus	13	Descending colon
5	Liver	14	Sigmoid colon
6	Gall bladder	15	Appendix
7	Stomach	16	Large intestine
8	Pancreas	17	Rectum
9	Transverse colon	18	Anus

The mouth leads to the throat (pharynx), which in turn leads to the oesophagus, the canal which passes through the midriff (diaphragm) to join the stomach. When food is taken into the mouth it mixes with saliva produced by the salivary glands, forming a thick paste which can be swallowed. The tongue pushes the food into the throat, squeezing it over the top of the larynx and into the oesophagus. The act of swallowing brings a small flap, the epiglottis, over the top of the larynx to stop the food going the wrong way.

Most of the digestive process takes place in the stomach, where gastric juices containing digestive enzymes and acid are secreted. From the stomach the food passes through the duodenum into the jejunum, then into the ileum. These three parts of the same canal make up what is called the small intestine. Ducts (small tubes) from the liver and the pancreas connect with the wall of the duodenum, allowing more digestive secretions to enter the intestine to continue the process of digestion.

The liver is the largest gland in the body and weighs about 3 lb (1.5 kg). It lies mainly under the right lower ribs but a small part overlaps the stomach. Its secretion, bile, is stored in the gall bladder which lies on the underside of the liver. The liver stores carbohydrate taken from the blood flowing to it, then redelivers it to the bloodstream as different sugars which the body can use as fuel. The bile neutralizes stomach acids and helps in the digestion of fats.

The pancreas lies behind the stomach and produces two secretions. One goes to the duodenum to help in the further digestion of proteins, carbohydrates and fats. The other goes directly into the bloodstream and plays a part in the utilization of sugar by the tissues and muscles. This is called insulin.

The small intestine is a narrow tube about 23 ft (7 metres) long, which occupies most of the remaining space in the abdominal cavity. By means of muscles in its walls the food is passed on by waves of contractions, a process called peristalsis, and eventually enters the large intestine. This part of the gut is of considerably wider bore and just under 7 ft (2 metres) long. It starts at the caecum, from which the appendix, a blind, narrow tube about 2–2½ in (5–7 cm) long, is attached. From the caecum the large intestine runs upwards along the right side of the abdominal cavity as the ascending colon. It then crosses the top part of the cavity as the transverse colon and finally goes down the left side as the descending colon, the sigmoid colon and finally ends as the rectum and anus.

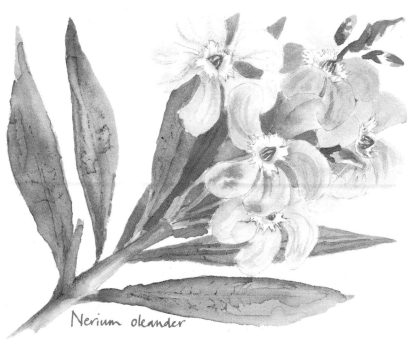

Nerium oleander

No digestion takes place in the large intestine, although water is absorbed from it. In passing through it, the undigested food takes a more solid form and becomes the characteristically smelling faeces which are passed out of the body through the anus. The faeces consist of undigested food, bile pigments, bacteria, water and sometimes mucus.

APPETITE, Loss of

In health the appetite becomes geared to a person's normal requirements and will allow a constant weight to be maintained. Loss of appetite occurs with many chronic physical diseases and may be significant in depression and anorexia nervosa. This latter condition is a serious psychological illness in which patients, usually young girls, starve themselves, take unnecessary laxatives or make themselves vomit to induce weight loss (see p. 58).

KEY FEATURES	TREATMENT
Total appetite loss in the morning Ravenous hunger after midday	ABIES NIG 6
No desire to eat Can swallow only small amounts Potatoes disagree	ALUMINA 6
Loss of appetite Desire for pickles and acidic foods	ANT CRUD 6
When overworked	CALC CARB 6
Appetite lost but enjoyment of cold drinks	COCCULUS 6
No desire to eat normal foods Craving for acidic and indigestible foods	IGNATIA 6
Bitter taste Aversion to all food	PICRIC ACID 6
When temperature is raised there is headache, diarrhoea, nausea and loss of appetite Thirstless	PULSATILLA 6
Aversion to meat Craving for bread and beer Loss of appetite generally	STRONTIA 6
Complete loss of, or excessive, appetite Acidity Milk disagrees	SULPHUR 6
Complete loss of appetite Dislike of meat, potatoes and onions	THUJA 6

DOSAGE

The selected remedy should be taken three times a day until an improvement occurs, then stopped. Repeat the treatment as and when necessary.

BELCHING/FLATULENCE

The sudden expulsion of gas from the stomach through the mouth occurs after eating certain foods, especially spicy foods, peas and beans, and food with a high carbohydrate content. It also occurs with digestive upsets, such as indigestion, or after swallowing excessive air through eating too quickly.

KEY FEATURES	TREATMENT
Sour belching with vomiting Violent stomach pain Cold sweat and cold skin	ACETIC ACID 30
Loss of appetite Craving for acidic foods Belches tasting of the food just eaten	ANT CRUD 30

With stomach upsets	ARG NIT 30
Pain over the stomach that radiates to all parts of the abdomen	
Belching, heaviness, fullness and sleepiness occur together	CARBO VEG 30
Worse when lying down	
Much flatulence, not relieved by the accompanying bitter vomiting	CHINA 30
Worse after eating fruit	

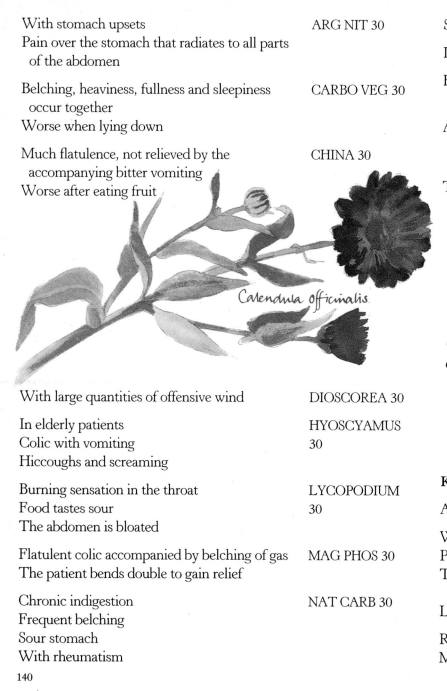

Calendula officinalis

With large quantities of offensive wind	DIOSCOREA 30
In elderly patients	HYOSCYAMUS 30
Colic with vomiting	
Hiccoughs and screaming	
Burning sensation in the throat	LYCOPODIUM 30
Food tastes sour	
The abdomen is bloated	
Flatulent colic accompanied by belching of gas	MAG PHOS 30
The patient bends double to gain relief	
Chronic indigestion	NAT CARB 30
Frequent belching	
Sour stomach	
With rheumatism	

Sour, bitter, difficult belches	NUX VOM 30
Large quantities of wind straight after eating	PHOSPHORUS 30
Hot, sour belching	PODOPHYLLUM 30
Alternating with hiccoughs	WYETHIA 30

DOSAGE

The selected remedy should be taken three times a day for 2–3 days.

COLIC

This is severe abdominal pain of variable intensity, with the spasms of pain seconds or minutes apart. In adults its commonest cause is constipation. It may also be due to partial or complete obstruction of the bowel. In babies it is from gas in the intestines associated with feeding problems (see p. 38).

If the colic does not settle within a short time after using homeopathic treatment, medical advice should be obtained.

KEY FEATURES	TREATMENT
Any attempt at eating leads to colic	CALC PHOS 12
With flatulence	CHAMOMILLA 12
Passing wind does not relieve the pain	
The abdomen is distended and sensitive to touch	
Local warmth helps the pain	
Restlessness	COLOCYNTH 12
Moaning between spasms	

Twisting and doubling up the body helps to
  relieve the pain

Better from walking about	DIOSCOREA 12
The pain radiates in all directions	
Worse bending forward or on lying down	
Violent colic relieved by vomiting	HYOSCYAMUS 12
After eating irritating food	
Relief from warmth, gentle pressure, rubbing and bending forward	MAG PHOS 12
Belching does not help	
Flatulence, constipation, irritability and anger	NUX VOM 12
From overeating	
Violent colic	PLUMBUM 12
Abdominal rumbling	
Obstinate constipation	
Flatulent colic with vomiting	PULSATILLA 12
Relieved by hard pressure	STANNUM MET 12
After anger	STAPHYSAGRIA 12
The abdomen is swollen, feels cold and is very sensitive to pressure	VERATRUM ALB 12

DOSAGE

The selected remedy should be taken every ten minutes until relief is
obtained.

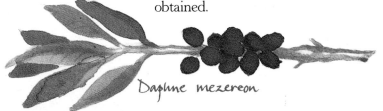

Daphne mezereon

COLITIS

*Inflammation of the colon causes diarrhoea, sometimes with
blood and mucus, and abdominal pain. The pain is usually
very slight but may be totally absent. This ailment may start
gradually and the diagnosis may not be made until there have
been several bouts of what appears to be a simple gut
inflammation. In fact, the early signs may not be related to the
colon at all. Sometimes a patient complains of mild depression
with a slightly raised temperature and some looseness of
the stools.
Several other conditions may be considered under the general
term of colitis. These are mucous colitis, ulcerative colitis,
spastic colon and irritable bowel syndrome.*

The symptoms of colitis must always be taken very seriously and
medical advice is essential.

KEY FEATURES	TREATMENT
Great distension of the stomach with much flatulence	ARG NIT 12
The motion is green, like chopped spinach	
Diarrhoea immediately after eating or drinking	
Loose motions made much worse by anxiety or fear	
Anticipation of an ordeal, such as an exam or interview, may produce the symptoms	
Diarrhoea alternates with constipation	ANT CRUD 12
The stool is slimy with much mucus, but also contains hard lumps	
Tongue coated thick and white	
Craving for acids and pickles	

Painless, yellow and frothy diarrhoea   CHINA 12
Worse at night and after eating
The patient becomes very weak and has much
   flatulence
Frequent belching does not ease the symptoms

Painful area just below the navel   COLOCYNTH 12
The stool is loose and like jelly
Severe colic pains in the abdomen are eased by
   bending double and pressing on the abdomen,
   or from local warmth, such as a hot-water
   bottle

The stool is either lumpy and covered with   GRAPHITES 12
   mucus, or very loose, brown and mixed with
   undigested food particles; it is very smelly and
   has a sour odour

Colic pains in both right and left sides of the IGNATIA 12
   abdomen
Painful constriction of the anus after passing a
   stool
Diarrhoea and pain after experiencing a shock
   or being frightened

Great urge to pass a stool, even immediately   MERC CORR 12
   after defaecation
The stool is hot, bloody, slimy and offensive
The abdomen feels bruised, and is bloated and
   very painful to the slightest pressure

Stabbing abdominal pains and the stool is   MERCURIUS 12
   greenish, bloody and slimy; all the symptoms
   are worse at night

Loose stools, more frequent during the   NAT SULPH 12
   morning, are yellow and watery
The amount passed is huge

Tight clothing around the waist causes burning
   sensations in the colon and abdominal pain as
   if bruised

Morning diarrhoea drives the patient out of bed   SULPHUR 12
The abdomen is very sensitive to pressure and
   colic occurs after drinking

DOSAGE

The selected remedy should be taken every hour until there is an
improvement. It may need to be repeated at intervals if a
deterioration occurs.

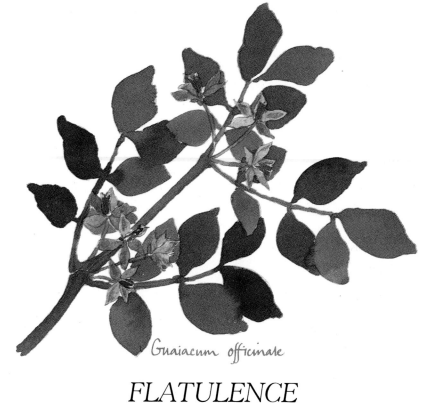

Guaiacum officinale

FLATULENCE

(see Belching, p. 139)

GALLSTONES AND GALL-BLADDER DISEASE

Multiple stones may form in the gall bladder as a result of previous infections, but occasionally a single stone forms due to the deposition of cholesterol and bile pigments. The stone may facilitate infection and the subsequent formation of multiple infected stones.

Gallstones and gall-bladder pain are serious and unpleasant conditions, both of which require medical/surgical attention.

KEY FEATURES	TREATMENT
Pain over the gall-bladder region, worse for pressure With constipation, or watery, pale diarrhoea	BERBERIS 30
Colicky gall-bladder pain Gallstones With jaundice	CHELIDONIUM 30
Gall-bladder colic Flatulence Better for bending double With jaundice	CHINA 30
Gallstones With jaundice Tenderness over the liver Food tastes bitter	HYDRASTIS 30

DOSAGE

The selected remedy may be taken at two-hourly intervals until an improvement occurs. Then take twice a day for three days.

HEARTBURN

If the acid gastric juices leak back from the stomach, they burn the lower end of the oesophagus and cause acidity, better known as heartburn. It is sometimes accompanied by a bitter, acid fluid in the mouth which is regurgitated stomach contents.

KEY FEATURES	TREATMENT
Pain in the pit of the stomach With nausea With chilliness	AMMON CARB 12
With loud belching Craving for indigestible things	CALC CARB 12
Nausea, acrid heartburn and acid belches Worse after going to bed and lying down Eating gives temporary relief	CONIUM 12
Indigestion in the elderly Burning acidity Bloating of the abdomen	KALI CARB 12
Acidity, nausea and gnawing pain Relieved by eating The patient cannot bear the slightest pressure on the abdomen	LITHIUM CARB 12
Acidity, flatulence and shortage of breath after eating With a profuse flow of saliva	LOBELIA 12
With palpitations	NAT MUR 12
Sour belches and taste With a yellow-creamy coating on the tongue	NAT PHOS 12

Acidity Frontal headache Sour belches, especially in children	ROBINIA 12
Great acidity Complete loss of, or excessive, appetite Milk disagrees The patient feels weak and faint at about 11 a.m., so must eat	SULPHUR 12
From sweet things	ZINC MET 12

DOSAGE
The selected remedy should be taken every two hours until an improvement is maintained.

INDIGESTION
Dyspepsia

This condition can be defined as discomfort in the upper abdomen after eating, sometimes accompanied by nausea or vomiting. It may signify no more than a disordered digestion due to bad eating habits, but it may indicate a stomach or duodenal ulcer, or even a hiatus hernia. Some indigestion has an emotional cause and can be related to stress and worry.

Indigestion which does not settle within a few days may require further investigation. (See also Ulcers)

KEY FEATURES	TREATMENT
In the elderly Worse after tea or smoking	ABIES NIG 12

Nervous indigestion	ALETRIS 12
Flatulent indigestion	AMMON CARB 12
Nervous indigestion relieved by food	ANACARDIUM 12
From fruit, acid foods and ice-cream or cold drinks	ARS ALB 12
In hot weather and from cold drinks taken when overheated	BRYONIA 12
With bad breath	CARBOLIC ACID 12
Acid indigestion	CAUSTICUM 12
Flatulent indigestion with vomiting	FERRUM MET 12
Poor digestion Bitter taste Feeling of weakness	HYDRASTIS 12
Flatulent indigestion in the elderly Acidity and sour belches	KALI CARB 12
Food tastes sour Distension and indigestion from eating carbohydrates	LYCOPODIUM 12

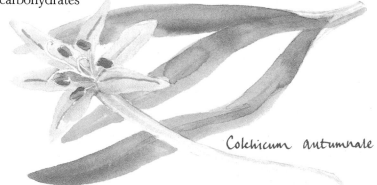

Colchicum autumnale

Great hunger but the stomach feels full after
   eating only a very small amount

Chronic indigestion and poor digestion   NAT CARB 12
With rheumatism

Heartburn, flatulence and vomiting   NAT SULPH 12
Acid indigestion

In nervous, debilitated patients   NICCOLUM 12
With frequent headaches
With constipation

With depression   NITRIC ACID 12
Huge hunger
Craving for fats and salt

Flatulent indigestion with hiccoughs   NUX
MOSCHATA 12

With a liking for highly seasoned foods and   NUX VOM 12
   coffee, all of which disagree
Preceded by a ravenous appetite

Distension after eating   PULSATILLA 12
Averse to fat, warm food and drink

Acid indigestion with a bloated abdomen   SEPIA 12
Sour belches
Nausea at the thought or smell of food
Faint, sinking feeling, not helped by eating

In those who eat very quickly   ZINC MET 12
With a ravenous hunger around 11 a.m.
Dislike of meat, sweets and warm food

DOSAGE

The selected remedy should be taken every hour until an
improvement is maintained.

JAUNDICE

*This is a condition in which the skin and the white of the eyes
become yellow to a variable degree. The motion may become
white and the urine dark brown. Jaundice indicates some
disorder of the liver or gall bladder. It may be caused by
inflammation of the liver (hepatitis), liver disease such as
cirrhosis, gallstones and certain blood disorders where there is
excessive destruction of the red blood-cells.*

Jaundice indicates that serious illness may be present which requires
immediate medical investigation and treatment.

KEY FEATURES	TREATMENT
Dull pain over the liver Pain may radiate to the navel area	AESCULUS 12
Pain over the liver, mainly on the left Swollen and sore gall bladder Yellow, or clay-coloured stools	CARDUUS 12
Pain under the right shoulder blade Nausea and vomiting Better for drinks of warm water Eating temporarily relieves the symptoms	CHELIDONIUM 12
Chronic jaundice Aching pain in and around the liver	CONIUM 12
The liver and spleen are enlarged Deep, severe jaundice Frothy, fatty stools	IODUM 12

Soreness over the liver	KALI CARB 12
Jaundice, coldness and distension of the abdomen	
Fluid retention elsewhere in the body	
Chronic liver disease	
Enlargement of the liver, which is sore to the touch	MERCURIUS 12
Perpetual hunger	
Dull pain in the liver region	MYRICA 12
Loss of appetite	
Loose, foul-smelling, light-coloured stools	
Deep jaundice	
Yellow, frothy urine	
Liver soreness, worse for deep breathing and lying on the left side	NAT SULPH 12
Vomiting of bile-stained fluid	
Yellow, spluttery, watery diarrhoea, worse in the early morning	
Frequent dark brown urine	
Acute hepatitis	PHOSPHORUS 12
Jaundice	
An enlarged, sore liver	
Light, clay-coloured, hard stools	
Jaundice in chronic alcoholics	RUMEX 12
Bilious attacks with headache, nausea, fatigue and jaundice	TARAXACUM 12
Severe pain in an enlarged liver	VIPERA 12
Jaundice and fever	
Pain radiates to the right shoulder and hip	

DOSAGE

For an acute illness take the selected remedy every four hours. For more chronic conditions it should be given twice a day. In both cases, once an improvement occurs, the remedy may be given less frequently.

ULCERS, *Gastric and Duodenal*

The patient often has a family history of stomach or duodenal ulcer, and in many cases there is a history of previous attacks. The other important symptoms are: pain in stomach region which is relieved by eating or antacids; pain right after eating (gastric ulcers); pain about one or two hours after a meal, which also often wakes the patient during the night (duodenal ulcers); heartburn, sudden and excessive salivation, especially with indigestion and nausea, and belching with abdominal distension; excessive vomiting, loss of appetite, loss of weight or black stools.

If an ulcer is suspected, medical advice and investigation are essential, urgently if any of the last symptoms above are present.

KEY FEATURES	TREATMENT
Dull pain radiating to the back two hours after eating	ANACARDIUM 12
Tasteless or sour belches	
Eating gives symptomatic relief	
Gnawing stomach pain	ARG NIT 12
Pain radiates in all directions and is worse from pressure and eating	

Flatulence may produce violent efforts to belch
Craving for sweets which disagree

Burning stomach pain   ARS ALB 12
Inability to digest food
Loss of appetite
Pains immediately after eating
Nausea and vomiting

Sharp, cutting pain soon after eating   BRYONIA 12
Pain extends to the shoulders and back
Food lies like a stone in the stomach
The mouth is dry
Bitter taste in the mouth
With constipation and frontal headaches

Burning, crampy, colicky pain   GRAPHITES 12
Better after eating
Hot drinks disagree
With an unpleasant taste of eggs in the
  morning
Great distension
Wind is rancid or putrid

Vigorous appetite   LYCOPODIUM
Full, bloated feeling after a few mouthfuls of 12
  food
Sleepy feeling after eating
Excessive flatulence may press upwards and
  cause difficulty with breathing

Pain about an hour after eating   NUX VOM 12
Pain after mental overwork
Nausea
Empty retching and sour belching
The patient is bad-tempered and worse in the
  morning

Craving for cold food and drink which give   PHOSPHORUS 12
  momentary relief before being vomited
Sour belching
The tongue is coated white

Dry mouth   PULSATILLA 12
Putrid taste in the morning
Sensation of food stuck under the breastbone
The tongue is thick, rough and white
Nasty taste of food eaten previously
Pain one or two hours after eating
Flatulence seems to move around
Worse in the evening

DOSAGE

The selected remedy should be taken four times a day until an improvement occurs, then stopped. Repeat the treatment as and when necessary.

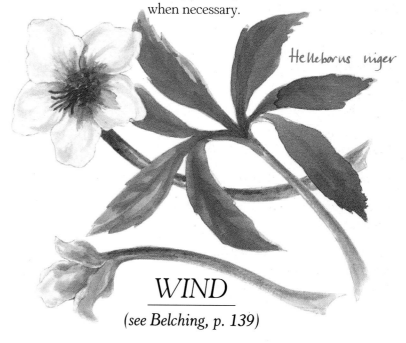

Helleborus niger

WIND

(see Belching, p. 139)

THE RECTUM AND ANUS

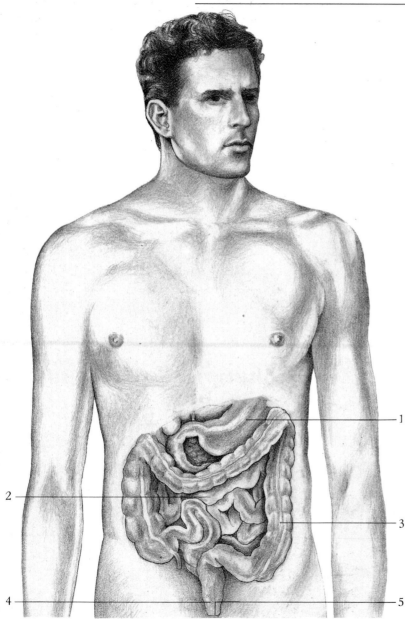

CONTENTS

Anal Burning	149
Anal Fissure	149
Anal Itching	150
Constipation	151
Diarrhoea	151
Piles	152
Stools, Difficulty with	153
Stools, Involuntary Passing of	154

*T*hese are the last two sections of the digestive tract. As undigested food, together with unused digestive chemicals and bacteria, passes through, it becomes more solid and acquires the characteristic smell of faeces. These remain in the rectum until expelled from the body during defaecation. At other times a ring of muscles, collectively called a sphincter, keeps the anus closed.

1 Stomach
2 Small intestine
3 Large intestine
4 Anal canal
5 Sphincter

ANAL BURNING

This sensation may occur on its own or following defaecation. It is usually associated with an anal fissure (split in the anal lining membrane) or piles.

KEY FEATURES	TREATMENT
With a sensation of pressure in the rectum and anus Rectal prolapse	ARS ALB 12
Diarrhoea followed by anal burning With piles	GRATIOLA 12
After defaecation Painful passage of faeces Swollen anal orifice	PAEONIA 12
Before defaecation and for hours afterwards The rectum feels as if full of broken glass With protruding piles	RATANHIA 12
Itching and burning of anus	SULPHUR 12

DOSAGE

The selected remedy should be taken every two hours until relief is maintained.

ANAL FISSURE

Overstretching of the anal sphincter by a hard motion may lead to the formation of a fissure (crack) in the lining of the anal tract. Defaecation thus becomes very painful and is often followed by a throbbing pain. Sometimes it is also accompanied by bleeding, especially in babies. The condition may occur in any age group and there is a history of constipation in about one third of all cases.

KEY FEATURES	TREATMENT
Constant desire to defaecate The anus burns and smarts	BERBERIS 30
The anus is sore and smarts The stools are covered in mucus With eczema	GRAPHITES 30

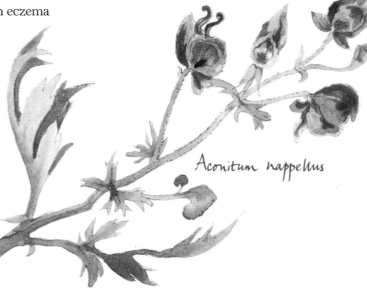

Aconitum nappellus

Burning, stitching pain after defaecation With anal bleeding The stool is dry and crumbly	NAT MUR 30
Sensation of splinters in the anus Burning, rawness and smarting Constant ooze of soft faeces Ineffectual urge to defaecate	NITRIC ACID 30

The anus is moist and sore Constant anal smarting Burning pain may last for hours after defaecation	PAEONIA 30
Cutting, lancing rectal pain Dryness of the anus Sudden, stitching anal pain Aching for hours after defaecation In very irritable patients	RATANHIA 30
Pain about thirty minutes after defaecation Pain lasts for several hours Slipping back of partially expelled stool	SILICA 30

DOSAGE

The selected remedy should be taken three times a day for four days.

ANAL ITCHING

Pruritis ani

This can be an early warning of the onset of sugar diabetes. Other causes are threadworms, piles, ringworm and vaginal discharge.

Continuous anal itching requires medical diagnosis.

KEY FEATURES	TREATMENT
Constant irritation With piles With constipation and flatulent indigestion	ALUMINA 12

Diarrhoea or constipation Irritation worse at night	ANT CRUD 12
Painful defaecation Severe irritation	IGNATIA 12
Painful piles Worse while urinating	MURIATIC ACID 12
Ineffectual desire to defaecate Painful defaecation Irritation and piles	NUX VOM 12

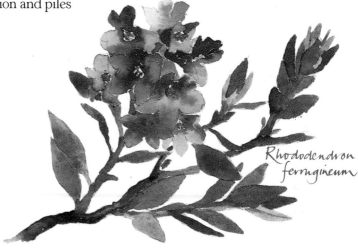

Rhododendron ferrugineum

Watery, gushing diarrhoea, daytime only Anal irritation	PETROLEUM 12
Burning, itching anus Redness around the anus Painless diarrhoea Desire to defaecate immediately on waking	SULPHUR 12

DOSAGE

The selected remedy should be taken every two hours until relief is obtained.

CONSTIPATION

Most cases of constipation (infrequent bowel movement) arise from poor dietary habits – too many refined foods, such as white bread and cakes. An increased intake of fibre will often cure the condition.

Any unexplained alteration in bowel habit requires medical attention

KEY FEATURES	TREATMENT
With soft, sticky, or hard, dry stool Defaecation is difficult	ALUMINA 6
A hard, dry, dark, lumpy stool Defaecation is difficult through lack of urge	BRYONIA 6
The stool is large, smelly and made up of many lumps stuck together with mucus Urge is lacking The stool is painful to pass	GRAPHITES 6
A hard, dry stool which is painful to pass	LYCOPODIUM 6
Light-coloured and crumbly stool	MAG MUR 6
Frequent ineffectual urging An incomplete stool is passed, so the rectum feels unemptied The patient is chilly and irritable	NUX VOM 6
Complete lack of desire to defaecate The stool is composed of hard little balls The appetite is very poor	OPIUM 6 *(prescription required in US)*
A hard stool which may slip back when partially expelled	SILICA 6

The stools are hard, dry, black and smelly Anal irritation Pain and burning with defaecation Reluctance to defaecate because of pain	SULPHUR 6

DOSAGE

The selected remedy should be taken three times a day until an improvement occurs. It may then be reduced to twice a day for three days, once a day for three days and then stopped.

DIARRHOEA

Simple diarrhoea is a self-limiting condition, requiring only a good intake of fluid to balance that lost in the diarrhoea. Homeopathic treatment will shorten the duration of the ailment, so may be used even if fluids only are recommended by your doctor.

Diarrhoea that does not settle within a few days may require investigation. A doctor should be consulted.

KEY FEATURES	TREATMENT
Following a fright or after cold drinks	ACONITE 12
From food poisoning With vomiting With restlessness and anxiety Worse during the night (12 a.m. to 3 a.m.) The rectum feels burned by watery diarrhoea Thirst for small, warm drinks	ARS ALB 12

Worse in the evening The stool is frothy, offensive and greenish The patient is restless and irritable	CHAMOMILLA 12
Painless, watery, offensive, yellow stools Extreme weakness After eating excessive fruit	CHINA 12
Painful, cramping colic relieved by pressure or bending double Thin, spluttery, copious, yellow stools Immediately after eating	COLOCYNTH 12
Painless, profuse, watery stools contain undigested food Of nervous origin	PHOS ACID 12
Profuse, spluttery, watery, pasty, yellowish diarrhoea Worse in the early morning and painless The stool is extremely offensive Followed by a weakness of the rectum	PODOPHYLLUM 12

With vomiting
The patient is icy cold with a cold sweat and
  asks for large amounts of cold drinks
Desire to be in the cold, fresh air
The patient may faint after defaecation
Profuse, watery stools preceded by abdominal
  pain
	VERATRUM ALB 12

DOSAGE

The selected remedy should be taken every thirty minutes until an improvement occurs. It may then be taken at increasing intervals until the improvement is maintained.

PILES
Haemorrhoids

Varicose veins occurring in the anal canal are called internal piles. Often, however, piles become external, and although these are painless, they may develop a clot within themselves which can be very painful until the thrombosed vein discharges the clot.

An early symptom is anal irritation. There may be a feeling of 'something coming down', particularly after defaecation, and in about half of all cases there is anal bleeding.

Although piles are not serious, any unexplained rectal/anal pain or bleeding requires early diagnosis.

KEY FEATURES	TREATMENT
Sensation of splinters in the rectum Aching in the lower part of the back Purple piles Burning, itching dryness of the anus With liver disease	AESCULUS 6
The piles protrude like a bunch of grapes and bleed easily Cold-water applications give relief Marked burning in the anus Tendency to diarrhoea	ALOES 6
Bluish-coloured piles Burning pain	ARS ALB 6
Bleeding piles Anal burning, itching, smarting and stinging during defaecation	CAPSICUM 6

Sensation of sticks in the rectum   COLLINSONIA 6
Constipation from bowel inertia
Itching around the anus
Piles during pregnancy

The piles protrude, burn and sting   GRAPHITES 6
Worse when sitting

Bellis perennis

With copious bleeding   HAMAMELIS 6
With excessive soreness
The anus feels raw

Sharp, stitching pain shoots up the rectum   IGNATIA 6

In the elderly   MURIATIC ACID 6
Extreme anal soreness and sensitivity

Large piles   NUX VOM 6
Burning, stinging, constricted sensation in the rectum

Bruised pain in the small of the back
With itching that prevents sleep
Cold-water applications relieve the itch
With bleeding and a constant desire to defaecate

For thrombosed piles   LYCOPODIUM 6

Anal oozing of soft faeces   SULPHUR 6
Itching and burning, with redness around the anus

DOSAGE
The selected remedy should be taken twice a day until an improvement is maintained.
For thrombosed, painful piles a dose may be taken every three hours.

STOOLS, *Difficulty with*

Colic, constipation and diarrhoea are conditions which alter the desire to defaecate. Psychological causes, such as fear and stress, may also be implicated. Any prolonged and unexplained alteration in bowel movement should be medically investigated.

KEY FEATURES	TREATMENT
No desire to defaecate for several days at a time	ALUMEN 12
Ineffectual desire	ANACARDIUM 12
The rectum seems powerless	
Even soft stools are passed with difficulty	

Hurried desire to defaecate	DIOSCORIA 12
Nausea accompanies the desire to defaecate	DULCAMARA 12
Bearing-down sensation with an urgent desire to defaecate	LILIUM TIG 12
Colic accompanies the desire to defaecate	NUX VOM 12
Constipation with no desire at all	OPIUM 12 *(prescription required in US)*
Desire to defaecate when lying on the left side	PHOSPHORUS 12
Desire immediately after eating	TANACETUM 12

DOSAGE

The selected remedy should be taken twice a day until an improvement is maintained.

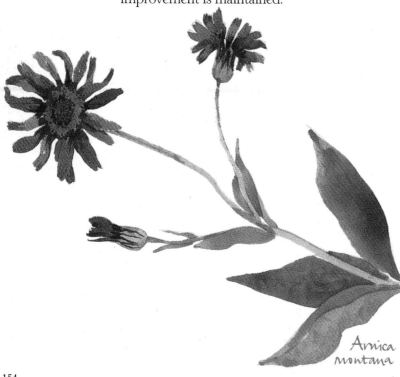

Arnica
montana

STOOLS, *Involuntary Passing of*
Faecal incontinence

The commonest cause of this distressing condition is old age when the sphincter (guard) muscle of the anus becomes weak and inactive. It can, however, occur at any age for psychological reasons. The main one in adults is fear or shock, while in children it can occur for a multitude of psychological reasons.

KEY FEATURES	TREATMENT
While asleep	ARNICA 30
Frequent involuntary, smelly stools Anal burning	CARBO VEG 30
Painless, involuntary stools from emotional excitement	GELSEMIUM 30
While urinating	MURIATIC ACID 30
While passing wind	NAT SULPH 30
Stools are black, offensive and frothy	OPIUM 30 *(prescription required in US)*
Stools are passed without any sensation, as the anus is wide open	SECALE 30

DOSAGE

The selected remedy should be taken three times a day for four days, then repeated as necessary.

THE URINARY SYSTEM

CONTENTS

Cystitis	156
Incontinence	157
Kidney Stones	158
Urine Retention	159

*T*he urinary system is responsible for the excretion of urine, one of the ways that the body rids itself of impurities and waste collected by the blood. The other routes of excretion are via the faeces formed in the bowel, the lungs, which rid the body of carbon dioxide, and the skin, which continuously produces sweat.

The two kidneys are found in the abdominal cavity on either side of the spinal column, the left kidney being slightly higher than the right. They both have large arteries and veins, the artery coming directly from the main blood vessel of the body, the aorta. A tube called the ureter runs from each kidney to the bladder where the urine collects.

The kidneys act as filters through which all the blood passes. They extract impurities, returning the clarified blood back to the circulation. The urine carries the impurities, the main one being urea, down to the bladder. This is an elastic and muscular pouch

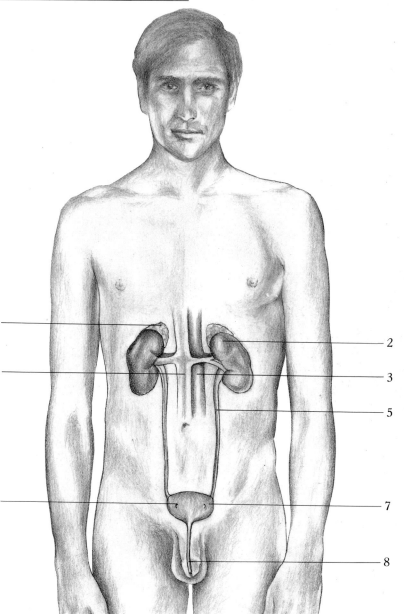

1	Adrenal gland	5	Ureter
2	Kidney	6	Opening of ureter
3	Aorta	7	Bladder
4	Inferior vena cava	8	Urethra

found in the pelvic cavity behind a part of the pelvic bone called the symphysis pubis. The bladder lies below all the intestines and rises into the abdomen only when it is quite full. At the lower end of the bladder is the urethra, the tube from which urine leaves the body. Urination, also known as micturition, occurs when the guard muscle between the bladder and urethra is relaxed and the bladder contracts, thus forcing urine along the urethra.

Around 2½ pints (1.5 litres) of urine are excreted each day, more being produced during the daytime than at night. More urine is excreted after increased consumption of food or drink, and after exposure to cold. The reverse also occurs, especially in hot climates, when more fluid is lost from the body by sweating.

KEY FEATURES	TREATMENT
Dribbling of high-coloured urine smelling offensively of ammonia	BENZOIC ACID 30
Constant desire to urinate Pain in the hips while urinating The urine is reddish with a red deposit Back pain with a tearing pain in the kidneys extending down the ureters to the bladder Cutting bladder pain extends into the urethra	BERBERIS 30

CYSTITIS

This condition, which is six times commoner in females than males, tends to recur. The main symptoms are frequency of urination (including during the night) and pain on passing urine, usually described as a burning sensation. Other, less common symptoms are pain over the bladder, fever and blood in the urine. One or more of these symptoms occur in about 20 per cent of all cases.

Recurrent attacks of cystitis should always be investigated by a doctor. In all cases a bacterial examination of the urine should be carried out to ensure complete eradication of infection.

Persistent and violent urging to urinate Intense burning sensation on urination The urine is passed only in drops The pain is worse immediately after urination Ineffectual urge to urinate	CANTHARIS 30
Throbbing bladder pain Intense desire to urinate increased on passing a few drops Ineffectual urging of the rectum The patient walks about, but is relieved by lying on his back	DIGITALIS 30

The bladder always feels full but this is not relieved by urination — **EQUISETUM 30**
Constant desire to urinate
The urine is scanty, high-coloured and contains much mucus

Violent ineffectual urge — **MERC CORR 30**
Extreme burning sensation when passing urine
Very little urine is passed
The urine may contain blood

Violent straining to urinate — **PAREIRA BRAVA 30**
The patient may have to kneel to urinate
The urine scalds and smells of ammonia
The pain extends down the thighs

Cystitis in pregnancy — **PULSATILLA 30**

'Honeymoon cystitis' — **STAPHYSAGRIA 30**
Burning sensation during urination, but also when not urinating
The bladder never feels emptied

The urine appears smoky, turbid and has a 'coffee-ground' deposit — **TEREBINTH 30**
Burning sensation during urination
Ineffectual urge to urinate
Slow, painful urination
Pressure in the bladder extends to the kidneys
Dull, aching pain in the kidney region
The urine smells like violets

DOSAGE

The selected remedy should be taken four times a day for four days. If an improvement does not occur within forty-eight hours, medical advice must be sought.

INCONTINENCE

Loss of normal bladder control leads to leakage of urine. This may happen both night and day, but in some patients the symptoms occur only during the night. In some cases incontinence may be due to a urinary tract infection.

KEY FEATURES	TREATMENT
Scanty, highly coloured urine In the elderly With prolapse in the female or enlarged prostate in the male	ALOE 12
Scanty urine Drowsiness, fluid retention, shortage of breath lying down and lack of thirst	APIS 12
Paralytic bladder conditions Involuntary urination when asleep, when coughing, blowing the nose or sneezing Difficulty in starting to urinate, with a slow stream and difficulty in passing the last few drops	CAUSTICUM 12

157

Incontinence day and night
Urine spurts with coughing — FERRUM PHOS 12

The urine is very yellow
With general debility — KALI PHOS 12

Involuntary urination when walking or when coughing
Inability to urinate if being watched — NAT MUR 12

Constant dribbling in the very old
Of nervous origin — RHUS AROMAT 12

With an enlarged prostate — SABAL SERR 12

Involuntary spurting of urine when coughing or sneezing
Pain over the bladder — ZINC MET 12

DOSAGE

The selected remedy should be taken twice a day until an improvement is maintained.

KIDNEY STONES

Renal calculi

Kidney stones, four times more common in men than women, develop for a variety of reasons. Recurrent infection may play a part, but other predisposing factors include prolonged bed-rest during chronic illness, congenital deformities of the renal tract, parathyroid tumours (very rare) and the pH (acid/alkaline) content of the urine. The passage of stones from the kidney down the ureter produces very severe pain (renal colic), which extends from one loin down into the flank. It may

radiate into the scrotum or even to the tip of the penis. The pain may last for several hours and is usually spasmodic. In some cases, however, it is continuous.

———

Medical help is required for this condition

———

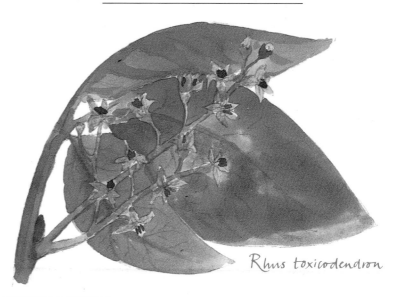

Rhus toxicodendron

KEY FEATURES	TREATMENT
Sticking, tearing pains in the kidney, worse from deep pressure	BERBERIS
Pain extends down the back and down the ureter to the bladder	
Acute kidney pain, usually left-sided	
Constant urge to pass urine	
Worse when standing	
The pain is usually right-sided	LYCOPODIUM
Severe backache relieved by passing urine which contains large quantities of red 'sand'	
Urination is very painful	

Frequent, painful urination due to the passage of red or yellow gravel Right-sided pain Pain in the ureter Nausea	OCIMUM CAN
The urine has a reddish clay-coloured sediment and an offensive smell Constant desire to urinate Dragging sensation in the bladder	SEPIA

DOSAGE

Take the selected remedy in the highest potency available every ten minutes until an improvement occurs. It should then be taken at increasing intervals until the improvement is maintained.

URINE RETENTION

If urine cannot be voided because of an obstruction to the urethra, or if the bladder is incapable of contracting and thus expelling the urine it contains due to some alteration to its nerve supply such as paralysis, multiple sclerosis or spinal injury, the patient will experience swelling in the lower part of the abdomen. If the nerve supply is intact and the retention is due to obstruction, extreme pain will also be present.

———————————

Medical help is required for this condition

———————————

KEY FEATURES	TREATMENT
With considerable pain Restlessness Any urine passed feels hot	ACONITE 12

The patient can only pass urine by attempting to open the bowels	ALUMINA 12
With urinary tract infections	BELLADONNA 12
Constant desire to urinate Spasmodic, painful urination The urine may contain clots of blood	CACTUS 12
After surgery Due to impaired nerve supply to the bladder	CAUSTICUM 12
With inflammation of the prostate gland Sensation of a ball in the perineum (the area between the scrotum and the anus)	CHIMAPHILA 12
Due to an enlarged prostate Slow and difficult urination	MORPHINUM 12 *(prescription required in US)*
After a fright The nerves affecting bladder-emptying are damaged and the patient is unaware that the bladder is full	OPIUM 12 *(prescription required in US)*

DOSAGE

The selected remedy should be taken every fifteen minutes while waiting for medical assistance.

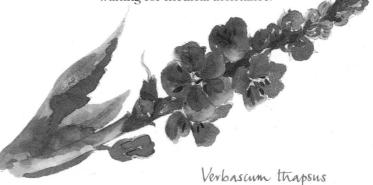

Verbascum thapsus

FEMALE HEALTH

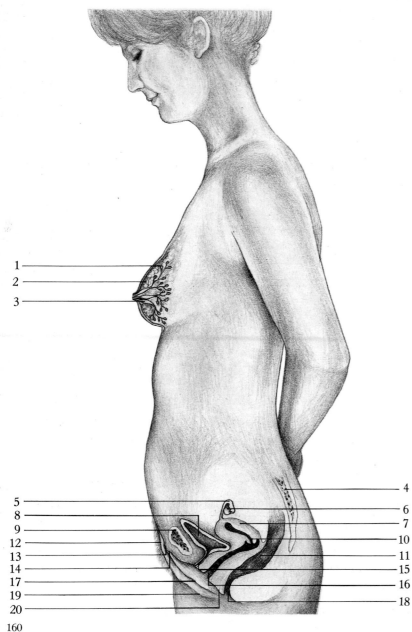

CONTENTS

Breast Conditions, including Mastitis	162
Frigidity	163
Genital Irritation	164
Intercourse, Painful	165
Menopause	165
Periods, Absence of	166
Periods, Heavy	167
Periods, Irregular	168
Periods, Painful	169
Premenstrual Syndrome (PMS)	170
Sexual Desire, Excessive	171
Vaginal Discharge	172

1 Lobules
2 Fatty tissue
3 Lactiforous sinus
4 Spine
5 Fallopian tubes
6 Ovary
7 Uterus
8 Bladder
9 Bone
10 Cervix
11 Rectum
12 Mons
13 Clitoral hood
14 Clitoris
15 Urethra
16 Vagina
17 Labia minora
18 Anus
19 Labia majora
20 Perineum

Many functions of the female body are related to reproduction, from providing a means of sexual arousal to the actual birth and subsequent feeding of a baby.

At puberty, which seems to be starting earlier and earlier and is now not unusual at ten years of age, several physical features of the female body alter in response to the production of female hormones. The breasts enlarge, the pelvic organs develop and mature, the typical female outline forms, the pubic and armpit hair appears, and the periods begin.

The beginning of a female's fertile life is known as the menarche (pronounced 'men-ar-kee'), and the end is known as the menopause. Between these events (30 – 40 years) a woman normally experiences vaginal bleeding lasting about 3–5 days every month, unless she becomes pregnant.

The menstrual periods or menses usually have a fairly regular pattern or cycle, which is often unchanged for many years. Sometimes, however, it may alter after a pregnancy or because of ill health, mental or physical. The menstrual flow consists of blood, mucus and fragments of the lining of the womb.

Alterations in the levels of female hormones produced at different times of the cycle sometimes cause unwelcome physical and mental symptoms to develop. These may include pain, fluid retention, weight gain, swelling of the breasts, irritability, depression, tiredness and headache.

The reproductive system of the female may be divided into two parts. The external genitalia, known collectively as the vulva, consist of several parts. At the entrance to the vagina, in an area called the vestibule, are folds of tissue called the right and left labia. The clitoris, found in front of the urethral opening, consists of sensitive erectile tissue and plays a major role in sexual arousal and the female orgasm.

The internal genitalia have five principal parts. The vagina is a canal which extends from the vestibule outside the body to the lower part of the uterus (womb) inside. The vagina is situated between the urethra and bladder in front and the rectum and anal canal behind. It has three main uses: to provide a passage into which the penis is inserted during sexual intercourse; to provide a passage through which a baby leaves the womb; and to allow the menstrual flow to leave the body.

The uterus is a pear-shaped organ lying in the pelvic cavity between the bladder and the rectum. The neck of the womb is called the cervix and opens into the vagina at the front and the uterine cavity behind. Attached to each side of the uterus are the fallopian tubes. These connect with the ovaries and allow the passage of the ovum (the egg) down the tubes to the uterus. The monthly release of an egg is called ovulation. If the egg is fertilized by a sperm it may implant into the uterine wall to develop as a baby.

During the reproductive part of a woman's life the vagina secretes a clear, semi-fluid, acidic secretion which mixes with a secretion from the cervix. During pregnancy the secretion thickens to plug the cervical canal and act as a defence against infection.

Of the millions of sperms a man produces in a single ejaculation, only a few reach the upper part of the fallopian tube, and of these, only one will fertilize the single mature egg produced at each ovulation. Unfertilized ova pass out through the uterus and vagina.

The ovaries are to be found on either side of the pelvic basin, held in place by ligaments. Besides ova, the ovaries also produce hormones named oestrogens which are responsible for the development of female sexual characteristics. Part of the ovary also produces the hormone progesterone, which prepares the uterine wall for the implantation of a fertilized egg, and the breasts for eventual milk production (lactation).

The female breast, which develops at puberty, has an erotic purpose in sexually arousing the male, but its primary function is to provide milk for the newborn child. Unfortunately, the breast is particularly prone to developing cancer, so self-examination should be performed regularly by all women as early detection can lead to a complete cure. Similarly, cancer at the neck of the womb may be completely cured if detected early enough. For this reason women should have a regular cervical smear as this can detect a pre-cancerous state which can be completely eradicated by a simple procedure using a laser.

Cucumis colocynthis

BREAST CONDITIONS, *including Mastitis*

The importance of regular self-examination has already been stressed (see above). Only by becoming familiar with the normal state of the breasts will you be readily able to identify the abnormal.

A tender lumpiness may arise in one or both breasts during early pregnancy or occasionally at the time of a period. This is usually caused by hormones and is not serious. If the breast becomes tender and redness develops over the painful area, this usually indicates that a breast abscess is about to form or, if the patient is lactating, acute mastitis is present.
Every woman fears finding a lump or cyst in her breast, but it is worth remembering that most are non-malignant. However, never ignore anything out of the ordinary.

Medical advice is essential for any lump in the breast that is present for seven days or more.

KEY FEATURES	TREATMENT
Mastitis after a chill	ACONITE 30
Red streaks radiate from a central point Pulsating pain with hardness of the breast Sudden mastitis, often with a headache	BELLADONNA 30
Pain due to bruising	BELLIS 30
The breast is hard, heavy and painful Mastitis after a chill Stitching pains and tense swelling	BRYONIA 30
Tender and swollen breasts before a period	CALC CARB 30

Piercing pain, worse at night
Tenderness in the uninflamed part of the
  breast which feels hard
The breast is painful, even from the touch of
  clothes or the jar of walking
	CONIUM 30

Painful, cracked nipples	GRAPHITES 30

The breasts are very sensitive during nursing and there is an excess of milk — PHYTOLACCA 30

Suppuration with crusting

Pain radiates from the nipple to all parts of the body, especially the arm

The patient is chilly, may have rigors, and aches all over the body

Chronic mastitis — SILICA 30

DOSAGE

The selected remedy should be taken four times a day for three days.

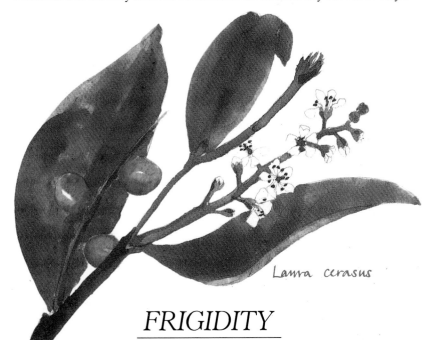

Laura cerasus

FRIGIDITY

This is the inability of the female to experience sexual pleasure and satisfaction. The causes are many, some psychological, others physical. It can occur with some drugs, particularly tranquillizers and high blood-pressure tablets and with certain diseases such as diabetes, pelvic disorders, multiple sclerosis, muscular dystrophy and an under-active thyroid. Painful intercourse may be an important factor. Psychological causes include inadequate sexual stimulation, anger, fear, guilt, marital discord, anxiety, stress and depression.

A poor technique in arousal and stimulation by the male can also lead to the woman's inability to experience sexual satisfaction and is a common cause of female frigidity. Medical advice should be sought if there is no prompt, satisfactory response to homeopathic treatment.

KEY FEATURES	TREATMENT
Abhorrence of intercourse Mental depression Generalized body itching, but especially of the eyes	AGNUS 12
Painful intercourse with vaginal burning and soreness In listless and apathetic women	BERBERIS VULG 12
Aversion to intercourse With a pale, thin, profuse vaginal discharge In fat, chilly and timid women	GRAPHITES 12
Total frigidity With great mood changes Sensitive and easily excited	IGNATIA 12
A dry vaginal wall makes intercourse painful	LYCOPODIUM 12
Complete lack of sexual desire The breasts ache, the nipples itch The patient often suffers from migraine	ONOSMODIUM 12

Painful vagina during intercourse Pelvic bearing-down sensation The periods are late, scanty and irregular The woman is sad, irritable and indifferent to her family	SEPIA 12

DOSAGE

The selected remedy should be taken three times a day until an improvement occurs. Thereafter, it should be taken if the symptoms recur.

GENITAL IRRITATION

Pruritis vulvae

Usually caused by a vaginal discharge, this condition may also arise from an allergy to soaps, bath products or even by washing powder not completely rinsed out of underclothes. Eczema and diabetes may also cause irritation.

An irritating vaginal discharge requires medical diagnosis.

KEY FEATURES	TREATMENT
Itching and pain after intercourse The nipples itch and burn Bearing-down pains	AGARICUS 12
Itching with soreness and swelling Bleeding between periods	AMBRA 12
Itching, swelling and burning Acrid vaginal discharge Great fatigue during periods	AMMON CARB 12
Burning and itching before and after periods, particularly in young girls	CALC CARB 12
Itching at the vaginal orifice	CONVALLARIA 12
Itching of the vulva and anus, with a bloody vaginal discharge	COPAIVA 12
Intense itching with pustular eruptions Scratching is painful	CROTON TIG 12
Itching and a yellow vaginal discharge seem worse when at rest In elderly women	FAGOPYRUM 12
Itching of the genitalia and nipples during periods	HEPAR SULPH 12

Burning itching within the vulva, with burning
    and swelling of the labia and violent itching
    between the labia and thighs
	KREOSOTE 12

Swelling and intense itching of the vulva Early, profuse, prolonged and acrid periods cause vulval soreness	RHUS TOX 12

Colchicum autumnale

Yellow-green, irritating discharge Intense bearing-down sensation in the pelvis	SEPIA 12
The vulva itches and the vagina burns because of an acrid, burning vaginal discharge	SULPHUR 12

DOSAGE

The selected remedy should be taken three times a day for five days.

INTERCOURSE, *Painful*

Dyspareunia

A number of women who suffer from this condition have no apparent physical abnormalities to account for it, so in these cases it is assumed that emotional factors are responsible. Fear of pregnancy is frequently the main cause, although other anxieties and general ill-health may be responsible. Some physical causes include an intact or tender hymen, a small vaginal canal, vulval inflammation or fissures, vaginal discharges, dryness of the vagina (usually menopausal) and tender prolapsed ovaries. Intercourse is often painful after childbirth, especially if a tear in the perineum has occurred.

Medical help is needed for this condition

KEY FEATURES	TREATMENT
Swelling of the labia relieved by cold water	APIS 30
The vagina feels tight	
Soreness and tenderness all over the lower abdomen and pelvis	
The vagina feels hot and dry	BELLADONNA 30
Sensation of the abdomen contents being about to drop out	
Low back pain	
Bleeding after intercourse	KREOSOTE 30
Burning and soreness of the vagina	
The pelvic organs feel sore and the vulva is itchy, burning and swollen	
The genitalia are hypersensitive, with an internal and external tingling sensation	PLATINA 30
Vaginal pain and spasm	
With great sexuality	
The vagina is painful during intercourse	SEPIA 30
Prolapse is present, or feels as if it is to the patient	

DOSAGE

The selected remedy should be taken four times a day for one week.

MASTITIS

(see Breast Conditions, p. 162)

THE MENOPAUSE

Sometimes called the 'change of life', the menopause marks the cessation of a woman's fertility and normally occurs between the ages of forty and fifty. During this time the body chemistry alters, producing a variety of symptoms: the periods may become heavier or lighter, irregular, or stop altogether, hot sweats and flushing may occur, sleep disturbances are common and symptoms of anxiety and depression may upset the normal lifestyle.

The desire for intercourse can alter considerably during the menopause. It usually reduces a great deal and the ability to reach orgasm may be lost. In some women, however, sexual desire is greatly increased, which may lead to promiscuity and

165

extra-marital affairs. Often coupled with the change in sexual appetite is a reduced or increased interest in day-to-day relationships and personal appearance.

Hormone replacement therapy (HRT) may be advised at this time, but it does not work for everyone and is far from being a cure-all. In cases where women cannot or prefer not to take HRT, or in cases where HRT does not relieve all the symptoms, homeopathic remedies can be taken alone or in conjunction to provide considerable relief.

KEY FEATURES	TREATMENT
Flushing followed by a hot sweat Frequent headaches with anxiety and palpitations	AMYL NIT 12
Excessive and permanent tiredness Backache	BELLIS 12
Irritability The patient is sad and restless Sinking feeling in the stomach accompanied by frequent headaches	CIMICIFUGA 12
A general unwell feeling With piles, vertigo, palpitations and headaches In women who have had frequent pregnancies The head may be flushed, the feet cold Worse after a sleep	LACHESIS 12
Hot flushes with right-sided headaches The skin burns and itches all over the body Offensive, acrid vaginal discharge The periods may be profuse and offensive The breasts become sore	SANGUINARIA 12

In spite of frequent flushes, the patient feels cold and sweats from the slightest exertion Worse towards the evening Intercourse is painful	SEPIA 12
Violent flushes of heat	VERATRUM VIR 12

DOSAGE

The selected remedy should be taken twice a day until an improvement occurs, then stopped. Repeat the treatment as and when necessary.

PERIODS, Absence of
Amenorrhoea

The most likely reason for periods to stop is pregnancy. However, wasting diseases like anorexia nervosa and cancer, and certain endocrine disorders such as an over- or under-active thyroid gland may be responsible. It is not unusual for young girls who have started regular menstruation sometimes to miss one or two periods before they start again. Women on the contraceptive pill occasionally develop very scanty periods, which may eventually disappear altogether. (Medical advice should be obtained if this happens.) Anxiety, fear and alcoholism may also cause periods to stop.

KEY FEATURES	TREATMENT
When the first periods are delayed In fair-skinned girls who perspire easily about the head and suffer indigestion With palpitations and headaches	CALC CARB 30

Throbbing, sudden headaches | BELLADONNA 30
The patient feels very cold
Sensation of fullness in the pelvis
With painful urination

Debility and palpitations | FERRUM MET 30
The ankles become swollen and puffy
The complexion is either flushed, or pale and
  livid with blue margins about the eyes

The periods flow by fits and starts and are very | PULSATILLA 30
  irregular
The patient dislikes exertion, has a poor
  appetite, faints easily and is very anxious

Very little loss, very slow to start | SEPIA 30
In tired girls with a dark complexion and
  delicate skin
Vaginal discharge instead of blood at the time
  the period is due

DOSAGE

The selected remedy should be taken four times a day for three days
before the period is due.
If there has been no previous period, the dose should be taken three
times a day for one week.

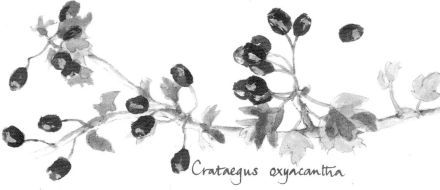

Crataegus oxyacantha

PERIODS, *Heavy*
Menorrhagia

*There are several causes of heavy bleeding at period time.
Fibroids (non-malignant growths in the uterus), polyps or a
hormonal imbalance may be to blame. However, heavy
bleeding may also signify more serious conditions, so if it recurs
each month, lasts more than seven days, or is excessive by your
normal standard, a doctor should be consulted.*

KEY FEATURES	TREATMENT
Early, profuse periods with pain like being in early labour With extreme fatigue With indigestion and constipation	ALETRIS 30
Bearing-down sensation, worse lying down Profuse, early, bright red periods Cramp-like back pain, cutting pelvic pain	BELLADONNA 30
Profuse, irregular, long-lasting periods The feet feel cold and damp	CALC CARB 30
Bearing-down pain going into the thighs Flooding	CALC FLUOR 30
Black, early, profuse periods Bladder irritation	CANTHARIS 30
When too frequent With spasmodic pain	CAULO-PHYLLUM 30
Early, profuse periods with wandering backache and muscle-ache With gloom and dejection	CIMICIFUGA 30

Early, profuse, long-lasting periods   KALI CARB 30
The body itches during the period and there is
  much backache

Abdominal bloating before the period   KREOSOTE 30
With headache and noises in the ears
Dragging back pain relieved by motion
Acrid, irritating discharge between periods

Dark, thick blood loss, chiefly at night   MAG CARB 30

Early, heavy period accompanied by morning   NUX VOM 30
  nausea and chilliness

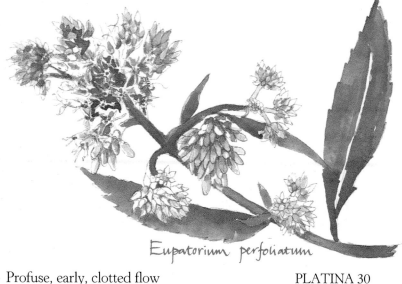

Eupatorium perfoliatum

Profuse, early, clotted flow   PLATINA 30
Great irritation of the genitalia
Bearing-down sensation in the womb
In haughty, melancholic females

DOSAGE

The selected remedy should be taken four times a day for four days,
starting two days before the period is due.
If the period is early, take the remedy at its start.

PERIODS, *Irregular*

Irregularity most commonly occurs at puberty, near the menopause and during or just after lactation. Although their cycle may not be exactly the same each month, most women menstruate within a few days of the expected date and their particular cycle is reasonably regular.

KEY FEATURES	TREATMENT
With pain Heavy vaginal discharge between periods	CALC SIL 30
Pain immediately before the period starts Profuse, dark period with pain across the pelvis and in the back With skin and rheumatic symptoms	CIMICIFUGA 30
Irregular, profuse, frequent periods with large clots Breast pain during the period With violent sexual excitement	MUREX 30
Irregular, profuse periods With a dry vagina and an acrid, watery vaginal discharge Severe headache after the period has finished	NAT MUR 30
The period is variable in both quantity and timing With fainting and tiredness	NUX MOSCHATA 30
Always irregular, with low back pain and a desire to defaecate The loss is very dark, almost black	NUX VOM 30

Slight, watery blood loss until the next period	SECALE 30
Pelvic pain with coldness but an intolerance of heat	
The loss is copious and dark	
Usually late and the loss is scanty	SEPIA 30
Great bearing-down sensation	
Rarely, the period is irregular, early and profuse	

DOSAGE

The selected remedy should be taken three times a day for four days, starting twelve days after the previous period has ended. This should be repeated each month until the periods become regular.

PERIODS, *Painful*

Dysmenorrhoea

Pain during periods is thought to be due to a tight cervix and should therefore be cured by childbirth or stretching the cervix. Unfortunately, this is not always the case and pain persists in some women, despite repeated pregnancies. Severe pain may occur with endometriosis, a condition in which tissue similar to that lining the uterus is found at other sites in the pelvis. It may also be caused by fibroids, chronic inflammation of the fallopian tube and pelvic disease. Over 75 per cent of cases involve young women who have not had a baby.

KEY FEATURES	TREATMENT
Pain precedes the flow	BELLADONNA 30
Sensation of pelvic heaviness relieved by sitting up straight	
The period starts and ends suddenly	
The vagina is hot and dry, the flow offensive and clotted	
Spasmodic, bearing-down pains felt in the groins, and sometimes in the chest and limbs	CAULO-PHYLLUM 30
The flow is scanty	
Tearing pains, with a dark, clotted flow	CHAMOMILLA 30
With excessive irritability and impatience	
Pain shoots across the pelvis from side to side and down to the thighs, starting just before the period commences	CIMICIFUGA 30
Sharp abdominal pains during a period make the patient double up	
Headache before the period starts	
Profuse, dark, irregular periods with colicky, spasmodic uterine pain	COCCULUS 30
Severe headache, nausea and a great feeling of weakness	
Severe, left-sided ovarian pain and pain extending down from the navel, helped by bending double	COLOCYNTH 30
Cramp-like pains start several hours before the period begins and continue throughout	MAG PHOS 30
Great relief from warmth, by bending double and from pressure	
Dark, delayed and intermittent periods	PULSATILLA 30
The more the pain, the chillier the patient feels	
The pain seems to move about, doubling the patient up so she becomes restless and tearful	

With extreme coldness and a cold sweat	VERATRUM ALB
The patient faints from the least exertion	30
Sexual activity is greatly increased just before the period is due	

Sudden, uterine, colicky pain before the period starts	VIBURNUM 30
The period is often late and very scanty, lasting only a few hours	
An ache in the lower back during the period extends down the thighs	
Occasional shooting pains in the ovaries	
Violent, bearing-down sensation ends in intense uterine cramp	

Agonizing, burning pain extending down the thighs	XANTHOXYLUM 30
The period is profuse	
Headache over the left eye the day before the period starts	
The patient is often delicate and nervous	

DOSAGE

The selected remedy should be taken twice a day for four days, starting one week before the period is due.

PREMENSTRUAL SYNDROME (PMS)

Many women find that for several days before their period starts they suffer from emotional upsets, such as depression, irritability, loss of libido, extreme anxiety, uncontrollable crying and loss of affection for their family. One or more of these symptoms may be accompanied by weight gain, sore and swollen breasts, swollen ankles and hands, and headache. Additionally they may have some pelvic discomfort and low back pain. As some of these symptoms are related to salt and water retention, it may help to cut down (but not eliminate) salt intake.

KEY FEATURES	TREATMENT
Headache, at its worst on waking	LACHESIS 30
The face appears and feels bloated	
Tight clothes cannot be tolerated, especially around the neck and waist	
Palpitations with a feeling of faintness	
The patient becomes jealous, vindictive, unreasonable and talks excessively	
Much better as soon as the period starts	
Blinding headache, with a pale face, nausea and vomiting	NAT MUR 30
Craving for salt	
The abdomen becomes distended	
With a 'fluttery' heart and palpitations	
Worse from noise, mental exertion and consolation, the worst time being about 10–11 a.m.	
Irritable, weary, selfish, withdrawn and moody	
Lack of thirst with a partial loss of the sense of taste	PULSATILLA 30
Shooting pain in the neck and upper part of the back	
Very moody and changeable, cries a lot and requires much sympathy	
Much better out of doors	

Severe headache   SEPIA 30
Food tastes too salty
Sensation of the pelvic contents being about to
  drop out
Cold, totally weary and tired, dislike of family,
  irritable and very sad, but enlivened with
  exercise and movement

DOSAGE

The selected remedy should be started ten days before the next period is due and taken three times a day for five days. It should be repeated in this manner each month until an improvement is maintained, and taken again only if the symptoms return.

SEXUAL DESIRE, Excessive

Nymphomania

The need to satisfy sexual feelings has no norm. It varies from person to person, so what is excessive for one person may be normal for another. Psychological factors may play a part, however; if the desire leads to promiscuity feelings of guilt may then develop.

KEY FEATURES	TREATMENT
Genital itching with soreness and swelling Blood-stained discharge between periods In nervous, hypersensitive women	AMBRA 30
Burning and itching of genitalia before and after menstruation Increased desire with easy conception	CALC CARB 30
Aching pain over the pelvic area Violent backache during periods In peevish, forgetful women	CALC PHOS 30
Fiery sexual desire Anxious restlessness ending in a rage Early, profuse periods	CANTHARIS 30
Heavy, frequent, lengthy periods Acrid, burning vaginal discharge The patient is indifferent and irresponsible	FLUORIC ACID 30
In suspicious, talkative, foolish women who laugh at everything and are very sexually excitable	HYOSCYAMUS 30
Violent sexual excitement easily brought on by the slightest touch In nervous, lively and affectionate women	MUREX 30
The external and internal genitalia tingle The patient is arrogant and contemptuous With vaginal spasm	PLATINA 30
Blood-stained discharge between periods Increased sexual drive The patient frequently aborts any pregnancies	SABINA 30
The vulva feels dry, hot and itchy Profuse periods accompanied by erotic sensations Immoral, moody, busy women who are sensitive to music	TARENT HISP 30

DOSAGE

The selected remedy should be taken three times a day for one week. It may need to be repeated at monthly intervals until an improvement is maintained.

VAGINAL DISCHARGE
Leucorrhoea

It is quite normal for women to have a vaginal discharge. However, if it becomes heavy, blood-stained, or causes burning or irritation, a doctor should be consulted.

Medical help may be needed for this condition

KEY FEATURES / TREATMENT

Very profuse and ropy, acrid transparent or yellow discharge
Mainly during the daytime — **ALUMINA 12**

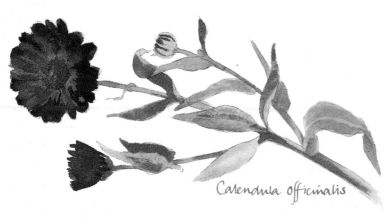

Calendula officinalis

Acrid, corrosive and yellow discharge
Mainly in the elderly and with chronic diseases — **ARS ALB 12**

Clear, copious, hot discharge, which is acrid and causes swelling of the labia and is at its worst mid-cycle — **BORAX 12**

Profuse, milky, itchy, burning discharge
In young girls before puberty
In women before periods — **CALC CARB 12**

Tenacious, thick, ropy discharge
The patient is weak and constipated — **HYDRASTIS 12**

Profuse, thin, white mucus discharge which comes in gushes with back and lower abdominal pain
More profuse in the morning on rising
The patient is constantly cold — **GRAPHITES 12**

Profuse, watery, acrid, irritating and burning discharge causes soreness, smarting and itching of the vulva
Worse before a period — **KREOSOTE 12**

Yellow, ropy, stringy discharge in fat, light-haired people — **KALI BICH 12**

Watery, yellow-brown burning discharge
The patient is depressed and has a bearing-down sensation in the pelvis — **LILIUM TIG 12**

Acrid, burning, greenish-yellow discharge, causing smarting and swelling of the vulva
Worse at night — **MERCURIUS 12**

Acrid, burning, creamy discharge with back pain — **PULSATILLA 12**

Yellow-green, offensive discharge
Worse before a period, with a bearing-down sensation in the pelvis — **SEPIA 12**

Profuse, bland discharge of white mucus, with great weariness and backache — **STANNUM MET 12**

DOSAGE

The selected remedy should be taken twice a day for ten days.

PREGNANCY

CONTENTS

After-pains	174
Backache and Muscle Pains	174
Cramps	175
Cravings	175
Emotional Upsets	176
False Labour	177
Labour, Preparing for	178
Lactation Problems	178
Miscarriage	179
Morning Sickness	180
Occasional Problems of Pregnancy	181

Far from being an illness, pregnancy and giving birth are normal, natural events. However, certain conditions peculiar to pregnancy, such as food cravings and morning sickness, may cause problems. In these cases homeopathic medicines may prove useful as they can be taken at any time with no fear of harming the foetus.

1	Lobules	8	Placenta
2	Fatty tissue	9	Umbilical cord
3	Lactiforous sinus	10	Rectum
4	Uterus	11	Bladder
5	Spine	12	Vagina (*Birth canal*)
6	Foetus	13	Anus
7	Small intestine		

None the less, always discuss home treatment with your doctor first.

This section covers some of the main problems associated with normal pregnancy. Other problems that may strike during pregnancy but are not specific to it, such as heartburn, will be found elsewhere in the book (see Index).

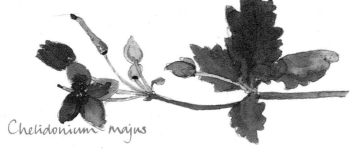

Chelidonium majus

AFTER-PAINS

These are abdominal pains which occur after childbirth and are caused by the uterus contracting. They are more likely to occur in women who are breastfeeding because this releases a hormone called oxytocin which causes uterine contractions.

KEY FEATURES	TREATMENT
Used routinely after labour	ARNICA 30
Soreness all through the pelvis, making walking and standing painful	BELLIS 30
Spasmodic pains which fly across the lower abdomen, especially after a prolonged and exhausting labour	CAULO-PHYLLUM 30
Intense pain in the groin, which the patient finds intolerable	CIMICIFUGA 30
Pains in the intestines rather than the uterus	COCCULUS 30

The pain appears to be in the rectum or bladder	NUX VOM 30
The pain shoots from behind forwards	SABINA 30
The pain shoots upward Sensation of a weight in the pelvis	SEPIA 30
If no other remedy fits	XANTHOXYLUM 30

DOSAGE

The selected remedy should be taken four times a day for two days after delivery.

BACKACHE AND MUSCLE PAINS

It is not uncommon for women to experience backache and muscle pain during pregnancy. These symptoms are due to the extra weight being carried, the relaxation of the pelvic muscles and the changed stance adopted by a pregnant woman (abdomen forward, upper back bent backward).

KEY FEATURES	TREATMENT
Severe, continuous, dull ache in the lower back and hips The back is worse when walking or stooping	AESCULUS 12
Muscular pains With vomiting	ALETRIS 12
Stiffness in the small of the back Better for complete rest lying on the back	BRYONIA 12

Back pain with vomiting in light-haired women	COCCULUS 12
Severe back pain, worse around 3 a.m., from cold and lying on affected side	KALI CARB 12
The back feels weak and stiff and causes great exhaustion	
Backache after delivery	PHOS ACID 12
Low back pain with tiredness	PULSATILLA 12
Stiffness with or without pain	RHUS TOX 12
Better for warmth and moderate movement	

In the hip region, better for firm pressure and warmth	COLOCYNTH 12
In the calves and feet	CUPRUM MET 12
The arms and legs go to sleep, with cramps in the lower part of the legs	NUX VOM 12
In the morning the arms and legs feel paralysed	
In the calves	VERATRUM ALB 12
The skin feels cold	
The patient faints from the least exertion	

DOSAGE

The selected remedy should be taken three times a day when the pain is present. Stop when the pain goes.

DOSAGE

The selected remedy should be taken at bedtime.

Veratrum album

CRAMPS

The pain of cramp is caused by the prolonged contraction of a muscle. It is especially prevalent in pregnancy due to poor posture.

KEY FEATURES	TREATMENT
In the calves	CALC CARB 12
With cold knees and cold, sweaty feet	

CRAVINGS

During pregnancy abnormal desires for certain foods often develop. Sometimes it can be for unusual mixtures of foods and on occasions even for indigestible substances like coal.

KEY FEATURES	TREATMENT
Meat, pickles, radishes, turnips, artichokes and coarse foods	ABIES CAN 12
Any food at noon and at night	ABIES NIG 12

175

Sweets, wants to eat very frequently	ALFALFA 12	Pickles and sour food and drink	SEPIA 12
Milk	APIS 12	Hot water	SPIGELIA 12
Sweets	ARG NIT 12	Sweet and fatty foods	SULPHUR 12
Tobacco	CALADIUM 12	Apples	TELLURIUM 12
Indigestible things, like chalk and coal, also for eggs, salt and sweets	CALCAREA 12		
Bacon, ham, salted and smoked meats	CALC PHOS 12		
Stimulants, such as coffee, alcohol and tobacco	CAPSICUM 12		
Salt and salty foods	CARBO VEG 12		
Anything and everything, but the smell of the food then nauseates	COLCHICUM 12		
Sour and strongly flavoured foods	HEPAR SULPH 12		
Wine	HYPERICUM 12		
Acidic foods	IGNATIA 12		
Alcohol and oysters	LACHESIS 12		
Chocolate and sweet things	LYCOPODIUM 12		
Meat	MAG CARB 12		
Salt	NAT MUR 12		
Highly seasoned foods	NUX MOSCHATA 12		
Iced water and frequent cold drinks	ONOSMODIUM 12		
Piquant foods	SANGUINARIA 12		

DOSAGE

The remedy should be taken twice a day until the craving goes.

EMOTIONAL UPSETS

Most pregnant women are concerned for the safety of their unborn child, but this anxiety is quite normal and does not interfere with their enjoyment of pregnancy.
However, in extreme (relatively rare) cases some women become very emotionally disturbed by pregnancy. They may show severe anxiety, agitation, unreasonable fears, or any number of 'hysterical' physical symptoms. A full-blown, acute depressive episode may develop and this requires urgent medical attention.

KEY FEATURES	TREATMENT
Depressed, morose and quarrelsome	AURUM 30
Everything seems a hardship	
Sleep is poor with nightmares and restlessness	
Threatens suicide	
All these symptoms require urgent medical help.	

In very nervous, almost hysterical women who feel there is a lump in the throat — IGNATIA 30

Nervous spasm of the throat makes swallowing difficult

Very rapid mood changes, with constant sighing

Desire for unusual and unhealthy food which, surprisingly, does not disagree

With many irrational fears — PHOSPHORUS 30

Lack of interest in the family, but needs a lot of sympathy from them

Desire for salt

Love of ices and cold drinks, but they are immediately vomited

Strong dislike of tea, coffee, meat and milk

Very moody and cries easily — PULSATILLA 30

Craves sympathy

Jealous and suspicious

Likes sour drinks but averse to milk, fat, butter and meat, especially pork

Total indifference to the family, with desire to get away and find peace and quiet — SEPIA 30

Depressed and hateful, but weeps if shown sympathy

Intolerance of noise and smells, especially of cooking smells, which lead to nausea

Great desire for vinegar, sour drinks and food

DOSAGE

The selected remedy should be taken four times a day for four days, then repeated when necessary if the symptoms reappear.

FALSE LABOUR

Pains rather like labour pains may occur in the last few weeks of pregnancy. These are said to occur when the womb is 'toning up' in preparation for the actual labour and birth. If the pains become very frequent or regular, or if there is a show of blood, a doctor or midwife should be called.

Medical help is needed for this condition.

KEY FEATURES	TREATMENT
Early in the pregnancy Pain shoots across the abdomen and doubles the patient up	CIMICIFUGA 12
In the last few weeks of pregnancy	CAULO-PHYLLUM 12

DOSAGE

The selected remedy should be taken every hour until the pains cease.

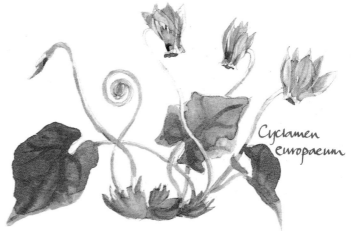

Cyclamen europaeum

LABOUR, Preparing for

A normal pregnancy lasts approximately forty weeks and for some time before labour becomes established occasional contractile pains may be felt in the abdomen. These are usually put down to the uterus 'toning up'.
Caulophyllum, taken for some weeks before the end of the pregnancy, may give an easier labour.

KEY FEATURES	TREATMENT
In early labour when the pains are frequent but irregular and the patient becomes restless, anxious and frightened	ACONITE 12
To reduce the bruising and bleeding of normal labour	ARNICA 30
Used routinely to help uterine contractions and leads to a smooth delivery	CAULO-PHYLLUM 30
Painful labour, the pain starting in the lower back and radiating to the inner part of the thighs The patient becomes over-excited and cross, and resents being examined	CHAMOMILLA 12
Early labour pains felt in the back	KALI CARB 12

DOSAGE

CAULOPHYLLUM 30 – three doses may be taken on the same day each week from the thirty-fourth week onwards.
ARNICA 30 – one dose should be taken at the beginning of labour, another just before delivery, then twice a day for two days after delivery.
The other remedies should be taken every hour until relief is obtained.

LACTATION PROBLEMS

Three main problems tend to occur in lactation: there is too much milk, not enough milk, or the milk produced is of poor quality and does not satisfy the baby. These problems respond well to the appropriate homeopathic remedy.

KEY FEATURES	TREATMENT
Too much milk which flows very freely The breasts become red, hot, swollen and tender and maybe rock hard The patient is flushed and feels hot	BELLADONNA 12

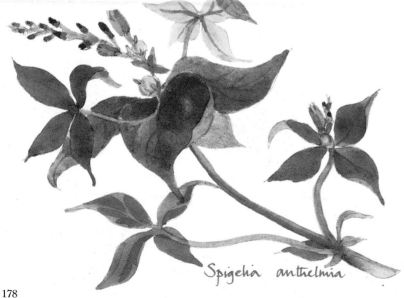

Spigelia anthelmia

Much watery, poor quality milk which the baby is reluctant to take

The patient feels chilly, anxious and fearful

Perspiration, mainly on the head, during the night

CALC CARB 12

Milk production stops

The patient becomes very depressed, develops a great thirst and forecasts her own death occurring within twenty-four hours

LAC DEFLOR 12

Excess milk is produced, the breasts become stone hard, lumpy and painful, and the nipples intensely sensitive

The patient hurts all over her body and is irritable and restless

PHYTOLACCA 12

Little milk, which is thin and watery

The patient cries when trying to feed the baby

The breasts feel sore and stretched

PULSATILLA 12

Little or no milk and the patient feels weak in mind and body

RICINUS COMM 12

Diminished flow of milk

The breasts become excessively swollen and tender

URTICA 12

DOSAGE

The selected remedy should be taken twice a day until an improvement occurs, then stopped. Repeat the treatment as and when necessary.

MISCARRIAGE

When a pregnancy ends at an early stage with the loss of the foetus, the mother is said to have miscarried. This most often happens during the first three months and tends to occur at the time when a period would have been due. Bleeding and regular lower abdominal pain are the usual symptoms, but not all threatened miscarriages result in a lost pregnancy. When miscarriage is feared, absolute rest should always be part of the treatment.

Medical help is needed for this condition.

KEY FEATURES	TREATMENT
Threatened miscarriage after anger	ACONITE 30
Threatened miscarriage after trauma	ARNICA 30
Profuse and hot-feeling blood discharge Backache and headache Labour-like pains come and go suddenly Feeling that everything might drop out of the pelvis	BELLADONNA 30

Chelidonium majus

179

Habitual miscarriage	CAULO-PHYLLUM 30
Severe pain in the back and sides of the abdomen	
Feeble uterine contractions with scanty blood loss	
With anger and great agitation	CHAMOMILLA 30
The pains go from side to side across the lower abdomen and double the patient up	CIMICIFUGA 30
With rheumatic tendency	

Cinchona perforatum

Around the third month	SABINA 30
Bleeding is the first symptom	
Pain in the small of the back which goes around and through to the front of the lower abdomen	
The blood is bright red and clotted	
In very early pregnancy	SECALE 30
The woman is often in poor health and pale	
Frequent labour-like pains	
Copious flow of very dark blood	
Tendency to miscarry late in pregnancy	

A preventive of miscarriage	SEPIA 30
In nervous and irritable women, with lax abdominal muscles and a tendency to rectal prolapse	
Pain starts in the back, goes round to the front, then down into the thighs	VIBURNUM 30
In frequent and early miscarriages	

DOSAGE

In threatened miscarriage the selected remedy should be taken four times a day until the symptoms cease.

As a preventive in patients with a previous history of miscarriage, the selected remedy should be taken three times a day on the same day of each week until the sixteenth week.

MORNING SICKNESS

This is a common problem in early pregnancy and does not always occur in the morning. If the condition persists or becomes excessive, a doctor should be consulted.

Medical help may be needed for this condition.

KEY FEATURES	TREATMENT
The most commonly used remedy	IPECAC 6
Constant nausea unrelieved by vomiting	
Despite vomiting, the tongue remains clean, but excessive salivation may develop	
The patient becomes irritable	

Nausea and a sour taste after breakfast	NUX VOM 6
The stomach is very sensitive to pressure	
In sullen, irritable, fault-finding patients who cannot bear noise or smells	
With much flatulence	
Nausea at the sight or smell of food, especially in the morning before eating.	SEPIA 6
Craving for sour foods	
The stomach feels empty, even after eating	

DOSAGE

The selected remedy should be taken three times a day until an improvement occurs, then stopped. Repeat the treatment as and when necessary.

MUSCLE PAINS

(see Backache, p. 174)

OCCASIONAL PROBLEMS OF PREGNANCY

Numerous inconvenient but non-threatening conditions may occur during pregnancy. The following respond well to homeopathic treatment.

KEY FEATURES	TREATMENT
Toothache from warm drinks	CHAMOMILLA 12
Toothache, worse at night and from cold	MAG CARB 12
Toothache and dry mouth but no desire to drink	NUX MOSCHATA 12
Itching of the vagina and vulva	CALADIUM 12
Itching all over the body	ICHTHYOLUM 12
Constipation and itchy piles	COLLINSONIA 12
Painful piles	MILLEFOLIUM 12
Bluish, hot, painful piles	MURIATIC ACID 12
Piles and anal prolapse	PODOPHYLLUM 12
Hot, sore, painful anus	ZINGIBER 12
Varicose veins, making walking difficult	BELLIS 12
Hiccoughs	CYCLAMEN 12
Dry cough, worse in the evening, at night, when lying down or talking	CONIUM 12
Dry, fatiguing, hacking night cough	KALI BROM 12
Insomnia	VALERIANA 12

Anemone pulsatilla

DOSAGE

The selected remedy should be taken up to three times a day when needed. It may be repeated as necessary.

MALE HEALTH

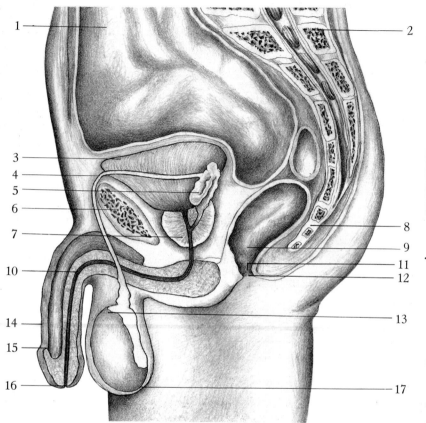

CONTENTS

Impotence	183
Intercourse, Aversion to	184
Premature Ejaculation	184
Prostate Disorders	185
Sexual Desire, Decreased	185
Sexual Desire, Increased	186

1	Large bowel	10	Urethra
2	Spine	11	Anus
3	Bladder	12	Sphincter
4	Vas deferens	13	Testes
5	Seminal vesicles	14	Penis
6	Bone	15	Glans penis
7	Prostate gland	16	Urethral opening
8	Coccyx	17	Scrotum
9	Rectum		

Problems specific to male health tend to relate to the reproductive system. Most of the male genitalia are found outside the body and consist of the two testicles, the scrotum in which they are found, the urethra and the penis. Internally are the prostate gland, the vas deferens and the seminal vesicles.

The urethra is the outlet for both urine and sperm, the latter carried in the semen.

From each testicle (right and left) a tubular vessel, the vas deferens, joins the urethra just outside the bladder at the point where the urethra goes through the prostate gland. Fluid from the testicles, containing the sperm, mixes at this point with the secretions of the seminal vesicles and prostate gland to form the semen.

The part of the male urethra outside the body is called the penis. Here it is surrounded by loose, spongy tissue which is extremely well supplied with blood vessels. Normally the penis is limp, but when the man is sexually aroused, the empty spaces in the spongy tissue fill with blood, making the penis erect and hard.

IMPOTENCE

Failure to achieve or maintain an erection tends to occur in middle-aged men and is frequently a symptom of anxiety, stress or tension. At least half the male population experiences temporary impotence at some stage of life. Among the many possible causes are illnesses such as diabetes, aortic aneurysm, multiple sclerosis, alcoholism and an underactive thyroid gland. Some high blood-pressure drugs, tranquillizers and sedatives may also lead to impotence.

Medical diagnosis is essential.

KEY FEATURES	TREATMENT
Physically impotent but strong sexual desire The testicles and penis feel cold to the patient With mental depression	AGNUS 12
Loss of sexual desire The erection fails on attempting penetration	ARG NIT 12
Diminished desire associated with enlargement of the prostate gland	BARYTA CARB 12
With premature and involuntary ejaculation	BUFO 12
The erection fails during foreplay Erections occur when half asleep and fail on wakening Emission of semen may occur at any time	CALADIUM 12
Increased sexual desire Involuntary nocturnal emission of semen occurs around 3 a.m. Weak erections	CALC CARB 12
Debility and impotence occur together, although sexual excitement may occur when half asleep	KALI BROM 12
Total inability to have an erection leads to great despondency Involuntary emissions of semen Enlarged prostate gland	LYCOPODIUM 12
Nocturnal emission of semen is followed by a feeling of weakness Enlarged prostate and urination becomes frequent and painful due to inflammation of the urethra	MEDORRHINUM 12
From psychological causes with total lack of desire	ONOSMODIUM 12
Imperfect or non-existent erections Loss of semen early in intercourse Sudden loss of the erection during intercourse The patient is distressed and anxious about his condition The testicles feel tender	PHOS ACID 12
Increased desire with decreased ability Semen dribbles involuntarily, especially during sleep Inability due to lack of confidence and the erection fails on attempting penetration	SELENIUM 12
The genitalia are relaxed, the penis flabby and cold Erections are infrequent Loss of semen at first contact With backache and depression	SULPHUR 12

DOSAGE

The selected remedy should be taken three times a day until an improvement occurs, then stopped. Repeat the treatment as and when necessary.

INTERCOURSE, Aversion to

Although this is mainly caused by psychological disorders, on rare occasions hormonal deficiency can be implicated. Sexual preferences, such as transvestism or homosexuality, may also be involved. (See also Impotence, p. 183)

KEY FEATURES	TREATMENT
Total aversion to intercourse	GRAPHITES 12
Premature ejaculation if intercourse is attempted	

DOSAGE

The remedy should be taken twice a day until an improvement occurs, then stopped. Repeat the treatment as and when necessary.

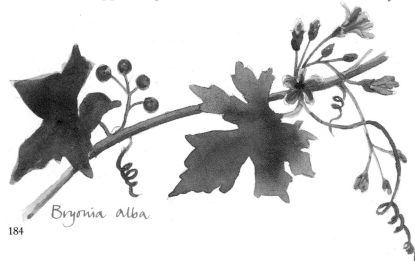

Bryonia alba

PREMATURE EJACULATION

This is a condition in which semen is released before or too soon after penetration. It is common in adolescent boys and is related to guilt feelings, anxiety over performance, and fear of venereal disease or Aids. Similar concerns may persist in adults.
In older men an enlarged prostate gland may be a cause, as may damage to the nerve pathways. Over 95 per cent of cases can be helped.

KEY FEATURES	TREATMENT
Partial impotence with premature and involuntary ejaculation	BUFO 12
Increased desire for intercourse Weakness and irritability follows intercourse Semen released too soon	CALC CARB 12
Total aversion to intercourse Premature or no ejaculation	GRAPHITES 12
Semen is discharged shortly after, or even before an erection occurs	PHOS ACID 12
Erections are infrequent Loss of semen at first contact	SULPHUR 12

DOSAGE

The selected remedy should be taken three times a day until an improvement is maintained. It should be repeated if a deterioration occurs.

PROSTATE DISORDERS

The prostate gland tends to increase in size after about the age of fifty. The vast majority of cases are benign, but as cancer of the prostate does occur, medical diagnosis is essential. Having to get up to pass urine during the night is one of the earliest symptoms and is quickly followed by difficulty in starting to pass urine and the development of a poor force to the stream.

Medical help is needed for this condition.

KEY FEATURES	TREATMENT
Incontinence in the elderly, with a bearing-down sensation and an enlarged prostate	ALOE 12
Enlarged prostate in the elderly, with a frequent urge to urinate The urethra burns on urination	BARYTA CARB 12
Great urge to urinate Straining necessary to commence urination The urine feels hot when passed	CHIMAPHILA 12
Enlargement of the prostate and difficulty in passing urine, which comes in stops and starts	CONIUM 12
Constant urging to pass urine, which comes in drops, with a cutting, throbbing pain in the bladder The urine is dark and feels hot Worse at night	DIGITALIS 12
Back pain before urinating, which goes afterwards The urine is slow in coming and the patient strains to pass it	LYCOPODIUM 12
The urine has a heavy red sediment Frequent need to urinate during the night	
Frequent urging with painful urination The urine flows slowly Worse during the night	MEDORRHINUM 12
Constant desire to urinate during the night Cystitis with enlarged prostate gland Straightforward prostate enlargement	SABAL SERR 12
Prostate condition with frequent urination and a burning sensation in the urethra when not urinating	STAPHYSAGRIA 12
Frequent and urgent desire to urinate Pain and burning between the rectum and the bladder The urine stream is poor	THUJA 12

DOSAGE

The selected remedy should be taken twice a day until an improvement occurs, then stopped. Repeat when necessary.

SEXUAL DESIRE, Decreased

Psychological factors, such as fear of pregnancy, dislike of partner and fear of an inadequate performance, can lead to decreased sexual desire, but it can also be a major symptom of depression. It does not necessarily accompany ageing.

KEY FEATURES	TREATMENT
Erections without any sexual desire	AMMON CARB 30

Diminished desire Impotence at an early age Enlarged prostate gland	BARYTA CARB 30
Loss of desire associated with debility and impotence	KALI BROM 30
Complete loss of sexual desire Impotence with involuntary discharge of semen when urinating	NUPHAR LUTEUM 30
Constant sexual excitement, but impotence leads to loss of desire	ONOSMODIUM 30
No desire and no ability	OXYTROPIS 30

DOSAGE

The selected remedy should be taken three times a day for four days. It may be repeated if necessary at monthly intervals.

SEXUAL DESIRE, Increased

Although there is no 'normal' in the sexuality of males in general, if the need for sexual intercourse becomes much increased for a particular individual, a homeopathic remedy may restore the balance.

KEY FEATURES	TREATMENT
Pleasant itching of the genitalia Discharge of semen when asleep Greatly increased desire	ANACARDIUM 30
Nervous and agitated, with increased sexual excitement	ASTERIAS 30

Frequent involuntary emissions of semen and premature ejaculations Increased desire, but weak and irritable after intercourse	CALC CARB 30
Painful erections Emission of semen at night	CAMPHORA 30
Strong desire with painful erections Constant desire to urinate	CANTHARIS 30
Desire increased, power decreased Nervousness from suppressing excess sexual desire	CONIUM 30

Atropa belladonna

Passion and desire greatly increased Erections while sleeping	FLUORIC ACID 30
Violent desire, involuntary emissions Nausea and vomiting after intercourse	MOSCHUS 30
Painful erections Itching of penis (prepuce) Sexual desire excitable	ZINGIBER 30

DOSAGE

The selected remedy should be taken four times a day for three days. It should not be repeated at less than six-weekly intervals.

THE BACK AND LIMBS

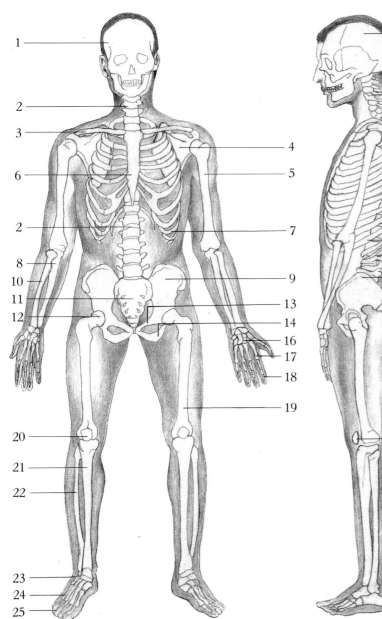

CONTENTS

Backache and Lumbago	189
Bunions	190
Corns and Calloses	190
Cramp, Hand and Arm	191
Cramp, Leg	191
Feet, Burning	192
Feet, Cold	192
Feet, Sweaty	193
Gout	193
Hands, Blue	194
Hands, Burning	195

1 Cranium (*Skull*)
2 Vertebrae
3 Clavicle (*Collar bone*)
4 Scapula (*Shoulder blade*)
5 Humerus
6 Sternum (*Breastbone*)
7 Ribs
8 Ulna
9 Ilium
10 Radius
11 Sacrum
12 Acetabulum
13 Pubis
14 Ischium
15 Coccyx
16 Carpus
17 Metacarpus
18 Phalanges (*Fingers*)
19 Femur
20 Patella (*Kneecap*)
21 Tibia
22 Fibula
23 Tarsus
24 Metatarsus
25 Phalanges (*Toes*)

CONTENTS *contd.*

Hands, Cold	195
Hands, Red	196
Hands, Weak	196
Heel Pain	196
Housemaid's Knee	197
Legs and Ankles, Weak	197
Legs, Restless	198
Nails, Disorders of	198
Rheumatism and Arthritis	199
Sciatica	201
Varicose Veins and Varicose Ulcers	202

The spine or vertebral column consists of thirty-three bones, each called a vertebra. These are arranged into five regions: the seven cervical vertebrae which form the neck, the twelve thoracic vertebrae, the five lumbar vertebrae, the five sacral vertebrae which are fused to form the sacrum, and the four coccygeal vertebrae which make up the coccyx.

The vertebrae vary a great deal in size and shape, becoming thicker and heavier the lower they are in the spinal column. The coccygeal vertebrae are the exception as they are relatively small. The sacrum and the coccyx together form the back wall of the pelvic cavity.

The thorax consists of the thoracic vertebrae, the ribs – twelve on either side – and the breastbone (the sternum). All the ribs are connected to the thoracic vertebrae at the back and, except for the lower two on each side, to the sternum in front.

The upper extremity has four principal parts. The shoulder consists of the clavicle (collarbone) and the scapula (shoulder blade). The arm consists of the humerus (upper arm bone), and the radius and ulna which make up the forearm. The wrist or carpus has eight carpal bones, while the hand is made up of five metacarpal bones and fourteen phalanges or finger bones.

The lower extremity has five principal parts. The hip or innominate bone is large and irregular, and is made up by the fusion of the ilium, the ischium and the pubis bones. It is attached behind to the sacrum and in front to its fellow of the opposite side, the junction being called the pubic symphysis.

The two hip bones and the sacrum make up the pelvis, a strong, bony semicircle forming a protective wall for the organs in the pelvic cavity (the bladder and rectum, plus the uterus in women). It also transmits the weight of the body to the lower limbs.

Where the three pelvic bones meet they form a socket, the acetabulum, into which fits the head of the femur to form the hip joint. The femur extends from the hip to the knee and is the strongest bone in the body. At its lower end it helps to form the knee joint, with the kneecap (the patella) in front.

The lower leg, from knee to ankle, consists of two bones, the larger inner one called the tibia and the outer one called the fibula.

The tarsus or ankle is formed by seven small, strong bones and is connected to the five long metatarsal bones which make up the sole of the foot. These are joined to the bones which make up the toes (phalanges), two for the big toe and three each for the others.

In all there are 206 bones in the adult human body.

ARTHRITIS

(see Rheumatism, p. 199)

BACKACHE AND LUMBAGO

Nearly everyone suffers from backache at some point in life. It may arise from poor posture or injury, but all cases will respond to some form of treatment. One of the many names for backache is lumbago, an incapacitating pain low down in the back. It is a symptom of several disorders, ranging from the common complaint fibrositis (inflammation of the muscles, usually in the back), to more serious conditions such as a slipped disc.

KEY FEATURES	TREATMENT
Relieved only by lying on the abdomen	ACETIC ACID 12
The back feels numb, stiff and painful, particularly in the neck region Bruised sensation between the shoulder blades	ACONITE 12
Severe, continuous, dull ache in the lower back region Worse when walking or stooping In pregnancy	AESCULUS 12
Lumbago alternating with headache	ALOE 12
Bruised pain in the coccygeal region when sitting Sensation of extreme cold between the shoulders, no better for local warmth	AMMON MUR 12
Painful stiffness in the neck and the small of the back brought on by sudden changes of weather Much worse for movement but better for pressure	BRYONIA 12
Burning pain in the lower part of the back Lumbago worse on beginning to move but relieved by continued movement Lumbago from a strained back	CALC FLUOR 12
Stiff neck, worse on the right side Pain under both shoulder blades but worse on the right	CHELIDONIUM 12
The thoracic spine (between the base of the neck and the lower back) is sensitive to touch Violent joint pains during periods General rheumatic pains throughout the body	CIMICIFUGA 12
The neck vertebrae crack on movement Severe bruised pain in the shoulders and arms	COCCULUS 12
Chronic pain, worse from continued motion Better for rest, especially if taken lying on the back	GNAPHALIUM 12
Dull, heavy, dragging pain with stiffness Pain mainly in the lumbar region Help is needed to get up from sitting	HYDRASTIS 12
The back feels stiff and weak, particularly in the small of the back Severe backache during pregnancy and after a miscarriage Lumbago with sudden, sharp pains Pain shoots up and down the back and into the thighs	KALI CARB 12

Pain and weakness in the back, worse when rising from a sitting position	KALI PHOS 12
Stiffness in the back after sitting for a long time	LEDUM 12
Lumbar pain, worse at night when lying in bed Cannot turn over in bed without first sitting up because of the pain	NUX VOM 12
Acute pain relieved by change of posture Pain and tenderness between the shoulders which extends to the arms	OXALIC ACID 12
Intense burning pain mainly between the shoulder blades The spine is tender to the touch	PHOSPHORUS 12
Pain on attempting to rise Rheumatic pains in the back Stiff neck from being in a draught Rheumatism, but not lumbago, is relieved by continued gentle movement	RHUS TOX 12
Pain all over the back, better for pressure Lumbago in the morning before getting up	RUTA 12
Backache associated with uterine disorders, worse when sitting Weakness in the small of the back when walking Sudden pain in the back, as if hit by a hammer Pain relieved by lying on something hard	SEPIA 12

DOSAGE

The selected remedy should be taken four times a day until an improvement occurs, then stopped. Repeat the treatment as and when necessary.

BUNIONS

This condition, ten times more common in women than in men, is a painful enlargement at the junction of the big toe and the foot. It is probably caused by wearing badly fitting shoes.

KEY FEATURES	TREATMENT
Tearing pain in the big toe The patient may also suffer from gout	BENZOIC ACID 30

DOSAGE

The remedy should be taken three times a day on one day each week. This helps the discomfort and appears to slow down the bunion's development.

BURSITIS

(see Housemaid's Knee, p. 197)

CORNS AND CALLOSES

These are hard, thick areas of skin which form when continual pressure or friction is applied to the skin. Corns are found mainly on the toes, while calloses appear on the soles of the feet and the hands.

KEY FEATURES	TREATMENT
Tender feet due to inflamed areas of hard skin	ANT CRUD 6

Corns with yellow discoloration	FERRUM PIC 6
Painful calloses on the soles of the feet The heel is also painful and the feet have an offensive, profuse sweat	LYCOPODIUM 6
Sensitive corns with many areas of hard skin on the feet	RANUNC BULB 6
Corns with burning and soreness, worse if the feet hang down	RANUNC SCELERATUS 6

DOSAGE

The selected remedy should be taken twice a day until an improvement is maintained.

CRAMP, Hand and Arm

Prolonged use of the hands and arms, as in writing or chopping wood, may lead to cramp. Similarly, fierce muscle action, as required to unscrew a tight lid, can also lead to cramp.

KEY FEATURES	TREATMENT
In both the hands and fingers, worse on trying to grasp something	AMBRA 6
In hands and feet Weakness in the right arm and a tearing sensation in the wrist and the fingertips	ARG MET 6
Specific for writer's cramp	BISMUTH 6
Trembling and weakness in all the limbs Cramp in the forearm muscles	GELSEMIUM 6

Weakness in the arms and hands The fingers feel stiff and numb Involuntary shaking of the hands	MAG PHOS 6

DOSAGE

The selected remedy should be taken twice a day and stopped when an improvement is maintained. Thereafter, provided it is still the indicated remedy, it should be taken if there is a deterioration.

CRAMP, Leg

Often worse in bed, cramp particularly affects pregnant women and the elderly. As it may also be a sign of diabetes, the urine should be tested for sugar.

KEY FEATURES	TREATMENT
In the lower leg while walking	CARB ACID 6
In the calves, worse after midnight and relieved by standing	CUPRUM ARS 6
Worse when cold	LATHYRUS 6
The legs feel numb and almost paralysed In the calves and soles	NUX VOM 6
In the calves The skin is blue, cold and clammy	VERATRUM ALB 6

DOSAGE

The selected remedy should be taken twice a day and stopped when an improvement is maintained. Thereafter, provided it is still the indicated remedy, it should be taken if there is a deterioration.

FEET, Burning

This symptom is experienced with some skin diseases, such as eczema, when it tends to be worse at night in bed. Blood-vessel abnormalities can also lead to a burning sensation in the feet.

KEY FEATURES	TREATMENT
Burning and swelling, mainly of the soles of the feet With a heavy, offensive sweat	ARUNDO 6
The soles of the feet burn and itch	CALC SULPH 6
Cold, sweaty feet with burning soles	CANTHARIS 6
One foot, usually the right, feels hot, while the other feels cold	LYCOPODIUM 6
The feet feel hot and tender and the soles feel sore The legs and feet become restless	MEDORRHINUM 6
Both the soles of the feet and the hands burn, especially during the night	SULPHUR 6

DOSAGE

The selected remedy should be taken twice a day until an improvement is maintained.

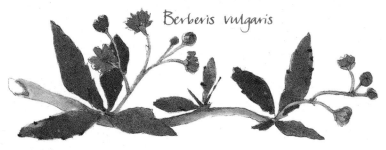

Berberis vulgaris

FEET, Cold

Poor circulation is often the cause of this condition. Smoking can have a bad effect on the arterial circulation in the legs, which can lead to coldness of the feet and in extreme cases may even lead to gangrene. Impaired blood supply to the feet is also found in some diabetics. The drugs known as beta blockers, which are used for the treatment of raised blood pressure, are another known cause of cold feet.

KEY FEATURES	TREATMENT
Numb, tingling and cold feet, often with the hands hot	ACONITE 6
Cold, clammy, smelly feet, with the toes and the soles of the feet feeling sore	BARYTA CARB 6
Cold legs and feet while the rest of the body is hot	BELLADONNA 6
Cold, damp feet with sour-smelling sweat Cramps in the calves; even the knees feel cold	CALC CARB 6
Icy-cold feet which feel sprained	CAMPHORA 6
Swollen, cold legs and feet	COLCHICUM 6
The feet feel icy cold during the day but burn at night	NAT PHOS 6
Cold, dry hands and feet in smokers, with tingling in the toes and violent cramps Worse for warmth	SECALE 6
Icy-cold feet with an offensive sweat The foot feels sore from the instep through to the sole	SILICA 6

Cold hands and cold, sore feet from standing too long   SQUILLA 6
The rest of the body feels warm

DOSAGE

The selected remedy should be taken twice a day until an improvement is maintained.

FEET, Sweaty

The degree to which the feet sweat differs from person to person. This uncomfortable and often offensive condition responds to homeopathic treatment but regular washing and changes of socks/stockings and shoes should not be neglected. Footwear made from synthetic materials can make the condition worse.

KEY FEATURES	TREATMENT
Copious and offensive foot sweat Fissures may develop, especially on the heel	ARUNDO 6
With a tendency to cramps The legs are cold from the knees downward	CARBO VEG 6
Cold hands and feet, with an acrid foot sweat	IODUM 6
Profuse foot sweat with pain in the heel when walking and painful calloses on the soles	LYCOPODIUM 6
Icy-cold feet with an offensive sweat The foot feels sore from the instep through to the sole	SILICA 6

DOSAGE

The selected remedy should be taken twice a day until an improvement is maintained.

GOUT

The deposition of monosodium urate crystals in a joint leads to this acute and very painful condition. The joint appears shiny and red. Although gout can occur in other joints, it is mainly found in the hands and feet, particularly the big toe. Small nodules called tophi are sometimes found in the external ears of gout sufferers.
Gout can become chronic, leading to deformed joints with typical gouty nodes forming.

Medical help may be needed.

KEY FEATURES	TREATMENT
At the start of an acute attack Red, shiny, swollen, very painful joint	ACONITE 30
In chronic cases rather than acute ones	AMMON PHOS 30
The patient fears someone will accidently touch the part affected, so tender is it Foot pain, worse towards evening Red, inflamed big toe joint	ARNICA 30
Typical acute gout symptoms Worse for the slightest touch or jar	BELLADONNA 30
With a large swelling	BRYONIA 30

Extreme tenderness to touch	COLCHICUM 30
The slightest movement is agonizing	
The patient feels weak and ill, and becomes very irritable	
All the symptoms are worse in the evening	
Gouty nodes form	GUAIACUM 30
Tearing pains and spasm of muscles	
Gout in the knee	
The ball of the big toe is swollen, sore and painful on walking	LEDUM 30
Gouty nodes develop in affected joints	
Worse for warmth, pressure and motion	
The pain travels upwards	
Acute and chronic gout, worse in a heated room	SABINA 30
Gouty nodes develop	
Acute attacks which end with the passage of urine containing a sand-like deposit	URTICA 30

DOSAGE

For an acute attack the selected remedy should be taken every hour until an improvement is maintained.
In chronic gout the selected remedy should be taken three times on one day every two weeks.

HANDS, *Blue*

If the circulation to the hands is poor, they may appear to become blue in cold situations and chilblains may develop. Occasionally, a condition known as Raynaud's disease may be present. This makes the arteries of the fingers go into spasm when the hands are cold, which leads to pallor, numbness and pain in the affected fingers.

KEY FEATURES	TREATMENT
Cold and blue	AMMON CARB 6
The veins in the hands are distended	
Chilblains, verrucae and bluish discoloration of the hands, especially in the elderly	CARBO AN 6
The arms and hands are swollen and blue	ELAPS COR 6
The skin on the fingertips peels off	
The hands sweat, especially on the palms	NITRIC ACID 6
The nails are discoloured blue	
The hands turn blue and cold	SAMBUCUS 6
Dry while asleep, profuse sweat when awake	

DOSAGE

The selected remedy should be taken twice a day and stopped when an improvement is maintained. Thereafter, and provided it is still the indicated remedy, it should be taken if there is a deterioration.

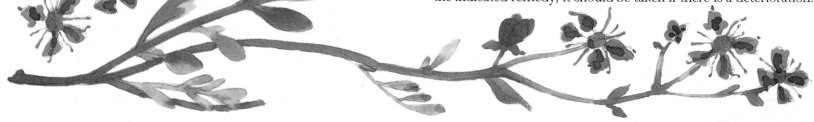

HANDS, *Burning*

If the nerves which dilate the blood vessels of the hands are overactive, the skin temperature of the hand will be raised. Similarly, in skin conditions such as eczema the hands may feel hot and burning to the patient.

KEY FEATURES	TREATMENT
Itching, burning, swollen hands	ARUNDO 6
Hands and feet feel burning The finger joints are enlarged and puffy The hands feel restless	MEDORRHINUM 6
The joints are hot, painful and swollen Cold, fresh air makes the skin painful	RHUS TOX 6
Hot, sweaty hands and feet, worse at night	SULPHUR 6

DOSAGE

The selected remedy should be taken twice a day and stopped when an improvement is maintained. Thereafter, and provided the remedy is still the indicated one, it should be taken if there is a deterioration.

Ruta graveolens

HANDS, *Cold*

Limitations in the circulation can make the hands become cold, or even icy cold. In this situation the skin may be easily damaged or chilblains develop.

KEY FEATURES	TREATMENT
Icy coldness and insensibility of both hands and feet, worse at night	ACONITE 6
Icy-cold and swollen hands which feel soft Numbness in the left arm	CACTUS 6
Extreme coldness of the fingertips The wrists and hands feel sore	CHELIDONIUM 6
The hands are alternately hot and cold	COCCULUS 6
Cold, dry hands and feet, especially in heavy smokers The fingers feel numb and are spread apart or bent backwards	SECALE 6
Cold hands and feet, but the rest of the body feels hot	SQUILLA 6
The hands and legs are cold and the arms feel weak	TABACUM 6

DOSAGE

The selected remedy should be taken twice a day and stopped when an improvement is maintained. Thereafter, provided it is still the indicated remedy, it should be taken if there is a deterioration.

HANDS, Red

Increased blood supply to the hands makes the skin become redder. This arises from warming the hands, as in a hot bath or in front of a fire.

KEY FEATURES	TREATMENT
Bright red palm surface at base of thumb	ACONITE 6
The hands and feet swell and become red after washing	AESCULUS 6

DOSAGE

The selected remedy should be taken twice a day and stopped when an improvement is maintained. Thereafter, provided it is still the indicated remedy, it should be taken if there is a deterioration.

HANDS, Weak

Rheumatism, arthritis and muscle disorders can all lead to weakness in the hands. It can also develop as a result of prolonged activity, especially after performing a repetitive movement, such as using scissors for a long period of time.

KEY FEATURES	TREATMENT
Rheumatism in the wrists and fingers leads to swelling from even slight movement and weakness in the fingers	ACTEA SPIC 6
Arthritic pains in the fingers, with brittle nails, and weakness and shaking of the hand	ANT CRUD 6

Clumsiness and objects are easily dropped Moist eczema on the back of the hand	BOVISTA 6
Weakness in the arms and hands The fingers feel stiff and numb Involuntary shaking of the hands	MAG PHOS 6

DOSAGE

The selected remedy should be taken twice a day and stopped when an improvement is maintained. Thereafter, provided it is still the indicated remedy, it should be taken if there is a deterioration.

HEEL PAIN
Calcaneal spur

Pain in the heel usually arises from a small projection of bone on the underside of the heel bone (calcaneum) called a calcaneal spur. It may make walking or standing painful, but may also be present without causing any symptoms at all. Only rarely does it need surgical removal.

KEY FEATURES	TREATMENT
Pain in the heel bone which feels swollen to the patient Worse in damp weather	ARANEA 12
Specific for calcaneal spur	HEKLA LAVA 12

DOSAGE

The selected remedy should be taken twice a day until an improvement is maintained.

BURSITIS

formerly known as 'Housemaid's Knee'

The bursae, of which there are several in the body, are closed sacs containing a minute quantity of clear, viscid fluid and are interposed between surfaces which glide on each other. Bursitis occurs when one of the bursae becomes inflamed. The amount of contained fluid increases and the part may become painful and hot. Housemaid's knee is just one example of bursitis and occurs after injury or excessive kneeling.

KEY FEATURES	TREATMENT
Specifically for housemaid's knee	KALI MUR 6
An inflamed swollen bursa, better for cold applications	RUTA 6
Inflammation and redness over a joint with shooting pains	STICTA 6
Bursitis at the knee or elbow	

DOSAGE

The selected remedy should be taken three times a day for ten days.

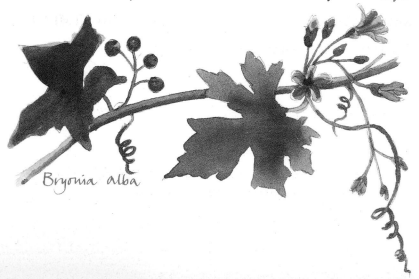

Bryonia alba

LEGS AND ANKLES, *Weak*

These symptoms are mainly due to under-use, which leads to poor muscle tone and diminished power. In greatly overweight people the legs and ankles literally 'give way' trying to support the rest of the body.

KEY FEATURES	TREATMENT
The hip and thigh feel lame, especially after lying down, the knee is unsteady and the ankle twists easily	ACONITE 6
The legs feel weak and trembling, especially going down stairs	ARG MET 6
Weakness in the knees, which feel icy cold and crack from time to time	CROCUS 6
Weakness in the legs followed by cramps in the abdominal muscles	LATRODECTUS 6
Great weakness of all the limbs, but especially in the morning	NAT CARB 6
The arms and legs feel weak, particularly at the knees and ankles	NAT MUR 6
The legs and back feel bruised and may be so weak that getting out of a chair is difficult	RUTA 6
The legs feel weak, twitch and jerk, and are constantly moving	TARENT HISP 6

DOSAGE

The selected remedy should be taken twice a day and stopped when an improvement is maintained. Thereafter, provided it is still the indicated remedy, it should be taken if there is a deterioration.

LEGS, Restless

Usually worse in bed, this condition (also known as Restless Leg Syndrome) particularly affects pregnant women and the elderly. As it may also be a sign of diabetes, the urine should be tested for sugar.

KEY FEATURES	TREATMENT
Worse after walking, climbing stairs and at about 1 a.m. and 11 p.m.	CACTUS 6
At night, better from the warmth of the bed	CAUSTICUM 6
The legs feel heavy, ache all night and cannot be kept still	MEDORRHINUM 6
Drawing pain in the legs, with restlessness, sleeplessness and chilliness	PULSATILLA 6
The legs feel weak, twitch and jerk, and are constantly moving	TARENT HISP 6
The feet move about constantly	ZINC MET 6

DOSAGE

The selected remedy should be taken twice a day until an improvement is maintained. Thereafter, provided it is still the correct remedy, it should be taken if there is a deterioration.

Solanum dulcamara

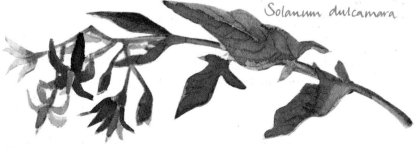

NAILS, Disorders of

These disorders may be broadly divided in two: the nails either become brittle, or the exact opposite occurs and they become thick and very overgrown. The first is often caused by over-washing, especially in detergents. The second may arise from three medical conditions: psoriasis, eczema and fungal infections. In all of these, the nails may become rough, thick and deformed.
Occasionally, the nail, usually of the big toe, becomes embedded in the skin at the top of the digit. This makes it particularly prone to bacterial infection, producing an infected ingrowing toenail.

KEY FEATURES	TREATMENT
Brittle, with a gnawing sensation beneath the nail	ALUMINA 6
Brittle nails that grow out of shape	ANT CRUD 6
Tingling sensation under the fingernails	COLCHICUM 6
Rapid overgrowth of fingernails	FLUORIC ACID 6
The fingernails are rough, thick and discoloured, the toenails brittle and they tend to crumple	GRAPHITES 6
The finger ends are cracked	
The skin beneath the toes cracks, with inflammation under the toenails	SABADILLA 6
White spots on the fingernails	SILICA 6
Ingrowing toenails	

Brittle nails and ingrowing toenails   THUJA 6
The tips of the fingers and toes become
swollen, red and feel dead

DOSAGE

The selected remedy should be taken three times a day until an improvement occurs. This may take several weeks or more. Thereafter, the remedy should be restarted if a deterioration occurs.

PHLEBITIS

(see Varicose Veins, p. 202)

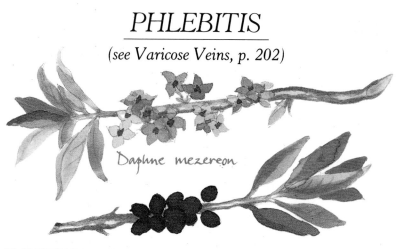

Daphne mezereon

RHEUMATISM AND ARTHRITIS

A recent classification of joint diseases and arthritis contained over 250 different disorders. From a homeopathic point of view we can lump most of these into the general classification of 'rheumatism' because the picture of these illnesses is very similar. This section therefore contains those remedies most suited to an illness which has joint, muscle or tendon pain, usually stiffness, and in some cases deformity of one or more joints.

The commonest form of rheumatism is osteo-arthritis, which is produced by the wear and tear that joints suffer during their use. It is over twice as common as rheumatoid arthritis, but if any doubt exists over the diagnosis or treatment, a doctor should be consulted.

Medical help may be needed for these conditions.

KEY FEATURES	TREATMENT
The smaller joints, such as the hands and feet, are those mainly affected The joints ache and swell, worse for walking	ACTEA SPIC 6
The affected part feels very stiff and sore to pressure The joints swell, making the overlying skin feel stretched and tight The swelling is pale Joints become swollen with fluid	APIS MEL 6
Rheumatism from exposure to damp and cold, with simultaneous muscle strain The part feels sore and bruised	ARNICA 6
Cutting, lightning-like pains run along the joints The joints are swollen, red and shiny, and pain radiates through them Often brought on by getting the head and neck wet, or sitting with them exposed to a draught	BELLADONNA 6
Rheumatism in the smaller joints, which develop nodular swellings	BENZOIC ACID 6

199

Acute rheumatism with hot, shiny, dark or pale red joints	BRYONIA 6	Relief from slow, gentle movement	LYCOPODIUM 6
Pain greatly aggravated by movement, external heat relieves it		Rheumatism in the right shoulder	MAG CARB 6
		Rheumatism worse in bed or after walking and better from warmth	
Rheumatism from working in water or damp surroundings	CALC CARB 6	Pain constantly moving from joint to joint	PULSATILLA 6
The upper back and shoulders are most affected		Worse in the evening, worse from warmth but relieved by cold	
Affected joints feel stiff and tight and lying on them makes them feel sore	CAUSTICUM 6	Severe pain that makes the patient move about to try to relieve it	
Pain worse from cold and relieved by warmth		With indigestion	
Restlessness at night, with drawing pains in the muscles		Rheumatism worse when there is a weather or temperature change	RANUNC BULB 6
With weak ankles		In the chest wall, which feels bruised although the pain is sharp	
Severe, almost intolerable pain, which makes the patient get up and walk about	CHAMOMILLA 6	Susceptibility to weather change, particularly cold, wintry weather	RHODODEN-DRON 6
Symptoms mainly in muscles	CIMICIFUGA 6	Chronic rheumatism affecting the smaller joints, which are worse during rest	
Pain worse in the evenings	COLCHICUM 6	The parts involved feel weak	
The affected parts are swollen and dark red		Muscle stiffness and soreness	RHUS TOX 6
The disease moves from joint to joint and typically occurs in debilitated and weak persons		Prominent body projections are tender	
		Pain worse on first starting to move, worse from sitting and worse rising from a sitting position	
Rheumatism worse in changeable weather, especially in damp, cold conditions	DULCAMARA 6	Relief from continued movement and warmth	
Chronic cases with distorted and nobbly joints	GUAIACUM 6	Damp weather and damp dwellings aggravate	
The joints are worse from movement and the tendons around them feel tight		The patient is continually restless	
Pain travels upwards, worse in a warm bed and affects the smaller joints	LEDUM 6	Soreness and lameness, as from a tendon sprain	RUTA 6
Any swelling is slight		Rheumatism of the wrists and ankles	
Nodes form			

200

Acute muscular rheumatism with shifting, sharp, stitching pains and soreness and stiffness in muscles, especially the back and neck, and right shoulder — SANGUINARIA 6

Chronic, often familial, rheumatism — SILICA 6
Pain worse at night and from uncovering, better from warmth
With weak ankles

Acute and chronic rheumatism — SULPHUR 6
Inflammation starts in the feet, then extends up the body
Pain worse in bed and at night
Jerking of the limbs while falling asleep

DOSAGE

The selected remedy should be taken twice a day and stopped when an improvement is maintained. Thereafter, provided it is still the indicated remedy, it should be taken if there is a deterioration.

SCIATICA

Sciatica refers to the pain that is felt down the back and outer side of the thigh, leg and foot as a result of pressure on the nerve roots which form the sciatic nerve. It is frequently brought about by an awkward lifting or twisting movement.

KEY FEATURES / TREATMENT

Sciatic pain worse on sitting, eased by walking, totally relieved by lying down — AMMON MUR 30

Electric shock-like pains shoot down the leg, which also develops cramps — CARB SULPH 30
Walking is difficult and the gait staggering

Sharp, cutting pain in the left hip, relieved by pressure, better sitting — CIMICIFUGA 30
The pain becomes so acute it can drive the patient out of bed

Sharp, spasmodic attacks of pain which shoot down the leg to the feet — COLOCYNTH 30
Crampy pains in the hip and knee
Pain worse on the right, at night and from movement
Relief from warmth

Intense pains along the sciatic nerve, which alternate with numbness — GNAPHALIUM 30
Pain extends as far as the toes
Relief from sitting in a chair

Darting, left-sided pains relieved by motion — KALI BICH 30

Pain worse at night lying on the affected side — KALI IOD 30

Right-sided sciatica, better lying down — LACHESIS 30

Darting, tearing pains, worse on movement — PHYTOLACCA 30

Chronic cases brought on by exposure to wet, from a strain or after heavy lifting — RHUS TOX 30
Pain worse at rest but relieved by movement, warmth and rubbing

DOSAGE

The selected remedy should be taken four times a day and stopped when an improvement is maintained. Thereafter, provided it is still the indicated remedy, it should be taken if there is a deterioration.

SPRAINS AND STRAINS

(see Emergencies and First Aid, p. 26)

TENNIS ELBOW

(see Housemaid's Knee, p. 197)

VARICOSE VEINS
AND VARICOSE ULCERS

Veins that become tortuous and distended are said to be varicose, and the surface leg veins are those most frequently affected. The commonest causes are pregnancy, excessive standing and constipation. Pain and skin discoloration frequently develop, and swelling around the ankle may come on after prolonged standing.

A common complication of varicose veins is phlebitis – inflammation of the wall of a vein, usually in the legs. The area affected is painful and tender, and the surrounding skin becomes red and feels hot to the touch. Occasionally the inflammation may occur in a deeper leg vein and go on to become a deep vein thrombosis, with pain and swelling.

Urgent medical help is needed for deep vein thrombosis, and varicose ulcers also require medical attention.

KEY FEATURES	TREATMENT
Varicose veins with a bruised, sore feeling	BELLIS 12
Specific for varicose veins and enlarged veins worse during rest but better for warm applications	CALC FLUOR 12
For varicose ulcers	CALC IOD 12
The veins are distended and itch, more so in the evening and in bed Burning varicose ulcers which are hard to heal	CARBO VEG 12
Varicose veins and ulcers which itch when lying down at night In heavy drinkers	CARDUUS 12
Varicose ulcers with enlarged, tender glands in the groin	CLEMATIS 12
Varicose veins, especially with small areas of 'spider veins'	FLUORIC ACID 12
The affected area feels bruised and sore Varicose veins and varicose ulcers Phlebitis	HAMAMELIS 12
Varicose veins in pregnancy	MILLEFOLIUM 12
Varicose veins and acute phlebitis The veins are swollen, sensitive and feel as if they will burst unless the leg is elevated	VIPERA 12
Large veins, sweaty and restless feet	ZINC MET 12

DOSAGE

The selected remedy should be taken twice a day and stopped when an improvement is maintained. Thereafter, provided it is still the indicated remedy, it should be taken if there is a deterioration.

THE SKIN

CONTENTS

Abscesses, Boils and Carbuncles	204
Acne	205
Allergy Rashes	206
Chilblains	207
Cracks and Fissures	207
Eczema	208
Infected Conditions (Cellulitis, Erysipelas, Impetigo)	209
Psoriasis	210
Rosacea	211
Sweat Rash	212
Swelling/Fluid Retention	212

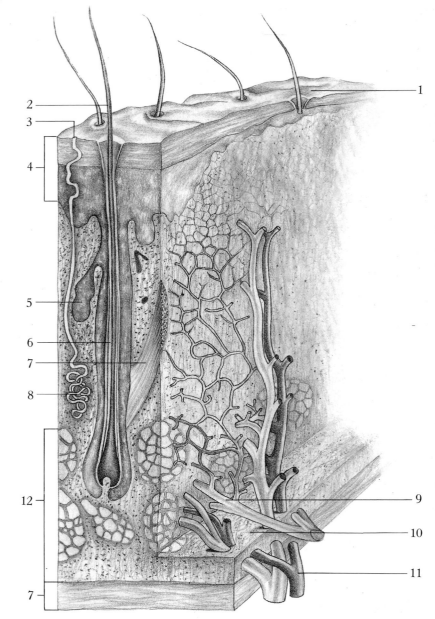

*T*he skin is the protective covering of the body. It has two layers. The epidermis or cuticle is the thin, semi-transparent outer layer. Its surface is waterproof and composed of flattened cells which are being constantly worn away and replaced by fresh cells from

1	Skin surface	7	Muscle
2	Hair	8	Sweat glands
3	Pore	9	Nerves
4	Epidermis	10	Collagen fibres
5	Sebaceous gland	11	Blood vessels
6	Hair follicle	12	Fat and subcutaneous tissue

below. It contains neither blood vessels nor nerves. The openings of the sweat glands, the pores, are found in the epidermis. The outer layer becomes cornified (horny) and is then able to protect the body surface against friction, water loss and the entry of bacteria. The nails are especially thick areas of epidermis.

The dermis consists of fibrous and elastic tissue and is freely supplied with nerves and blood vessels. It also contains the sweat glands, which secrete the sweat (a mixture of water and impurities from the blood) and the sebaceous glands, which produce an oily secretion which prevents the outer horny layer of the skin and the hairs from becoming dry and brittle. Beneath the dermis is a further layer consisting of looser connective tissue, and fat deposited in adipose cells. This is called the subcutaneous layer.

Apart from acting as a protective covering, the skin also helps with temperature control. As much as 8 pints (4 litres) of fluid (in the form of sweat) may be lost each day. On reaching the skin surface, it evaporates and thus helps to prevent the body from overheating. When large quantities of fluid are being lost in this way, less water is excreted in the urine and a thirst develops to ensure that the fluid is replaced.

The small blood vessels in the skin also influence temperature control. When the body becomes overheated, they dilate and bring more blood to the surface, causing a flushed appearance and having a cooling effect. The exact reverse occurs when the body is exposed to cold situations. The skin blood vessels constrict, causing a paler appearance and ensuring less heat is lost.

The third and last major function of the skin is its sensitivity to touch and pain. It contains many sensory nerve endings which send messages to the brain, telling it what the skin is in contact with. For example, it distinguishes between hot and cold, rough and smooth, thus helping to protect the body from injury.

204

ABSCESSES, BOILS AND CARBUNCLES

An abscess is a collection of pus under the skin enclosed by damaged and inflamed tissue. It is usually painful. Boils are inflammatory conditions surrounding a hair follicle. Carbuncles are inflammatory conditions involving several hair follicles and the surrounding tissue. They may have several discharging 'heads'.

KEY FEATURES	TREATMENT
Crops of boils all over the body Sore at first before the pus forms Boils which only partially come to a head	ARNICA 30
Carbuncles with cutting, burning pains Worse after midnight, relieved by heat	ARS ALB 30
Throbbing, redness and pain which all come on quickly	BELLADONNA 30
Recurrent boils and carbuncles	ECHINACEA 12
Throbbing with prickling pains Easy discharge The patient feels chilly	HEPAR SULPH 30
Intense, shiny redness with throbbing and stinging pains Abscesses in glands Use after Belladonna to help the rapid formation of pus	MERCURIUS 30
The area is very sore Slowly developing abscesses with a purplish colour to the skin and thin, dark pus	LACHESIS 30

Pus, intense pain and dark red swelling	RHUS TOX 30
Boils occur in crops	SILICA 12
Discharge continues and the boils are slow to heal	
The discharge is thin and watery	
Chronic abscess with a profuse discharge	SULPHUR 12
The patient may be emaciated	
The patient appears ill and toxic	TARENT CUB 30
The carbuncle is very painful and quickly develops a black core	

All these symptoms require medical help.

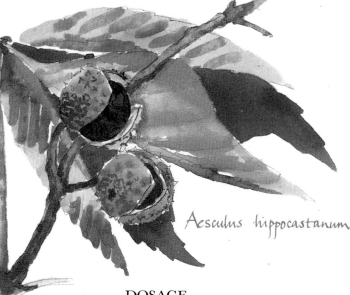

Aesculus hippocastanum

DOSAGE

For an acute inflammatory condition the selected remedy should be taken in the 30 potency every two hours until the abscess/boil/carbuncle bursts and starts to discharge its pus.

When the condition is more chronic and slowly developing, take the selected remedy in the 12 potency four times a day until an improvement is maintained.

ACNE

This skin condition is most common in adolescents and the typical eruption is found mainly on the face, neck and upper chest and back. It is caused by inflammation of the small sebaceous glands which open into hair follicles. The glands become blocked and the acne rash develops. Infection occurs in some of the spots and these are likely to feel sore.

KEY FEATURES	TREATMENT
Small red pimples on the face	ANT CRUD 6
Frequent indigestion with a white-coated tongue	
With great thirst	
Very rough skin and persistent acne	BERBERIS 6
On the face, neck and shoulders	KALI BROM 6
Especially in very sensitive and nervous girls	
Red, pimply eruptions on the face and small pimples at the root of the nose	LEDUM 6
In girls who have scanty periods	SANGUINARIA 6
Chronic acne with rough, hard skin	SULPHUR 6
The lesions are red, sore and often infected	
Water and washing aggravates the spots	

DOSAGE

The selected remedy should be taken twice a day until an improvement occurs, then stopped. Repeat the treatment as and when necessary.

ALLERGY RASHES

Urticaria

Skin eruptions are often allergic in origin and may develop quite quickly in response to the causative agent. The rash, which may cover the whole body, consists of multiple, very itchy pink weals which are smooth and slightly raised. This condition is sometimes called hives or nettle rash because the rash produced is similar to that produced by nettles.

KEY FEATURES	TREATMENT
Typical nettle rash with intense itching In very irritable people	ANACARDIUM 6
Resembles measles	ANT CRUD 30
With burning and restlessness From eating shellfish	ARS ALB 30
With diarrhoea, after excitement Develops overnight Worse from bathing	BOVISTA 30
Chronic rash, worse from drinking milk	CALC ARB 30
With fever and constipation Chronic rash in children	COPAIVA 30
Chronic rashes which become worse at the start of winter Extreme itching on exposure to cold air	DULCAMARA 30
From strawberries	FRAGARIA 30
Chronic and recurring rashes	HEPAR SULPH 30
'Nerve rash' from stress and anxiety	KALI BROM 30
More itchy after exertion	NAT MUR 30
From pork or fruit With diarrhoea and chilliness	PULSATILLA 30
Red, swollen and intensely itching Better from warmth	RHUS TOX 30
From milk or milk products Worse in the warmth of bed	SEPIA 30
From shellfish	TEREBINTH 30
Intense, intolerable itching, often related to temperature changes Itching swellings of the fingers Blotchy face	URTICA 30

DOSAGE

The selected remedy should be taken every three hours until an improvement occurs, then stopped. Repeat the treatment as and when necessary.

BOILS AND CARBUNCLES

(see Abscesses, p. 204)

CELLULITIS

(see Infected Conditions, p. 209)

CHILBLAINS

Although they occur most commonly on the toes, chilblains may also develop on the fingers and other parts of the body. They form on the skin as a reaction to cold, causing considerable congestion and swelling, with severe itching and a burning sensation. The skin surface can become damaged and in severe cases ulceration may occur.

KEY FEATURES	TREATMENT
Burning, itching, redness and swelling from exposure to cold Pustules may develop	AGARICUS 12
On the soles of the feet	ANTHEMIS 12

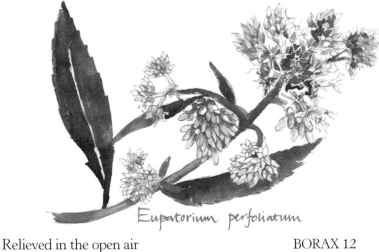

Eupatorium perfoliatum

Relieved in the open air	BORAX 12
Worse from water or washing Ulcerate easily	CALC CARB 12
Worse in the evening and in bed, as well as from the cold	CARBO AN 12

Of bluish coloration Worse in warm, moist air	HAMAMELIS 12
Moist, itchy, burning chilblains which crack and bleed easily	PETROLEUM 12
Bluish discoloration Pricking pain made worse in the warmth	PULSATILLA 12
Dark red discoloration, with intense itching relieved by hot bathing	RHUS VEN 12
Potentially gangrenous *This patient requires medical help.*	SULPH ACID 12
With intense itching and pulsating pains	TEREBINTH 12

DOSAGE

The selected remedy should be taken four times a day until an improvement occurs, then stopped. Repeat the treatment as and when necessary.

CRACKS AND FISSURES

These often occur in the skin as a result of conditions such as eczema. However, people doing heavy manual work may also find that the skin cracks easily.

KEY FEATURES	TREATMENT
In the fingers and on the heels Burning and swelling of the soles The feet sweat copiously	ARUNDO 12
In the palms of the hands and in hard skin	CALC FLUOR 12

The hands have hard, thick skin which is dry and deeply cracked
The hands become swollen and itchy — CISTUS CAN 12

In the finger ends which become infected easily — GRAPHITES 12
Brittle and deformed fingernails

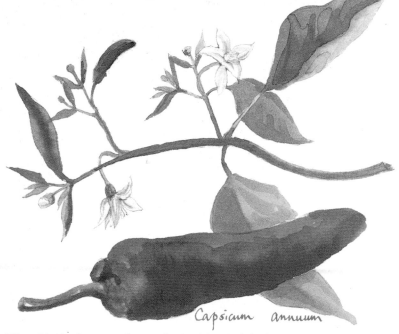

Capsicum annuum

The skin is dry, rough, cracked and painful; the cracks bleed easily — PETROLEUM 12

The skin is dirty, greasy, brownish and wrinkled — SANICULA 12
Eczema on the hands, complicated by deep cracks on both the hands and fingers

DOSAGE

The selected remedy should be taken three times a day until an improvement occurs, then stopped. Repeat the treatment as and when necessary.

ECZEMA

This condition starts with the affected area of skin showing a greater degree of redness than the surrounding skin. Small blisters then develop and as these rupture, they leave crusts or pits which ooze serum. As they heal they become scaly and very itchy, especially at night in the warmth of the bed. Eczema may be due to a constitutional defect and if this is the case, a constitutional remedy (administered by a professional) may be required to cure the condition. However, symptom treatment as follows will help.

KEY FEATURES	TREATMENT
With violent itching In irritable patients	ANACARDIUM 6
Honey-coloured crusts The skin cracks easily and thick, horny calloses form	ANT CRUD 6
In chronic eczema where the skin itches, burns and swells	ARS ALB 6
On the scalp, extending to the face The crusts are white and very itchy	CALC CARB 6
Moist, scabby eruptions on the scalp, face, bends of joints, between the fingers and behind the ears The corners of the mouth and eyes become cracked and ooze a gluey, thick, tenacious, honey-like discharge Extreme itching The rest of the skin may be dry and horny, and the hair is dry and falls out	GRAPHITES 6

Moist eczema, especially of the scalp, which has become chronic	KALI MUR 6
Chronic eczema, worse during periods and at the menopause	MANGANUM 6
Great itching, worse when warm or wrapped up Small blisters quickly form scabs and crusts from which an acrid, thick pus emerges	MEZEREUM 6
Moist eczema without much itching	NAT MUR 6
Thick scabs which ooze pus The skin is harsh and dry The fingertips crack and the hands chap	PETROLEUM 6
Mainly on the head and face, cheeks and ears The skin looks dirty, greasy and unwashed	PSORINUM 6
With numerous small blisters which itch and tingle Worse at night and in damp weather	RHUS TOX 6
The skin is rough and coarse, with soreness in the folds and violent itching everywhere The scalp is dry and hot, with intense itching, especially at night Scratching causes soreness and burning Water aggravates, particularly causing great burning	SULPHUR 6

DOSAGE

The selected remedy should be taken twice a day until an improvement occurs, then stopped. Repeat the treatment as and when necessary.

ERYSIPELAS

(see Infected Conditions, below)

Coffea arabica

HIVES

(see Allergy Rashes, p. 206)

IMPETIGO

(see Infected Conditions, below)

INFECTED CONDITIONS
Cellulitis/Erysipelas/Impetigo

Cellulitis is a diffuse inflammation of the subcutaneous tissue of the skin. It shows as redness, swelling and pain, with a raised temperature.
Erysipelas is very similar, but is an inflammation caused by a bacteria called the streptococcus, which spreads through the skin and subcutaneous tissues.

Impetigo is an inflammatory, pustular skin disease, usually caused by bacteria called the staphylococcus. Honey-coloured crusts which form on the skin are typical.

Medical help is needed for these conditions.

KEY FEATURES	TREATMENT
Bluish-red pustular eruptions	ANT TART 30
Starts as a light red discoloration, but the affected skin soon becomes livid, purple and swollen and has a bruised, sore feeling The tissue swelling appears early in the disease	APIS 30
The skin appears bright red and rapidly swells, making it appear smooth, shiny and tense Sharp, throbbing pain With headache, fever and swollen glands	BELLADONNA 30
The infection starts on the nose and spreads to the right cheek, with the formation of large blisters which burst and discharge an acrid, burning fluid	CANTHARIS 30
Large yellow blisters High temperature Pain extends from the gums to the ear	EUPHORBIUM 30
Recurring and chronic cases involving the nose and face The slightest irritation to the skin brings on an attack	GRAPHITES 30
Mainly left-sided, the area is at first bright red, then becomes dark blue or even purple The patient feels drowsy and weak	LACHESIS 30

Infection of the skin around joints In the early stages of cellulitis	MANGANUM 30
Cellulitis with many blisters The skin looks dark red and swollen, with great itching and tingling For skin infections of the scalp, face and genitalia	RHUS TOX 30

DOSAGE

The selected remedy should be taken every two hours until an improvement occurs and is maintained.

NETTLE RASH

(see Allergy Rashes, p. 206)

PSORIASIS

This is a chronic skin complaint in which red areas covered with scales develop. It is to be found most frequently on the knees and elbows. If the scales are scraped off they produce a shiny, silver sheen which is typical of this disease. As constitutional treatment is also necessary for this condition, the help of a homeopathic physician should be sought.

KEY FEATURES	TREATMENT
With itching and burning, worse for cold and scratching The skin is dry, rough and scaly	ARS ALB 6

Dry, scaly, itchy skin The scales peel off easily, leaving a raw surface exposed In the emaciated and elderly	ARS IOD 6
Pimply, dry, rough, scaly skin On the scalp, extending to the face and neck	BERBERIS AQUIFOL 6
The skin is unhealthy and any injury tends to become infected and discharge pus Better in cold weather	BORAX 6
Dry, scaly eruption, especially around the eyes and ears	CHRYSA- ROBINUM 6
Rough, thickened skin which may crack Involving the finger and toenails Much worse in winter	PETROLEUM 6
Yellowish-brown spots on the skin Itching, redness and rawness	SEPIA 6
Well-established psoriasis in considerably overweight people The skin is dry, the hands and feet cold	THYROIDINUM 6

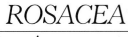

Bryonia alba

DOSAGE

The selected remedy should be taken twice a day until an
improvement occurs, then stopped. Repeat the treatment as and
when necessary.

ROSACEA
Acne rosacea

*A skin complaint which appears on the flush areas, rosacea
develops particularly in women at the menopause. The small
blood vessels (capillaries) near the skin surface dilate and the
sebaceous follicles increase in size. Rosacea is often complicated
by an acne-type eruption.*

KEY FEATURES	TREATMENT
With violet pimples on the nose Worse in the spring	ARS BROM 6
The skin feels dry and hot but may alternate between redness and paleness	BELLADONNA 6
The rash is more copper-coloured than red	CARBO AN 6
Purple rash, worse for warmth	KALI IOD 6
A brownish rash involving the cheeks and nose (a saddle-like distribution)	SEPIA 6
Scanty periods and poor circulation Hot flushes and red cheeks, both worse for warmth	SANGUINARIA 6

DOSAGE

The selected remedy should be taken twice a day until an
improvement occurs, then stopped. Repeat the treatment as and
when necessary.

SHINGLES

(see Infectious Diseases, p. 48)

SWEAT RASH

Intertrigo

This is a superficial inflammation occurring in moist skin folds. It appears mainly in the groin and under the female breast.

KEY FEATURES	TREATMENT
The inner thighs become red and sore when walking, as the patient perspires very freely	AETHUSA 6
Soreness in skin folds, especially between the thighs In teething babies	CAUSTICUM 6
Rawness due to a moist eruption Washing aggravates the condition	CLEMATIS 6
The skin between the thighs and in the bends of limbs becomes sore, red, moist and cracked Aggravation at night when warm in bed	GRAPHITES 6
With psoriasis of the hands Better in warm, dry conditions	PETROLEUM 6

DOSAGE

The selected remedy should be taken twice a day until an improvement occurs, then stopped. Repeat the treatment as and when necessary.

SWELLING/FLUID RETENTION

Oedema/Dropsy

Abnormal infiltration of tissues with fluid may be due to one of several causes. It can occur in diseases of the heart, the liver, the lungs and the kidneys, but it also develops in malnutrition because of protein deficiency.
However, swelling of the feet and ankles may occur in normal adults if they stand for too long, or sit for long periods in cramped conditions, such as in an aeroplane. Overweight, middle-aged women are particularly prone.

Medical diagnosis is required for this condition.

KEY FEATURES	TREATMENT
The skin becomes waxy-looking With great thirst and stomach upsets	ACETIC ACID 30
Transparent, waxy-looking skin Thirst is absent Urine is scanty and may contain a dark deposit	APIS 30
Great thirst but drinking upsets the stomach Feeling of pressure in the chest and abdomen Indigestion is frequent	APOCYNUM CAN 30
Great thirst but for a small amount very frequently Shortage of breath on exertion, but may also disturb sleep	ARS ALB 30

DOSAGE

The selected remedy should be taken each morning until an improvement occurs, then stopped. Repeat when necessary.

HOLIDAY REMEDIES

CONTENTS

Cramps after Swimming	213
Immunization After-Effects	213
Injuries and Accidents	214
Insect Bites and Stings	214
Muscle Aches and Pains	214
Stomach Upsets	215
Sunburn and Overheating	215
Travel Sickness	216
Various Holiday Problems	216

Homeopathic remedies can be of great value in treating the annoying illnesses that may ruin a holiday. They can be taken by young and old alike, and there are no unpleasant side-effects such as the sedation and confusion that can be produced by conventional medicines. Why not take a copy of this section on holiday with you?

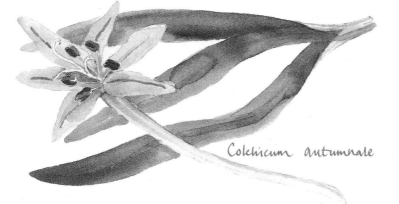

Colchicum autumnale

CRAMPS AFTER SWIMMING

KEY FEATURES	TREATMENT
If cold and chilly	ACONITE 12
With much muscle spasm	NUX VOM 12

DOSAGE
Take the selected remedy hourly for three doses.

IMMUNIZATION AFTER-EFFECTS

KEY FEATURES	TREATMENT
Sore, enlarged glands Headaches General tiredness	THUJA 30

Pain, swelling and redness over
  the injection site
The patient feels very cold and finds
  it hard to get warm
	SILICA 30

DOSAGE
Take the selected remedy three times a day for two days.

INJURIES AND ACCIDENTS

KEY FEATURES	TREATMENT
For all accidents, blows and bruises	ARNICA 30
For overtired, fractious children who can't get off to sleep	
For counteracting hard hotel beds	
Crushed fingers or toes	HYPERICUM 30
Sprains and strains	RUTA 30

DOSAGE

Take the selected remedy every two hours for three doses.

LOCAL TREATMENT

KEY FEATURES	TREATMENT
Cuts and scrapes	CALENDULA CREAM
Irritable piles	HAMAMELIS CREAM
Bruised legs and varicose veins	
Other bruises, whether the skin is intact or not	
Insect bites	LEDUM TINCTURE
Burns, including sunburn	URTICA TINCTURE FRESH ALOE VERA GEL

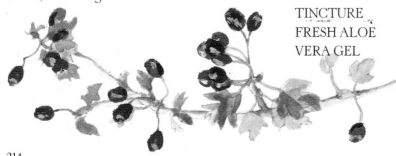

INSECT BITES AND STINGS

KEY FEATURES	TREATMENT
Wasp and bee stings	APIS 12
Other stings, especially when there is much itching and swelling	
Horsefly bites	BELLADONNA 12
These often become septic and may need medical attention	
Bites in general, especially when there is much irritation	ECHINACEA 12
Bites in general and those which feel better for a cold application	LEDUM 12

DOSAGE

Take the selected remedy every hour until an improvement is maintained

MUSCLE ACHES AND PAINS

KEY FEATURES	TREATMENT
From unaccustomed exercise and carrying heavy suitcases	BELLIS 30
Lumbago which is worse on first movement but improves with continued movement	RHUS TOX 30

DOSAGE

Take the selected remedy three times a day for three days.

214

STOMACH UPSETS

Remember – it is very easy to become dehydrated in hot climates, so drink large amounts of fluid if you have diarrhoea and/or vomiting.

KEY FEATURES	TREATMENT
Constipation from change of food and water	ALOES 12
Diarrhoea and sickness often occurring at the same time	ARS ALB 12
The patient feels very cold and ill	
Diarrhoea and vomiting, with extreme lethargy	BAPTISIA 12
Colic, especially that from cold drinks	COLOCYNTH 12
Constipation because away from home	LYCOPODIUM 12
After over-indulgence or unaccustomed rich food	NUX VOM 30

DOSAGE

DIARRHOEA AND SICKNESS – take the selected remedy every three hours until an improvement occurs.
CONSTIPATION OR OVER-INDULGENCE – take the selected remedy twice a day.
COLIC – take the remedy every two hours until an improvement occurs.

SUNBURN AND OVERHEATING

Medical advice should be obtained for all but simple cases. Sweating may lead to a disturbance of the body's fluid balance, which should be corrected by drinking large amounts of liquid.

KEY FEATURES	TREATMENT
The patient becomes very fearful and restless	ACONITE 30
For sunburn and burns generally	CANTHARIS 30
Nausea and headache from overheating	CARBO VEG 30
In children who become very listless after being in the sun	
Extreme lethargy and much shaking	GELSEMIUM 30
Severe headache from being in the sun for too long	GLONOINE 30
Persistent headache from too much sun which only comes on several weeks later	NAT CARB 30

DOSAGE

Take the selected remedy every two hours for four doses. Local treatment with Urtica tincture and fresh Aloe Vera gel is soothing. Calendula cream can be used for lip sores caused by the sun.

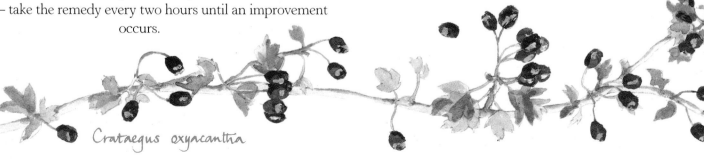

Crataegus oxyacantha

TRAVEL SICKNESS

KEY FEATURES	TREATMENT
Headache in the back of the head Dislike of the sight or smell of food Dry throat Swollen abdomen	COCCULUS 30
Increased salivation Better for eating, warmth and lying down with the head raised Irritable and quarrelsome	PETROLEUM 30
Nausea from smells such as engine fumes, even from seaweed	SEPIA 30
Pale face, cold sweat Better in the cold, fresh air	TABACUM 30

DOSAGE

The selected remedy should be taken the night before the journey, and immediately before the journey starts if to a known sufferer. Repeat at approximately three-hourly intervals.

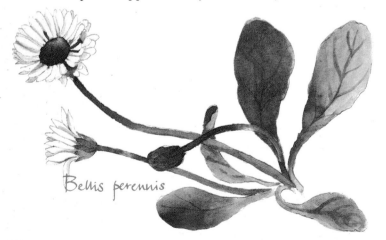

Bellis perennis

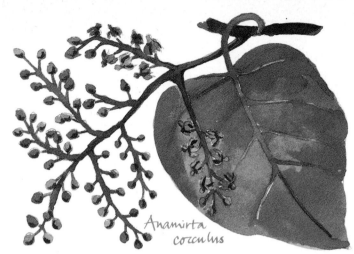

Anamirta cocculus

VARIOUS HOLIDAY PROBLEMS

KEY FEATURES	TREATMENT
Sudden chills from inadequate clothing	ACONITE 30 – three doses over three hours
Hysteria in children from a sudden, unexpected ducking	BELLIS 30 – one dose
In fair-skinned people who overreact to sun and/or glare	CANTHARIS 30 – twice a day for one week before going away
Teething infants	CHAMOMILLA 30 – as often as necessary
Hot day, cold nights, leading to a stuffy nose and sore eyes	DULCAMARA 30 – twice a day
Prickly heat	URTICA 12 – four times a day

MATERIA MEDICA

Ailments mentioned in Main Medical Uses, but not discussed
elsewhere in this book, are not suitable for home treatment.
In these cases, and any others where you are uncertain of diagnosis
and treatment, always seek professional advice.

It has been recently estimated that there are about 2000 homeopathic remedies available – a number that would appear to make remedy selection for a particular illness rather a daunting task. Fortunately, the number of remedies in constant use (even among doctors) is much smaller, so this section of the book restricts itself to describing 100 of them.

You will notice that some remedies have much fuller descriptions than others. This is because several of them are polycrests – remedies which have a particularly wide range of action.

THE ORIGINS OF HOMEOPATHIC MEDICINES

The so   varied –
animal   the same
manne

Fr   venoms,
whole   al secretions,
such a   are
homeo

Re   out half of
those   art of them;
leaves,   ds and roots
all hav   llected at the
optimu   ies of
extract   rm which is
known as a mother tincture.

Minerals and ores, plus organic and inorganic chemicals both natural and synthetic, also yield useful remedies. In a process called trituration, these substances are ground in a mortar while being diluted with lactose. After three such dilutions, the substance becomes soluble and is put into solution.

THE MANUFACTURE OF HOMEOPATHIC MEDICINES

Whatever their source, all homeopathic remedies are prepared in a special way that was originally described by Dr Samuel Hahnemann. On discovering that conventional remedy strengths produced unwanted side-effects, he began to dilute the medicines, vigorously shaking them each time. He called each of these dilutions 'potencies' and found, to his surprise, that the more dilute the preparation, the more potent its effect. (Studies subsequently carried out some years later at the Royal London Homeopathic Hospital showed that remedies made by dilution without succussion (shaking) do not produce the desired results.)

POTENCIES

The potency of a particular remedy is expressed mainly in two scales: the X (or D) scale, which works on a base of ten (decimal), and the C (or CH) scale, which works on a base of 100 (centesimal).

In preparing a remedy on the decimal scale, one drop of the mother tincture is succussed with nine drops of diluent (alcohol/water solution) and this becomes the 1x potency. One drop of this is then succussed with nine drops of diluent to become the 2x potency. The process continues in exactly the same way until the required potency is reached.

In preparing a remedy on the centesimal scale, one drop of mother tincture is succussed with ninety-nine drops of diluent to become the 1c potency. One drop of this succussed with ninety-nine drops of diluent becomes the 2c potency and so on.

With solid, insoluble substances, such as zinc, one part of the substance is ground in a mortar for one hour with ninety-nine parts of lactose to produce the 1c potency. This process is repeated until the 3c potency is reached and this is now soluble in alcohol to make the 4c potency. The process then follows the method of liquid succussion described earlier.

TYPES OF PREPARATION

Homeopathic remedies are usually dispensed in five different forms.

POWDERS are individually wrapped and taken dry on the tongue. One powder is the correct dose for both children and adults.

TABLETS are supplied in glass or plastic containers which hold either a specific number or weight. One tablet may be chewed or allowed to dissolve in the mouth. The dosage is the same for both children and adults because it is the potency, not the quantity, that counts.

PILLS are tiny round balls which tend to dissolve more quickly than tablets. They are taken in the same way and quantity as tablets.

GRANULES are available in glass containers and about half a capful is the correct dose for children and adults.

LIQUIDS are supplied in dropper bottles, the smallest containing 5 ml. The dose, for both children and adults, is 3–5 drops directly on to the tongue or in a little water.

If you are treating a baby and the only preparation you have is in tablet form, it can be crushed between two folds of paper (using the container as a rolling-pin) to make it easier to administer. It can then be given dry or dissolved in a little water. If, during the crushing process, you lose a few fragments, don't worry; it is the potency and not the quantity that counts in homeopathic treatment.

(Theoretically, each particle of a remedy is as powerful as the whole, so administering the smallest quantity possible will have no less an effect than the largest.)

Ointments are available in a few remedies for local application. These are:

ARNICA (for bruises, provided the skin is intact)
CALENDULA (for cuts and grazes)
GRAPHITES (for broken, discharging skin conditions)
HAMAMELIS (for bruises with broken skin, and for piles)
HYPERICUM (for crush injuries)
PAEONIA (for piles and violent itching conditions)
RHUS TOX (for stiff arthritic joints)
RUTA (for sprains and strains)
SULPHUR (for eczema and similar skin complaints)
TAMUS (for chilblains)
THUJA (for warts)
URTICA (for burns, sunburn and allergy rashes resembling nettle rash)

Tinctures (soothing lotions) diluted for local use are Arnica, Calendula, Hypercal and Urtica.

CHOOSING A POTENCY

Throughout this book the decision of what potency to use has been made for you. However, as you become more experienced and confident in the use of homeopathic remedies, you may well choose to employ different potencies that strike you as more appropriate.

Even within the medical profession there is far from universal agreement on which potency to use for any specific complaint.

While it is true to say that the choice of potency comes with experience, there are some general rules which can be applied.

Three potency ranges are in use in Great Britain, the USA and most other countries:

LOW up to 6c (for purely physical symptoms or severe changes, internal or external, arising from the disease)
MEDIUM 12c–30c (for mixed mental and physical symptoms)
HIGH 200c and above (when symptoms relate to the mind, the illness goes back many years, or in severe, acute illness)

France has a slightly different range:

LOW 4 or 5c
MEDIUM 7 or 9c
HIGH 15 or 30c

Despite this difference of opinion as to what constitutes a normal range, there is basic agreement as to how the low, medium and high potencies are used.

Home prescribers are advised not to go above the medium range. High potency prescribing should be left to the professional as it requires great accuracy in matching symptoms to a remedy and a knowledge of homeopathy far beyond the scope of this book.

U S READERS

Certain remedies, such as Cocaine, Morphine and Opium, which are based on narcotic substances, are not available over the counter in the United States. The Federal Drug Administration has strict rules about the distribution of these drugs, even in the safe homeopathic form. If your ailment requires one of these restricted substances, you will need to get it on prescription from a homeopathic doctor.

Remember – it is better to give the correct remedy in the 'wrong' potency than the reverse. This is because the correct remedy will always work eventually, whatever the potency given. The wrong remedy will never work.

A HOMEOPATHIC MEDICINE CABINET

It is worth keeping a small selection of remedies to treat everyday ailments. For the beginner with small children in the family the following range should be sufficient.

Aconite	Chamomilla	Nux vom
Arnica	Gelsemium	Phosphorus
Ars alb	Hepar sulph	Pulsatilla
Belladonna	Mercurius	Rhus tox
Bryonia	Nat mur	Sulphur

For the more experienced home prescriber, some additional remedies should be stocked. These might be:

Allium cepa	Colocynth	Ipecac
Ant crud	Drosera	Kali bich
Ant tart	Euphrasia	Ledum
Apis	Ferrum phos	Lycopodium
Arg nit	Graphites	Ruta
Camphor	Hamamelis	Sepia
Cantharis	Hypericum	Thuja
Carbo veg	Ignatia	Urtica

STORING REMEDIES

Homeopathic medicines require special handling and storage so that they do not lose their power as a result of contamination.

• Always keep them in the container in which they are supplied.

• Store away from bright light, great heat and strong odours, particularly mint, camphor, menthol, tee tree and Eucalyptus oil.

• Keep handling to a minimum. The dose should be tipped on to a clean palm and transferred directly to the mouth. Powders should be tipped straight on to the tongue.

• Discard tablets or pills dropped on the floor. If returned to the container, they will contaminate the rest of the remedy.

HOW TO TAKE HOMEOPATHIC MEDICINES

• The dose should be put into a 'clean mouth', i.e. one that has been free of food, drink, tobacco and toothpaste for ten minutes. The mouth should also be kept clean for ten minutes after taking a dose.

• Do not 'wash down' pills or tablets with water. They should be chewed or allowed to dissolve under the tongue.

• If a remedy must be taken in water, mix it in a clean glass with a plastic spoon.

NOTE

Manufacturers of homeopathic remedies give varying advice about dosage which may lead to confusion for beginners to homeopathy. Always follow the dosage advice given in this book as it has been tailored to specific conditions.

One tablet constitutes one dose, but it has become established practice for manufacturers to suggest two tablets per dose for adults and one tablet per dose for children under twelve. Adhering to the smaller dose will prove cheaper and just as effective.

WARNING

Ailments mentioned in Main Medical Uses, but not discussed elsewhere in this book, are not suitable for home treatment. In these cases, and any others where you are uncertain of diagnosis and treatment, always seek professional advice.

ACONITE
Aconitum napellus

This remedy is for conditions that come on quickly after exposure to dry, cold winds. If used in the early stages of such illnesses, it will often stop them developing further.
Patients needing Aconite typically show extreme anxiety, apprehension and impatience, and have a vivid imagination with many fears, for example, fear of death, fear of crowds, etc.

MAIN MEDICAL USES

Angina	Palpitations
Anxiety, fear, restlessness	Piles
Colds	Rheumatism
Conjunctivitis	Shock after an accident or operation
Croup	Sudden chills after being in a
Earache	cold, dry wind or draught
Facial neuralgia	Tension, emotional and physical
Fevers in general	Toothache
Headache	Urinary retention

MAJOR SYMPTOMS

HEAD   Throbbing headache with giddiness and nausea after rising.

FACE — Feels red and hot, or one cheek is red the other pale. Both cheeks became pale on rising. Left-sided facial pain with severe toothache.

EYES — Inflamed, with red swollen lids, profuse tears and intense dislike of light.

EARS — Earache with a hot, red, swollen external ear and great sensitivity to noise.

NOSE — Dry and blocked, with an acute sense of smell.

THROAT — Red and dry.

LARYNX — Sudden spasmodic croup with hoarseness, especially in children; in both adults and children it is accompanied by a dry, distressing cough.

CHEST — Coughing produces shooting pains in the chest, with a bruised sensation over the breastbone and a sensation of breathlessness – all worse in the evening, particularly after midnight.

HEART — Extreme anxiety about having heart disease. The blood pressure may be raised. Palpitations with a hard, rapid pulse and tingling pains in the left shoulder and arm.

STOMACH — Vomiting with profuse sweating and increased urination lead to a great thirst for cold water.

RECTUM/ANUS — Bleeding piles with shooting pains in the rectum on defaecation.

STOOLS — Green stools resembling chopped spinach.

URINE — Scanty, hot urine which is painful to pass. However, profuse urination with excess sweating and diarrhoea can occur, as can urinary retention causing pain and restlessness.

BACK — Stiffness down the spine with a bruised feeling and numbness extending to the legs.

LIMBS — Feeling of numbness and heaviness in the joints with pain and/or swelling, worse for movement. Numbness, tingling and shooting pains down the limbs. The hands become hot while the feet remain cold.

SKIN — Hot, dry skin with an intolerance of warmth and a great thirst.

BETTER

For being in fresh air
For rest

WORSE

In the evening and at night
In a warm room
Lying on the left side

AESCULUS

Aesculus hippocastanum

The patient is despondent, irritable and cannot concentrate. The mind feels dull.

MAIN MEDICAL USES

Colds
Constipation
Low back pain
Pharyngitis

Piles
Vaginal discharge
Varicose veins

MAJOR SYMPTOMS

NOSE — Feels dry and full. Frequent sneezing.

MOUTH	Feels scalded. Metallic taste. The tongue is thickly coated and yellowish.
THROAT	Painful, dry and raw. Swallowing is difficult.
ABDOMEN	Soreness, fullness and tenderness in the liver region.
RECTUM	Sensation of the rectum being full of splinters. It feels hot, dry and swollen.
ANUS	Intense burning pain for some time after defaecation. Constipation with painful piles which tend not to bleed.
GENITALIA	Yellow, sticky vaginal discharge with low back pain.
BACK	Severe, dull, low back pain involving the lower back and hips, worse for walking or stooping. The back is tender from the neck downwards.

BETTER	WORSE
In the summer	From walking or stooping
In the open air	In cold air
	In the winter

ALLIUM CEPA

Allium cepa

MAIN MEDICAL USES

Catarrh	Neuralgic pains after surgery or dental work
Colds	Urinary incontinence
Conjunctivitis	Whooping cough
Hay fever	
Laryngitis	

MAJOR SYMPTOMS

HEAD	Dull frontal headache from catarrh, better in the open air.
EYES	Sensitive to light. Very watery with bland tears.
NOSE	An acrid, watery discharge burns the nose and upper lip. Bouts of violent sneezing.
CHEST	Acute laryngitis with a tickling, painful laryngeal cough. Early whooping cough with vomiting and flatulence.
BLADDER	Constant dribble of urine, especially in the elderly.
LIMBS	Fine shooting pains after injuries or after amputation. Ulcers on the heel.

BETTER	WORSE
In the open air	In the evening
In a cold room	From warm air

ALOE

Aloe

The Aloe patient dislikes mental or physical effort. This remedy is of particular use in the elderly.

MAIN MEDICAL USES

Bowel incontinence	Lumbago
Diarrhoea	Nosebleeds
Headache	Piles
Itching associated with jaundice	

MAJOR SYMPTOMS

HEAD	Headache with pain above the forehead and a sensation of pressure in the eyes and nose. The eyes feel better if closed.
NOSE	Morning nosebleeds.
STOMACH	Nausea with a frontal headache and flatulence.
ABDOMEN	The abdomen feels full, hot and bloated, with soreness in the sides and over the liver. Colicky pains before and during defaecation.
RECTUM/ ANUS	Bleeding, itching piles, which may protrude and look like a bunch of grapes. Wind, when passed, may be accompanied by faecal leakage.
STOOLS	Spluttery diarrhoea in the early morning, or straight after eating or drinking.
BACK	Lumbago alternating with headache and piles.
SKIN	Itching associated with jaundice.

BETTER	WORSE
In the open air	In hot, dry weather
For cool applications	In the early morning

ALUMINA
Alumina

The patient is chilly, wakes up feeling depressed, is moody, has a poor memory and is always weary. Talking tires him out, there is a general tremulousness and involuntary limb movements may occur. Time passes slowly. The sight of knives and blood can depress him.

MAIN MEDICAL USES

Conjunctivitis, chronic	Outer-ear infection
Constipation due to rectal inactivity	Period problems
	Toothache
Depression	Vaginal discharge
Dryness of mucous membranes and skin	Vertigo
	Weakness and poor muscle coordination
Eyelid inflammation	
Mouth ulcers	

MAJOR SYMPTOMS

HEAD	Vertigo on opening the eyes in the morning.
EYES	The eyelids burn, itch and stick to each other.
EARS	Discharge of pus with a sensation of cracking while chewing.
NOSE	Sore, scabby and blocked.
MOUTH	Dry, although there is increased salivation. Mouth ulcers. Toothache on chewing.
THROAT	Dry and raw with difficulty in swallowing, relieved by warm food and warm drinks. Sensation of a lump

in the throat, and another is felt in the middle of the chest after swallowing food.

STOMACH   Craving for indigestible foods. Potatoes in particular disagree. Dislike of meat.

RECTUM   The bowels become inactive and even soft stools require great effort and straining; however, the stool tends to be hard and dry and bleeding may occur after its passage.

BLADDER   The patient cannot pass urine without straining as if to open the bowels.

GENITALIA   Acrid, profuse, clear vaginal discharge.

PERIODS   Delayed and scanty, but they exhaust the patient physically and mentally.

LIMBS   Sensation of heaviness, numbness and weakness in the arms and legs, which may lead to a staggering gait. The soles of the feet and the heels become numb and the nails brittle.

SKIN   Dry and wrinkled, with intolerable itching when warm in bed.

BETTER	WORSE
In the open air	On waking
For moderate	In the morning
movement	In the afternoon
In the evening	From warmth

AMMON CARB
Ammonium carbonicum

Patients tend to be unclean in their bodily habits, always tired, take cold easily and are restless. Very sensitive to cold, they have a constant desire to stretch and the body feels bruised. They dislike water and may be apathetic, indolent and neurotic. Any discharges are acrid and cause rawness.

MAIN MEDICAL USES

Asthma	Laryngitis
Colds	Menstrual problems
Chronic bronchitis and	Nosebleeds
emphysema	Piles
Diarrhoea	Restless leg syndrome
Gout	Snuffles in babies and young
Headache and migraine	children
Indigestion	Toothache and gum disease

MAJOR SYMPTOMS

HEAD   Throbbing frontal headaches and chronic headaches with nausea, worse walking in the open air.

EYES   Burning sensation with dislike of bright light.

NOSE   Feels obstructed during the night and the patient breathes through the mouth when asleep. Colds with a dry nose at the start but becoming acrid and watery. Nosebleeds after washing and after eating.

MOUTH   The gums swell and bleed easily and the teeth hurt on biting. Swelling on the inside of the cheeks, with blisters in the mouth and on the tongue. Increased salivation with a sour taste.

225

CHEST	Laryngitis and hoarseness, shortage of breath, palpitations and a spasmodic cough which is especially troublesome at 3–4 a.m.
HEART	Nocturnal cardiac asthma (difficulty in breathing with palpitations and a cold sweat).
STOMACH	The appetite is easily satisfied but there is a constant thirst with a desire to drink while eating. Heartburn and nausea with a need to loosen clothes come on after eating. Desire for sugar.
RECTUM	Bleeding, itching piles, worse during periods.
PERIODS	Frequent and heavy, accompanied by great fatigue. Profuse diarrhoea and colic at the beginning of a period. Constipation afterwards.
LIMBS	The right arm feels heavy and weak. Bruised pains in the hips and thighs. The big toe becomes swollen and painful, worse at night.

BETTER	WORSE
In dry weather Lying on the stomach and on the painful side	From cold wet weather During periods From water Between 3 and 4 a.m.

ANT CRUD

Antimonium crudum

The patient shows excessive irritability and fretfulness, is often sulky and peevish, and dislikes being looked at or touched. There is a tendency to fatness. The heat of the sun is unbearable. Especially useful at the extremes of life – babies and geriatrics.

MAIN MEDICAL USES

Allergy rashes
Arthritis
Bad temper in children and adults who hate being touched
Constipation alternating with diarrhoea (This must be referred to a doctor for investigation.)
Corns, calloses, crusts and cracks

Eczema
Eyelid inflammation, chronic
Headache
Impetigo
Indigestion from overeating and eating unwisely
Laryngitis
Warts

MAJOR SYMPTOMS

HEAD	Headaches after overeating and after bathing.
FACE	Crusts and cracks around the nostrils and lips. Yellow, crusted eruptions on the cheeks and chin.
MOUTH	Cracks at the corners of the mouth. The tongue is thickly coated white.
LARYNX	The voice becomes quite harsh or is completely lost.
CHEST	A cough, worse going into a warm room, is associated with an itchy chest wall.

STOMACH — Loss of appetite but a desire for pickles and acidic foods. Tendency to vomit, with constant belching. Wind tastes of the food last eaten. The stomach may become grossly bloated after eating.

RECTUM — Piles which constantly ooze mucus.

STOOLS — Hard and mixed with a watery discharge.

LIMBS — Arthritic pains in the fingers. Brittle fingernails. Horny warts on the hands and soles of the feet, which become red and tender.

SKIN — Allergy rashes and warts. Eczema accompanied by an upset stomach.

BETTER

In the open air
During rest
From moist warmth

WORSE

In the evening
From heat, acids, wine
From water and washing
From extremes of cold and heat

ANT TART
Antimonium tartaricum

Patients are very despondent and fear being left alone. As the symptoms below suggest, they may be critically ill. They dislike consolation. Suited to fractious children who do not like being touched but want to be carried.

MAIN MEDICAL USES

Acne
Asthma
Bronchitis, acute and chronic
Emphysema
Headache

Indigestion
Loss of sense of taste and smell
Pustular skin eruptions
Trembling head

MAJOR SYMPTOMS

HEAD — Dull frontal headache with an inclination to close the eyes and sleep. Chronic trembling of the head.

FACE — Pale, covered in a cold sweat; the chin and lower jaw tremble.

NOSE — A running cold with loss of smell and taste.

TONGUE — Thick white coating on the tongue but the edges remain red. It becomes very dry.

CHEST — Great rattling of mucus, but with very little expectoration. Coughing with paroxysms of suffocation and vomiting. These are accompanied by a cold sweat on the forehead. Fluid may form in the lungs with eventual respiratory failure

STOMACH — Nausea, retching/vomiting with great anxiety after food. Desire for small amounts of cold water taken very frequently. Aversion to milk and a craving for apples, other fruits and acidic foods.

BACK — Lower-back pain. Feeling of heaviness in the coccygeal region.

LIMBS — General weakness.

SKIN — Pustular eruptions, such as acne, are frequent and may be widespread.

SLEEP — When ill the patient is very drowsy most of the time.

BETTER	WORSE
For sitting erect	In the evening
After belching	Lying down at night
After coughing up	From warmth
phlegm	In the damp cold
After vomiting	After sour drinks
	and food
	After drinking milk

APIS

Apis mellifica

The patient is awkward and drops things, also restless, apathetic, indifferent, whining and tearful. General drowsiness, a high temperature, fever without thirst and an afternoon aggravation are all typical.

MAIN MEDICAL USES

Allergy rashes	Rheumatism
Conjunctivitis and styes	Swelling due to fluid retention
Dental conditions	(oedema)
Erysipelas	Thirstless fevers
Genital inflammation	Throat infections
Insect bites that cause blisters	Vertigo
Painful periods	

MAJOR SYMPTOMS

HEAD	Vertigo with a confused headache, better for walking. The head feels hot and heavy.
FACE	Swollen and red.
EYES	The eyelids are swollen, hot and red, and the tears burn and sting. Sudden piercing pains on using the eyes. Eye infections with pus formation.
NOSE	Red, swollen and inflamed.
MOUTH	The gums are sore and bleed easily, the tongue feels swollen, dry and sore. The whole mouth feels as if scalded.
THROAT	The uvula may be swollen and the tonsils are swollen, puffy and bright red. Swallowing is difficult. Complete lack of thirst (on rare occasions there may be a thirst).
CHEST	The larynx is hoarse. Cough worse for lying down and after sleep, with extreme shortage of breath.
ABDOMEN	Feels sore and bruised and is very tender in all areas.
STOOLS	Frequent, profuse diarrhoea with faecal leakage.
URINE	Scanty and of high colour; the last drops burn.
GENITALIA	Swelling and inflammation of the external genitalia in both male and female. Ovarian pain with painful periods and a puffy face in females.
LIMBS	The knees are swollen, shiny, sensitive and sore, with stinging pains. Fluid retention leads to swollen ankles and feet.
SKIN	Sore and very sensitive, with stinging or pricking pains all over the body.
SLEEP	The patient becomes very drowsy, with sudden starting during sleep.

BETTER	WORSE
In the open air	For heat of any form
When uncovered	From the slightest touch
For cold bathing	In the late afternoon
	After sleeping

ARG NIT
Argentum nitricum

Apprehension is the key. Patients are fearful, nervous and melancholic, impulsive and want to do things in a hurry. Time passes slowly for them. They are intolerant of heat.

MAIN MEDICAL USES

Apprehension before examinations and interviews
Conjunctivitis and eye infections
Diarrhoea from stress and emotional upsets
Facial neuralgia
Flatulence
Headache
Hiatus hernia
Laryngitis
Palpitations
Peptic ulcer
Pharyngitis
Tinnitus (noises in the ears)
Vertigo looking downwards from a height

MAJOR SYMPTOMS

HEAD — Dull, aching headache relieved by tight binding, or a congested, throbbing headache; both may be accompanied by weakness and trembling. Vertigo with buzzing in the ears. The scalp feels tender, the hair as if pulled and one side of the head feels larger than the other.

FACE — Pale and sickly-looking. Left-sided facial neuralgia.

EYES — Eye infections with profuse discharge of pus, and swelling and redness of the lids.

EARS — Vertigo with buzzing noises in the ears.

NOSE — Simultaneous catarrh, loss of smell and headache.

MOUTH — General sensitivity to cold. Toothache from cold or sour things. The gums are tender and bleed easily. The tongue has a red tip.

THROAT — Thick mucus causes hawking. Sensation of a splinter in the throat on swallowing.

CHEST — Hoarseness and a suffocative cough are both aggravated by tobacco smoke. Palpitations worse when lying on the right side.

STOMACH — Belching is difficult but it relieves pain in the pit of the stomach. Extreme flatulent distension of the stomach. Great desire for sweet things.

ABDOMEN — Colic with flatulent distension.

STOOLS — Watery, spluttering and white, or green like chopped spinach. Chronic diarrhoea from emotional disturbances.

BACK — Backache relieved by standing or walking.

LIMBS — Trembling, twitching and weakness of the muscles.

BETTER	WORSE
After belching	From warmth
From fresh air	At night
From the cold	From cold foods
From pressure	After eating
	From emotional events

229

ARNICA
Arnica montana

Arnica patients want to be left alone and deny that there is anything wrong with them. They are nervous, despondent, morose and over-sensitive.

MAIN MEDICAL USES

After trauma, physical or mental	Bruises
Agoraphobia	Diarrhoea
Angina	Gout
Bad breath	Septic conditions
Before childbirth, surgery or dental work	Tinnitus with vertigo
	Whooping cough

MAJOR SYMPTOMS

HEAD Feels hot, but the rest of the body is cold. Vertigo on the least movement.

EYES Tired eyes after close work.

EARS Sharp pain in and behind the ears with a roaring noise in the ears.

MOUTH The breath is foul (smells of bad eggs).

CHEST Sore, bruised feeling with a spasmodic, dry cough and an inability to cough up phlegm. Chest pains which radiate to the left arm.

STOMACH Loss of appetite. Craving for vinegar. Foul belching with nausea and vomiting. Cramp-like pains in the stomach extend to the spine.

ABDOMEN Very distended and hard. Pain after lifting. Colic with retention of urine.

STOOLS Offensive diarrhoea with incontinence of faeces.

LIMBS Bruised, sore feeling all over the body makes the bed or couch feel too hard. Great fear of being touched in case it increases the pain.

SKIN Feels bruised and becomes black and blue after any injury. Crops of small boils.

BETTER	WORSE
Lying down with the head low	From the least touch
In clear, cold, stimulating weather	From motion
	In the evening and at night

ARS ALB
Arsenicum album

Patients are exceptionally fastidious and chilly, showing great anguish and restlessness with a fear of death. They become exhausted after the slightest exertion and even with minor illnesses. Any pain present is burning, showing the unusual feature of being better for a hot application (the headache is the only exception to this). Symptoms tend to recur at regular intervals and are generally worse after midnight.

MAIN MEDICAL USES

Anxiety and depression	Dry eye
Asthma, acute	Eczema
Conjunctivitis	Food poisoning (acute gastro-enteritis)
Dandruff	Hay fever
Diarrhoea	

Headache
Middle- and outer-ear
  inflammation
Migraine

Mouth ulcers
Nausea and vomiting
Psoriasis
Vaginal discharge

MAJOR SYMPTOMS

HEAD	Headache relieved by cold applications. Severe irritation of the scalp, with dandruff and hair loss.
FACE	Appears sunken, pinched and very red. The lips become sore and cracked with burning pains.
EYES	Sensitivity to light. The eyes become inflamed and burn with acrid tears, the lids swollen. Dry eye may also develop.
EARS	Thin, watery, offensive burning discharge. Middle-ear pain.
NOSE	Thin, watery, burning nasal discharge, but the nose feels blocked. Sneezing spasms.
MOUTH	Teeth grinding during sleep. Profuse mouth ulcers; the tongue is brown and dry, sore and blistered.
THROAT	Inflammation with burning pains and a feeling of constriction in the throat.
CHEST	Asthma, which is worse after midnight, with scanty, frothy sputum. Pain in the upper, right side of the chest. Dry cough, worse in the evening.
STOMACH	Burning pains. The sight or smell of food induces nausea. Great thirst for frequent small amounts of cold water. Nausea with retching and vomiting after any food or drink. Fruit, vegetables, ices and vinegar disagree. The patient shows extreme irritability and profound distress about these symptoms.
RECTUM	Burning pains with burning piles, both relieved by local heat.
STOOLS	Thin, watery, acrid, burning and offensive. Especially frequent during the night and after eating or drinking.
GENITALIA	A copious yellow, thick and corrosive vaginal discharge.
PERIODS	Frequent and heavy.
LIMBS	Trembling, twitching, weakness and heaviness in the legs can appear as cramps or sciatica.
SKIN	Itching, burning, dry, rough, scaly eruptions.

BETTER	WORSE
For heat	In wet weather
With the head elevated	Between midnight and 3 a.m.
For warm drinks	From the cold

ARUNDO
Arundo mauritanica

MAIN MEDICAL USES

Catarrh
Colds
Eczema

Fluid retention
Hay fever
Sweaty feet

MAJOR SYMPTOMS

EARS	Eczema behind the ears.

MOUTH/ NOSE	Itching of the nostrils and the roof of the mouth. Loss of sense of smell. Colds with much sneezing.
LIMBS	Itching and burning with swelling of the hands and feet due to fluid retention. The soles of the feet burn and there is copious foot sweat.
SKIN	Eczema with cracks in the fingers and heels. The irritation is mainly on the chest and arms.

AURUM
Aurum metallicum

Patients are deeply depressed, often with suicidal thoughts, and they fear they are totally worthless. These individuals require medical help. Aurum types are oversensitive to noise of any sort and to contradiction. They are also hypersensitive to pain.

MAIN MEDICAL USES

Depression	Raised blood pressure
Bad breath	(hypertension)
Headache	Sinusitis
Mastoiditis	Toothache
Outer-ear infection	

MAJOR SYMPTOMS

HEAD	Severe headaches, worse at night and after mental exertion.
EYES	Very sensitive to light. Visual field defect (inability to see the upper half of objects).

EARS	Offensive, runny discharge which can lead to mastoiditis.
MOUTH	Foul breath. Toothache and ulceration of the gums, worse when cold air enters the mouth.
HEART	Occasional missed heartbeats, rapid irregular pulse. Raised blood pressure.

BETTER	**WORSE**
In the summer	From cold damp
From fresh air	weather
From cold	From sunset to
applications	sunrise

BAPTISIA
Baptisia

Patients show great mental confusion with difficulty in concentrating; they may fall asleep while being spoken to or even while answering questions. Weakness makes them incapable of physical or mental effort. There is a general intolerance of pressure.

MAIN MEDICAL USES

Diarrhoea	Oesophageal constriction
Heavy periods	Offensive breath, sweat, faeces
Influenza	or urine
Miscarriage, threatened	Tonsillitis
Muscular soreness	Sciatica
ME (chronic fatigue syndrome)	Severe infectious illnesses

MAJOR SYMPTOMS

HEAD	Feels heavy and numb. The skin of the scalp feels tight.
FACE	Has a besotted appearance.
EYES	The eyes and lids feel sore.
MOUTH	The tongue feels burnt and has a yellow-brown centre with dark red edges. Foul breath.
THROAT	Dusky redness of the tonsils with a painless sore throat. Can swallow only liquids. The throat feels constricted.
CHEST	Sense of suffocation at night in bed; fears going to sleep.
STOMACH	Sinking feeling with tenderness over the stomach, worse from beer.
ABDOMEN	Distended and rumbling. Tender over the liver.
STOOLS	Offensive, frequent, dark and acrid, mainly in the morning.
PERIODS	Early and profuse.
PREGNANCY	Threatened miscarriage after a shock.
BACK/ LIMBS	Sore, bruised feelings with numbness and weakness. Stiff neck. Pain in the lower back travels down the right leg.
SKIN	Feels hot. Livid spots all over the body.

BETTER	WORSE
No influencing factors	In humid heat
	In fog
	Indoors

BARYTA CARB
Baryta carbonica

This remedy is especially useful in infancy and old age. Patients may be shy, bashful and upset by strangers. They have mental weakness with a poor memory.

MAIN MEDICAL USES

Bleeding gums	Nasal catarrh
Colds	Nosebleed
Colic	Prostate enlargement
Dandruff	Raised blood pressure (hypertension)
Deteriorating hearing	Senile dementia
Flatulent indigestion	Sweaty feet
Hiccoughs	Tonsillitis (sometimes with an abscess behind the tonsil)
Mental and physical retardation in children	

MAJOR SYMPTOMS

HEAD	Dandruff and hair loss.
EARS	Deterioration of hearing. Tinnitus. Swollen lymph glands behind the ear.
NOSE	Colds with swelling of the upper lip and nose. Thick yellow mucus.
MOUTH	Retracted, bleeding gums. Toothache before a period. Inflamed mouth blisters. The tip of the tongue smarts.
THROAT	Colds which extend to the throat causing tonsillitis. Smarting pain on swallowing, can swallow only liquids. Swollen lymph glands in the back of the neck. Sore throat from overuse of the voice.

233

LARYNX	Mucus produces hoarseness and voice loss.
CHEST	Dry cough, worse for weather changes. Palpitations, worse lying on the left side. Raised blood pressure.
STOMACH	Flatulence and indigestion. Hiccoughs. Tenderness over the stomach. Worse for warm food.
ABDOMEN	Hard and distended. Pain after eating. Colic and hunger at the same time but the patient will not eat.
BACK	Swollen neck glands. Bruised pain between the shoulder blades.
LIMBS	Foul-smelling foot sweats. Cold clammy feet. The toes and soles of the feet feel sore.

BETTER	WORSE
Walking in the open air	From the slightest exposure to cold/damp

BELLADONNA
Belladonna

Illnesses are typically of sudden onset and any pain tends to be throbbing. The patient may live in a world of his own with vivid, visual hallucinations. Delirium occurs during febrile illnesses and all the senses become acute, so any stimulus is intolerable.

MAIN MEDICAL USES

Acne rosacea
Acute fevers of sudden onset

Acute illnesses such as middle-ear infection, mastitis (breast infection) and tonsillitis

Boils
Chest infections
Congestive headaches
Delirium and hallucinations
Dental abscess
Erysipelas
Facial neuralgia
Febrile convulsions in children

Laryngitis
Nosebleeds
Restless and disturbed sleep
Urinary tract infections
Scarlet fever
Sciatica
Vertigo

MAJOR SYMPTOMS

HEAD	Throbbing frontal headache of sudden onset, worse lying down, from light, noise and jarring, and in the afternoon. Better for pressure. Vertigo, falling to the left or backwards.
FACE	Red, flushed and hot. Facial neuralgia with twitching muscles and flushing.
EYES	Dilated pupils, staring eyes. Red conjunctiva, dry, burning eyes with dislike of bright light.
EARS	Throbbing, very painful earache, with a fever.
NOSE	Frequent nosebleeds. Acute sense of smell.
MOUTH	The mouth and lips are dry. A typical 'strawberry' tongue develops. Grinding of the teeth, especially when asleep. Dental abscess.
THROAT	Red, dry and inflamed, worse on the right. Constricted feeling and swallowing is difficult.
LARYNX	Painful laryngitis.
CHEST	Dry, irritating cough, worse at night.
BREASTS	Mastitis with a throbbing, red, heavy and painful breast. Red streaks radiate from the nipple.

STOMACH	Great thirst for cold water but dread of drinking. Loss of appetite.
ABDOMEN	Distended and tender, worse for touch or jarring.
RECTUM	Piles.
STOOLS	Thin and green.
BLADDER	Normally frequent, profuse urination but the exact opposite (urinary retention) may occur.
GENITALIA	Dry, hot vagina.
PERIODS	Bearing-down sensation. The periods are early with a bright red, hot, profuse loss.
SKIN	The skin feels hot and dry and may show alternate redness and pallor. Pustular eruptions, tender to the touch. Burning, steaming heat of the body. No thirst, the feet feel icy cold. Sweats on covered parts of the body only.

BETTER

Resting in a semi-recumbent position

WORSE

For touch, jarring, noise
In a draught
Lying down
In the afternoon

BELLIS

Bellis perennis

This remedy, which resembles Arnica, is especially useful after major surgery involving the deeper tissues of the body.

MAIN MEDICAL USES

Acne	Diarrhoea
Boils	Sprains and bruises
Bruised soreness of the scalp, the breast and the pelvic region	Varicose veins in pregnancy
	Vertigo in the elderly

MAJOR SYMPTOMS

HEAD	Bruised soreness of the scalp with itching, worse from heat. Headache which radiates from the neck to the top of the head. Vertigo.
ABDOMEN	Soreness of the abdominal wall.
STOOLS	Yellow, painless diarrhoea with a foul odour, worse at night.
PREGNANCY	Difficulties in walking because of varicose veins. The womb feels sore, as if squeezed. Engorged breasts.
SKIN	Frequent boils. Acne. Varicose veins with a sore, bruised pain.

BETTER

No influencing factors

WORSE

From a hot bath or a warm bed
Before a storm
From cold winds
From cold bathing

BERBERIS
Berberis vulgaris

Pains tend to radiate. There is often a rapid alternation of symptoms, such as hunger alternating with loss of appetite, or thirst alternating with lack of thirst.

MAIN MEDICAL USES

Anal fissure, chronic
Eczema on the hands and
  around the anus
Gall-bladder disease
Gallstones
Gout, chronic
Headache
Kidney pain (renal colic,
  predominantly left-sided)

Kidney stones
Laryngeal polyps
Lumbago
Painful intercourse
Piles
Rheumatism
Vertigo
Warts

MAJOR SYMPTOMS

HEAD	Painful sensation of a tight cap pressing on the scalp. Frontal headaches. Cold sensation in the back of head and the spine. Vertigo with fainting.
FACE	Pale, sickly complexion with sunken cheeks and blue rings around the eyes.
EARS	Hard, gouty material forms in the external ear.
MOUTH	Diminished saliva. Sticky sensation in the mouth. The tongue feels scalded.
LARYNX	Hoarseness with polyps forming.
STOMACH	Nausea in the early morning.
ABDOMEN	Pain over the gall bladder, worse for pressure. Gall-bladder inflammation with jaundice and constipation.
STOOLS	Constant urge to defaecate. Painless, clay-coloured, burning and acrid diarrhoea. Anal fissure.
KIDNEYS	Colic with stitching and cutting pains that follow the course of the ureter into the bladder and urethra.
URINE	Burns when being passed, leaving a sensation immediately afterwards that some urine still remains in the bladder. Pains in the thighs and loins when urinating. The urine has a thick mucus and bright-red sediment.
GENITALIA	Burning and soreness in the vagina producing pain on intercourse.
BACK	Stitching pains in the neck and lower back. Numb, bruised sensation leading to difficulties in rising from sitting position.
LIMBS	Rheumatic pains in the shoulders, arms, hands and fingers, legs and feet. Neuralgic pain under the fingernails. The legs become extremely tired after walking only a short distance.
SKIN	Round, pigmented, itchy, eczematous patches, worse after scratching, better for cold applications. Eczema of the hands and anus. Flat warts.

BETTER	WORSE
In the open air	For motion and standing

BORAX
Borax

Patients have a great fear of downward motion and are generally extremely nervous and sensitive to sudden noises. They find it difficult to remain asleep after waking during the night because all the body, but especially the head, feels too hot. There is a fear of sudden noise, such as thunder.

MAIN MEDICAL USES

Chilblains
Dental abscess
Diarrhoea, especially in children
Erysipelas
Fear of downward motion, such
  as a plane landing or
  descending in a lift
Genital herpes
Genital itching in women
  (vulval pruritis) and eczema

Headache
Ingrowing eyelashes
Mouth ulcers
Painful periods
Psoriasis
Sterility
Vaginal discharge

MAJOR SYMPTOMS

HEAD — Headache with nausea and trembling.

EYES — The eyelashes grow inward, making the eye sore and red.

EARS — Great sensitivity to the slightest noise.

NOSE — Crusty and inflamed, with a bright red, shiny and swollen tip.

MOUTH — Ulcers make the mouth hot and tender; they may bleed when eating. Painful gumboil.

CHEST — Right-sided stitching pains, worse for coughing and deep breathing, Violent, hacking cough.

STOOLS — Loose, offensive, yellow or green, often preceded by colic.

URINE — Hot and burning. Urination is accompanied by shooting pains which make the patient (often a child) scream before passing water.

GENITALIA — Warm, profuse vaginal discharge which looks like the white of an egg. Vulval itching and eczema. Sterility.

PERIODS — Early and heavy, producing griping, nausea and stomach-ache which radiates to the small of the back.

SKIN — Wounds easily become infected. Psoriasis. Erysipelas, particularly on the face. Chilblains which feel better in the open air.

BETTER	WORSE
For pressure	With downward
In the evening	motion
For cold weather	From noise
	In warm weather
	After a period

237

BRYONIA
Bryonia alba

Patients are irritable and get angry over small matters; after losing their temper they feel cold. They become anxious very easily and worry about the future. There is a great desire for stillness, as all their complaints are made worse by movement. Typically, pains are stitching and mucous-membranes are dry. Bryonia children dislike being picked up and carried.

MAIN MEDICAL USES

Arthritis
Bronchitis, with or without
  pleurisy
Colds
Constipation
Feverish illness
Headache

Indigestion
Laryngitis
Mastitis
Nosebleeds
Sinusitis (especially frontal)
Tinnitus (noises in the ear)
Vertigo

MAJOR SYMPTOMS

HEAD — Right-sided, splitting headache, worse for any movement, even of the eyes. Frontal headache with sinusitis. Vertigo and nausea on rising. Greasy hair.

EARS — Tinnitus.

NOSE — Frequent bleeding when the period should start, but may also bleed in the early morning, relieving any headache that may be present. Colds with an aching forehead.

MOUTH — Parched, dry and cracked lips. The mouth and throat are dry, the tongue yellow or brown and coated. Foul, bitter taste in the mouth.

THROAT — Dry pain on swallowing. Tough mucus in the larynx and trachea which is difficult to shift. Worse going into a warm room.

CHEST — Dry, hacking cough with stitching chest pain relieved by firm pressure on the chest wall. The pain is worse for any movement, even breathing. The cough is worse on entering a warm room and from eating or drinking. Better if sitting upright.

STOMACH — Great thirst for long drinks. Nausea and faintness on rising. Vomiting after eating and after warm drinks. The stomach is tender and feels as if a stone is in it. Summer indigestion.

ABDOMEN — Tenderness over the liver, worse for pressure, coughing and deep breathing.

STOOLS — Constipation with dry, hard, dark, crumbling stools. Diarrhoea can occur in hot weather and after cold drinks.

PERIODS — Early, profuse and worse for movement. Suppressed periods lead to a headache. Pain in the right ovary. Accompanying breast pain that makes the breasts feel hot, hard and sore. Pain between periods.

BACK — Stiffness and stitching pains in the neck and lower back.

LIMBS — Red, swollen and hot joints, with stitching pains, worse on the slightest movement, and painful to pressure.

SKIN — Raised, itchy red rash all over the body.

BETTER	WORSE
Lying on the painful side	For any movement
For pressure on the pain	For warmth and in hot weather
For peace and quiet	For touch
With rest	Sitting up
For cold drinks	In the morning
For cool air and applications	

CACTUS

Cactus grandiflorus

There is an intermittent raised temperature which occurs at the same time every day, usually at its worst by midday. Patients may be melancholic, taciturn, sad and ill-humoured. Any pain that develops is so severe that it makes them scream and they are constantly frightened of dying. The tendency to bleed can affect any organ.

MAIN MEDICAL USES

Angina	Painful periods
Colds	Palpitations
Constipation with piles	Piles
Facial neuralgia	Restless leg syndrome
Headache	Tendency to bleed
Heart conditions	Thyroid gland over-activity
Nosebleeds	Urine retention
Painful intercourse	Vaginal spasm

MAJOR SYMPTOMS

HEAD	Headache if a meal is missed. Congestive headache, making the head feel as if about to burst.
FACE	Right-sided facial pain at the same time each day.
NOSE	Frequent and profuse nosebleeds.
THROAT	Sensation of constriction in the throat.
CHEST	Feels constricted and breathing becomes difficult. Palpitations with left-sided chest pain that radiates to the left arm and is accompanied by a cold sweat and a feeling of suffocation. The heart is weak due to smoking, over-exertion in athletes and arteriosclerosis in the elderly. Violent palpitations with vertigo, flatulence and shortage of breath, worse lying on the left side and before a period.
STOOLS	Morning diarrhoea, or constipation with hard, black stools and swollen, painful piles.
BLADDER	Retention of urine due to constriction of the bladder neck. Urgent desire to pass urine at night.
GENITALIA	Vaginal spasm leads to pain on intercourse.
PERIODS	With pulsating pain. The period is early, the loss, very dark.
LIMBS	Icy-cold hands, restless legs and numbness in the left arm. Swollen hands and feet.

BETTER	WORSE
In the open air	About noon
	Lying on the left side
	For exertion

CALC CARB
Calcarea carbonica-ostrearum

Patients are apprehensive and fear mental illness; they can be forgetful and confused. Anxiety may bring on palpitations. Children who need this remedy are usually slow to develop, slow to learn and may be characterized as 'fair, fat and flabby'.

MAIN MEDICAL USES

Anxiety and nervous apprehension	Gall-bladder colic due to stones
Bed-wetting	Growth disorders in children
Circulatory disorders	Kidney stones and pain
Colds	Middle-ear infection
Corneal ulcers	Piles
Diarrhoea in children	Polyps (nose, ears, uterus, etc.)
Digestive disorders	Premature ejaculation
Enlarged lymph glands	Rheumatism
Fatigue (mental or physical) due to overwork	Teeth eruption delayed
	Tonsillitis
	Vaginal discharge

MAJOR SYMPTOMS

HEAD — Headache from mental exertion or overlifting, with cold hands and feet, better after sneezing. An icy-cold sensation both in and outside the head, mainly on the right. The head sweats excessively at night in bed and soaks the pillow.

EYES — Corneal ulcers with light sensitivity and itchy, dry lids. The eyes tire easily.

EARS — Discharge containing mucus and pus, with enlarged glands, worse in the cold. Deteriorating hearing. Cracking noises in the ears. Polyps, which bleed easily, form in the ear.

NOSE — Sore and ulcerated nostrils. Frequent colds with every weather change. Nasal polyps.

MOUTH — Sour taste with hot, offensive breath. The tongue is dry at night and the tip burns. Bleeding gums. Toothache worse for hot or cold. Delay in the teeth erupting in children.

THROAT — Frequent tonsillitis. Swallowing is difficult and painful. Painless hoarseness, which is worse in the morning.

CHEST — Shortage of breath, much worse climbing stairs. The chest wall is sensitive to touch or pressure. Tickling night cough.

STOMACH — Heartburn with loud belching. Stomach cramp, worse for pressure and cold drinks. Craving for indigestible things (such as chalk or coal) and for eggs, salt and sweets. Frequent sour belching with the vomiting of sour fluid. Dislike of fat. Milk disagrees. Overwork leads to loss of appetite.

ABDOMEN — Distended with intolerance of tight clothes around the waist. Gallstone colic.

RECTUM/ANUS — Burning, stinging piles. Anal prolapse.

STOOLS — Large, hard, white, watery and sour, or diarrhoea with undigested food particles in it.

GENITALIA — *Men:* Premature ejaculation.

Women: Vulval burning and itching, with tender swollen breasts before a period. White milky vaginal discharge.

PERIODS   Early and the loss is profuse and prolonged. Vertigo, toothache and cold, damp feet accompany the period.

LIMBS   The feet are cold and damp and the soles raw. Rheumatism with sharp, sticking pains after exposure to the wet. Cold knees. Cramps in the calves. Fevers start with a temperature rise and stomach symptoms around 2 a.m. and are accompanied by sweating. Profuse night sweats particularly on the head, neck and chest.

BETTER	WORSE
In a dry climate	From any exertion
Lying on the painful side	From anything cold
If constipated	From anything wet

CALC PHOS
Calcarea phosphorica

Patients can be peevish and forgetful. They always seem wanting to go elsewhere and their symptoms are worse when they think about them.

MAIN MEDICAL USES

Adenoid and tonsil enlargement
Adolescent acne and headaches
Anaemia in children
Colic
Debility after an acute illness

Non-union of fractures in the elderly
Teething disorders in babies
Tiredness and irritability

MAJOR SYMPTOMS

HEAD   Headaches in school children, worse at weather changes, often with abdominal distension.

MOUTH   The teeth develop slowly and decay easily. The mouth becomes painful to open.

THROAT   The tonsils and adenoids become enlarged.

STOMACH   Babies and older children have frequent vomiting attacks. Flatulence can become excessive. Craving for bacon, ham and salted or smoked meats. Great hunger and thirst relieved by sour belching.

ABDOMEN   Colic occurs every time the patient attempts to eat. The abdominal wall appears sunken and flabby.

STOOLS   Diarrhoea with teething, the stool is green, hot and spluttering with offensive, fetid wind. Hard stools can also occur and lead to rectal bleeding.

GENITALIA   A vaginal discharge, like the white of an egg, is heaviest in the morning.

PERIODS   The periods are either early and profuse, or late and dark, with severe backache.

LIMBS   Stiffness and pain in the limbs, with a cold, numb feeling, worse if the weather changes.

BETTER	WORSE
In the summer	After cold, damp weather
In a warm, dry atmosphere	

CALENDULA
Calendula officinalis

Calendula is a superb antiseptic and healing agent and may be used locally, either in ointment form or as a mother tincture, which should be diluted before application.

MAIN MEDICAL USES

Bleeding after tooth extraction
Erysipelas
Infected and discharging ulcers

Lacerations, especially of
  the scalp
Superficial burns and scalds
Wounds of all kinds

CAMPHOR
Camphora

This remedy is useful in cases of collapse with icy coldness and pain, which improves for thinking about it.

MAIN MEDICAL USES

Asthma
Cholera
Colds or flu (first stages)
Collapse
Measles, after-effects

Persistent nosebleeds
Prolonged erection without
  stimulation
Urine retention
Vertigo

MAJOR SYMPTOMS

HEAD	Vertigo with a feeling of dying. Headache, with catarrh and sneezing, in influenza. The nose is icy cold. Stitching pains behind the eyes and in the temple region. Throbbing pains occur at the back of the head.
FACE	Blue with cold, covered in a cold sweat and with an anxious expression.
NOSE	Colds with sudden weather changes. Nosebleeds, especially when the patient is cold.
CHEST	Violent, dry, hacking cough with suffocative shortage of breath. The exhaled breath feels cold.
LIMBS	Numbness with tingling coldness. The body feels icy cold. Cramps in the calves. Icy-cold feet. Rheumatic pains may develop between the shoulder blades.
SKIN	Cold, pale and blue, but the patient cannot bear to be covered up.
SLEEP	Insomnia because of feeling so cold.

BETTER	WORSE
For warmth	For motion
	At night
	From cold air

CANTHARIS
Cantharis

Patients may show marked anger and irritability. Acute mania associated with sexual overtones can develop. Paroxysms of rage and crying with a barking cough occur, especially after drinking water.

MAIN MEDICAL USES

Blistery skin eruptions	Dysentery
Burning sensations anywhere in the body	Fainting tendency
	Gastric upsets in pregnancy
Burns and scalds	Mouth ulcers
Cystitis	Sunburn

MAJOR SYMPTOMS

HEAD — Burning sensation in the mouth, throat and pharynx, with difficulty in swallowing liquids.

TONGUE — Furred and covered in small blisters.

STOMACH — Burning thirst but with an aversion to all drinks. Food and drink disgust.

ABDOMEN — Inflammation anywhere in the digestive tract, but especially in the lower bowel.

STOOLS — Bloody, hot and loose, with shivering after defaecation.

URINE — An intolerable, constant urge to urinate. The urine scalds, may be blood-stained and is passed drop by drop.

GENITALIA — *Men:* Strong sexual desires and painful erections.

Women: Nymphomania.

SKIN — Blistery eruptions. The skin itches and burns.

BETTER

For warm applications and rubbing

WORSE

When drinking, especially water or coffee
While urinating
From being touched

CARBO VEG
Carbo vegetabilis

There is a well-marked fear, or strong dislike of, the dark and a fear of ghosts. Patients are typically sluggish, fat and lazy, and may be subject to sudden memory losses.

MAIN MEDICAL USES

Asthma, especially in the elderly	Headache from over-indulgence in food or drink
Bedsores	Hoarseness
Chilblains	Mouth ulcers
Collapse (blue and cold with cold sweat)	Nosebleeds
	Piles
Extreme debility following a previous illness	Spasmodic cough
	Stomach ulcers
Flatulence and indigestion	Varicose veins
Gums bleed when cleaning teeth	Whooping cough (very early stages)
Hair loss	

MAJOR SYMPTOMS

HEAD — The scalp itches when warm in bed. The head feels heavy and constricted, the scalp sore and hair loss occurs.

FACE — Puffy, pale or mottled; feels cold, with a cold sweat.

EARS — Ear discharge, particularly after measles.

NOSE — Regular daily nosebleeds eventually produce pallor and anaemia.

MOUTH — The tongue is white or yellow/brown and covered in ulcers. The teeth feel sore while eating and the gums bleed easily.

CHEST	Hoarseness and voice loss, worse in the evening and from talking. Cough, with a burning sensation in the chest. Itching feeling in the larynx. Wheezing and rattling of mucus and a feeling of suffocation, worse in the evening, in the open air, after eating and from talking. The patient feels unable to get enough air and consequently likes to be fanned.
STOMACH	A faint feeling when hungry is not relieved by eating. Cramp and pain, relieved by bending double, comes on about half an hour after eating. Sour or putrid belching as digestion is slow. Aversion to milk, meat and fat.
ABDOMEN	Distension, with much wind being passed.
LIMBS	Tendency to feel heavy and 'go to sleep'. The legs feel cold from the knees downwards. Cramps in the soles of the feet. Chilblains of the toes, which become red and swollen.
SKIN	Blue and cold (marble-like). Itching, worse in the evening and when warm in bed. The sweat feels hot.

BETTER	WORSE
For being fanned	In the evening and at night
	In the open air
	From fat food, coffee and wine
	In warm, damp weather

CAULOPHYLLUM
Caulophyllum

Given in the last few months of pregnancy, Caulophyllum tones the uterus and may lead to an easier labour.

MAIN MEDICAL USES

During the later stages of pregnancy	Rheumatism, especially in the smaller joints
Painful periods	

MAJOR SYMPTOMS

HEAD	Headache associated with a period, worse on stooping.
STOMACH	Vomiting associated with the periods.
GENITALIA	Acrid vaginal discharge, especially in young girls.
PERIODS	Pains are cramping and violent. The loss is slight.
LIMBS	Rheumatism in the small joints (fingers, toes, ankles, wrists), with aching, drawing or cutting pains.

CAUSTICUM
Causticum

Causticum patients tend to be morose, apprehensive, absent-minded people. Children are slow in learning to walk and talk, while the elderly are weak and anaemic, having no desire or ability to undertake anything either mental or physical.

MAIN MEDICAL USES

Bed-wetting in children	Rheumatism
Bell's palsy	Sciatica
Constipation	Skin scars after burns or wounding
Eyelid inflammation	Stress incontinence (involuntary
Incontinence of urine	passing of urine)
Laryngitis, chronic and acute	Tinnitus (noises in the ear)
Paralysis of the upper eyelid	Verrucas
Piles	Vertigo
Restless leg syndrome	

MAJOR SYMPTOMS

FACE	Rheumatism of the lower jaw makes eating difficult. Facial neuralgia from cold air.
EYES	The lids close involuntarily, as the upper lids feel heavy. Weakness or paralysis of the upper lids, especially after, or even with, a cold. The lids become inflamed and there is a sensation of sand under them.
EARS	Deterioration of hearing, with roaring sounds in the ear and re-echoing of words spoken.
NOSE	Dry catarrhal conditions, with frequent sneezing and a stopped-up feeling.
THROAT	Total or partial inability to speak due to paralysis of the vocal cords. Hoarseness, worse in the morning and in the evening. Mucus is difficult to get up, so it is swallowed.
CHEST	Nervous cough, with involuntary spurting of urine, worse in a warm bed, better for sips of cold water.
RECTUM	Frequent, sudden, piercing rectal pain. Frequent and ineffectual urging to defaecate; it is easier to pass the stool when partially standing. Piles which produce sore pain on walking.
URINE	Bed-wetting in children immediately after falling asleep. Involuntary passing of urine when coughing, sneezing, blowing the nose and during sleep. Retention of urine after labour or an operation.
BACK/ LIMBS	Drawing, bruised pain in the region of the coccyx. Tearing pains in the joints which flit from joint to joint. Weakness and trembling in the limbs.

BETTER	WORSE
From cold drinks	In cold, dry winds
From draughts	In a humid, hot environment
	At 3–4 a.m.

CHAMOMILLA

Chamomilla

Patients needing Chamomilla are peevish, impatient, angry, whining, changeable and restless. Any pain they get seems intolerable.

MAIN MEDICAL USES

Anal fissure	Insomnia
Angry, intolerant adults	Piles
Colic	Teething in children
Diarrhoea	Tinnitus (noises in the ear)
Fever	Unbearable pain
Headache	

245

MAJOR SYMPTOMS

HEAD	Throbbing headache, with a hot, clammy sweat on the forehead and scalp.
FACE	Convulsive movements of the face and lip muscles, with stitching pain extending to the ear. One cheek is hot and red, the other cold and pale.
EARS	Violent shooting pains in the ears. Hearing is acute. Ringing tinnitus.
NOSE	Nasal irritation, causing frequent sneezing. The nose feels blocked.
MOUTH	Intolerable toothache made worse by warm drinks but better for ice-cold water.
LARYNX	Feels raw and produces tough mucus which is hard to move.
CHEST	Whistling, wheezing and rattling in the trachea, which produces a dry, night cough, worse around midnight.
STOMACH	Stitching pain in the pit of the stomach, with frequent, foul belching. Acute indigestion brought on by anger. Nausea after coffee. Sweats after eating or drinking.
ABDOMEN	Cutting pains with marked flatulence may extend into the chest. Griping, tearing pain in the navel area goes through to the small of the back. Flatulent colic with flushed cheeks and hot perspiration.
RECTUM	Piles and anal fissure.
STOOLS	Diarrhoea from anger and at teething. Hot, green, slimy, watery stools.
BLADDER	Women feel a frequent urge to urinate.

GENITALIA	*Men:* Increased libido.
	Women: Yellow, acrid, vaginal discharge.
PERIODS	With labour-like pain and profuse, dark clots of blood. Suppression of the period brought on by anger.
LIMBS	The joints feel sore and bruised and there is cracking in the joints, especially the legs. The hands and feet feel weak. Violent rheumatic pains during the night.

BETTER	WORSE
When being carried	Lying in bed
In warm, wet	From anger
weather	In the evening

CHELIDONIUM
Chelidonium majus

The patient is sluggish, bilious and lazy, with weariness and weakness.

MAIN MEDICAL USES

Liver complaints, including jaundice

MAJOR SYMPTOMS

HEAD	Right-sided headache which extends down the neck to the shoulder. The head feels heavy.
FACE	Yellow discoloration, worse around the nose and cheeks.

EYES	Neuralgic pain over the right eye with profuse tears. The whites of the eyes look dirty and yellow.
MOUTH	The tongue is yellow, with a red margin which has an imprint of the teeth. The saliva tastes bitter, as do food and drink.
CHEST	Cough soon after waking. Much sputum, which is difficult to get up.
STOMACH	Indigestion, nausea and vomiting relieved by hot water. Hot drinks and hot food are preferred. Pain from the stomach goes through to the back and the right shoulder blade, temporarily relieved by eating.
ABDOMEN	Jaundice due to liver and gall-bladder disease. The liver is tender and pain goes through to the right shoulder blade, then down and across the navel area. Discomfort is worse from the pressure of clothes.
STOOLS	Copious and bright yellow, with much mucus. They may also be pasty, watery, slimy, or hard and grey. Diarrhoea or constipation may occur.
URINE	Varies from dark yellow to dark brown.
BACK	Sticking pain beneath the right shoulder blade goes through the chest to the breastbone.
LIMBS	The tips of the fingers are icy cold. Rheumatic pains in the hips and thighs. Painful heels.
SKIN	The whole body itches. The skin is dry and yellow. Painful red pimples and pustules.

BETTER

For eating hot food

WORSE

For motion
For weather change
At 4 a.m. and 4 p.m.

CHINA
(or Cinchona)

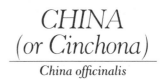

China officinalis

Patients are excitable, have an intolerance of noise, and sudden screaming bouts may interrupt a more cheerful mood. They worry over trifles, are discouraged easily, discontented, disinclined to mental work and have a slow flow of ideas. Hands and feet are cold, as is the skin, which is very sensitive to touch, although hard pressure helps. They sweat excessively during sleep and their illnesses return at regular intervals.

MAIN CLINICAL SYMPTOMS

Debility following feverish illnesses	Headache
	Hearing defects
Debility following fluid loss (e.g. haemorrhage, diarrhoea)	Indigestion
	Night sweats
Distension	Nosebleeds
Gallstone colic	Tinnitus (noises in the ear)
Gout, chronic	

MAJOR SYMPTOMS

HEAD	Throbbing, violent, bursting headache, worse in the temples and aggravated in the open air, by bright light, noise and odours. It is helped by binding the head tight. The scalp is hypersensitive to touch.
EARS	Defective or deteriorating hearing. Tinnitus, ringing or roaring in the ears.
EYES	Deterioration of vision.
NOSE	Acuteness of smell. Nosebleeds. Violent, dry sneezing.

LARYNX	Feels as if full of mucus.
CHEST	Cough caused by laughing and after eating. Suffocative attacks, worse towards evening.
STOMACH	The appetite varies but generally there is an indifference to eating and drinking, or a ravenous hunger. Indigestion after eating, with belching, distension and drowsiness. Craving for sour, pungent, spicy food. The distension is so marked that palpitations and shortage of breath may occur. Digestion is very slow.
ABDOMEN	Distension after eating fruit. Rumbling, with offensive wind, worse 6–10 p.m. Pressure over the liver when standing improves when bending forward. Gall-bladder colic from stones.
STOOLS	Painless diarrhoea after eating. Frequent, ineffectual urging with biting, burning rectal pain.
PERIODS	Profuse and early, with pain, dark clots and abdominal distension. Blood-stained vaginal discharge between and before the periods. Fainting may accompany the period.
BACK	Pain as if there is pressure on the lower back. Cramp-like pain in the small of the back, much worse on movement. The spine is very sensitive to touch and the pain shoots into the head.

BETTER	WORSE
For hard pressure	For the loss of any
In the open air	body fluids
For warmth	If touched gently
	For draughts

CICUTA
Cicuta virosa

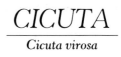

Between epileptic attacks patients may be melancholic, mistrustful and indifferent. After an attack there may be confusion about time and laughter for no apparent reason.

MAIN MEDICAL USES

Chronic effects of concussion
Convulsions
Eczema without itching
Epilepsy

Neck pain with restricted movement due to disc degeneration

Convulsions and epilepsy require medical attention.

MAJOR SYMPTOMS

HEAD	Jerking movements of the head accompanied by vertigo. Stupefying pain in the forehead, worse for rest. Tearing pain in the back of the head (occiput) followed by a feeling of exhaustion.
FACE	Red face accompanied by violent hiccoughs, which make breathing difficult.
EYES	Staring gaze, with large, dilated pupils.
STOMACH	Stomach-ache may precede an epileptic attack.
BACK	During convulsions the back may be bent backwards. Pain in the coccygeal area at the start of a period, especially if it comes late.
LIMBS	Violent, convulsive, distorted movements.
SKIN	Eczema without itching, particularly on the scalp. Hard, bright yellow crusts form.

BETTER	WORSE
For warmth	For even a light
For quiet	touch
	For smoking
	From a draught

CIMICIFUGA
(or Actaea racemosa)
Cimicifuga racemosa

Patients are incoherently loquacious, passing from subject to subject without stop. A restless body and a restless mind. They may be grieved, troubled, sighing, miserable or dejected but these emotions alternate with joy and playfulness. Subjects tend to be fearful of death and insanity, and visual and tactile hallucinations may occur.

MAIN MEDICAL USES

Angina	Periods, heavy, irregular
Muscular rheumatism	or painful
Pains during and after labour	Tendon inflammation

MAJOR SYMPTOMS

HEAD — Headache starting in the back of the head and extending to the top, made worse by bending the head forward. The headache can occur with the periods, the menopause or with a hangover.

EYES — Pain in the eyeball. The eyes become congested during a headache.

HEART — Pain over the heart, with palpitations and pain radiating to the left arm. Often associated with rheumatism or uterine disorders.

GENITALIA — Pain in the uterus shoots across the pelvis, and upwards.

PERIODS — May be profuse and early, or scanty and delayed. The pain is worse with a heavy loss, but better with a slight loss.

BACK — Rheumatic pains in the neck and back, with stiffness and tightness. Tenderness over the first three dorsal vertebrae, especially in the morning.

LIMBS — Muscular pains feel like an electric shock, or are cramp-like, with stiffness and twitching. Pain in the Achilles tendon at the ankle.

BETTER	WORSE
For warmth	During periods

CINA
Cina

Often the patient is a sullen, cross, obstinate and ill-humoured child who refuses to be touched or looked at. Typically, he wants something, but throws it away when received and demands something else.

MAIN MEDICAL USES

Abdominal migraine	Bulimia which may alternate
Anal itching	with anorexia
Behaviour disorders, children	Convulsions
Bronchitis	Whooping cough
	Worms

MAJOR SYMPTOMS

HEAD — Severe frontal headache, worse in the open air, extends from over the eye into the skull. May alternate with abdominal pain.

FACE — Alternately flushed and pale, with a bluish pallor around the mouth and dark rings around the eyes.

NOSE — Itching is so bad, that attempts to relieve it by picking result in a nosebleed.

MOUTH — Grinding of the teeth during sleep.

CHEST — Violent, hoarse, hacking cough, worse in the morning after rising. In the evening the cough comes in paroxysms and gurgling may be heard going down the throat. The patient is pale, anxious and clutches at his throat.

STOMACH — Considerable hunger, even after eating. Likes a very varied diet. Indigestion on waking and before a meal.

ABDOMEN — Cramp-like or pinching pains after eating, especially around the navel. Helped by lying on the stomach.

LIMBS — Convulsions, especially at night.

BETTER	**WORSE**
Lying on the abdomen	At night
	If touched or looked at

COCCULUS
Cocculus indicus

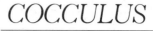

This remedy is suited to sad, sensitive individuals, offended by everything. They are absorbed in themselves, their minds seem benumbed, they cannot think or express themselves and cannot bear contradiction. Time passes too quickly.

MAIN MEDICAL USES

Flatulent colic during pregnancy	Period pain
Insomnia	Rheumatism
Nausea and vomiting during pregnancy	Travel sickness
	Vertigo
	Weakness and debility

MAJOR SYMPTOMS

HEAD — Sick headache, with vertigo as a constant accompaniment, caused by worry, loss of sleep, overworking and travelling. Vertigo from any cause is often associated with a dull pain across the forehead.

STOMACH — Aversion to food, even to the smell of it. Eating and drinking aggravate all other symptoms.

ABDOMEN — Distension and flatulence cause pain and wake the patient around midnight. Relief from lying on either side. Flatulent colic, especially during pregnancy.

PERIODS — Cutting, contracting pelvic pain, with a feeling of overall weakness.

BACK/ LIMBS — Trembling of the hands when eating, worse the higher the hand is raised. The arms and hands 'go to sleep'. The knees threaten to give way due to weakness and the patient totters when attempting to walk. Paralytic pains develop in the small of the back. The shoulders and arms hurt, as if bruised.

MAJOR SYMPTOMS

HEAD	Sharp piercing pain, worse in the open air.
FACE	Dry with red cheeks.
MOUTH	Intolerable toothache relieved by cold water.
STOMACH	Unable to wear tight clothes around the waist.
PERIODS	Prolonged with dark clots, especially on the first day.
PREGNANCY	After-pains in nervous, excitable women.

BETTER

No influencing factors

WORSE

From loss of sleep
From emotional disturbance
From cigarette smoke
From the motion of travel
In the open air
After eating
From touch, noise and jarring

BETTER

For lying down
For warmth

WORSE

From noise, touch and mental exertion
From cold
In the open air
From narcotics, alcohol, coffee
From excessive emotional stimulation

COFFEA
Coffea cruda

The ability to think seems enhanced, ideas flow, the memory is improved but great anguish may also be present. Restlessness and sleeplessness due to the activity of the brain occurs, thoughts can be pleasant but may sometimes be sad. Hysteria, with repeated attacks of weeping alternating with laughter, may result from pleasurable emotions.

COLOCYNTH
Colocynthis

Typical of this remedy is the person who is easily angered and has a quick, irritable temper, sedentary women with heavy periods and those of either sex who are overweight. Most symptoms relating to this remedy are in the head and abdomen, and severe neuralgia is prominent among them.

MAIN MEDICAL USES

After-pains in pregnancy
Headache
Insomnia

Toothache
Vulval and vaginal hypersensitivity

MAIN MEDICAL USES

Diarrhoea	Kidney pain
Facial neuralgia	Period pain
Gall-bladder pain	Sciatica
Headache	Vertigo
Intestinal colic	

MAJOR SYMPTOMS

HEAD Severe headache, which may be a boring, burning pain in the right temple region or in the left orbit, relieved by warmth and pressure. Vertigo on turning the head quickly.

FACE Neuralgia, especially on left, relieved by pressure.

EYES Cutting pains in the eyeballs made worse by stooping. The lids may twitch.

ABDOMEN Distension, with agonizing colic relieved by pressure and bending forward, passing a stool or the discharge of wind. Eating fruit and walking make the pain worse.

STOOLS Fluid and aggravated by eating and drinking. Thin, frothy, yellow, musty and offensive diarrhoea from anger, from fruit and from ice-cold drinks taken when the body is overheated.

URINE Frequent urges to urinate but only small quantities are passed. Left-sided kidney pain (very occasionally right-sided).

GENITALIA Cramp-like pains in the left ovary and the uterus, which feel as if clamped in a vice.

PERIODS Suppressed, with cramping pain helped by bending double.

BACK Paroxysms of acute pain in the pelvis, lower back and hips, relieved by flexing the thighs or the pelvis.

LIMBS Cramp in the left thigh and pains from the hip to the knee, better for sitting, lying on the left side and warmth.

BETTER	WORSE
For rest	From anger and
For hard pressure	indigestion
For warmth	From motion
For bending forward	From eating and
	drinking
	In the evening and at
	night

CONIUM

Conium maculatum

Patients suffer an inability to sustain mental effort, difficulties in understanding, loss of memory, an aversion to being near people and anxiety with great guilt. Excitement may lead to depression.

MAIN MEDICAL USES

Coughs	Impotence with increased
Complaints associated with	sexual desire
old age	Mastitis
Headache	Vertigo

MAJOR SYMPTOMS

HEAD — Headache on waking in the morning, feeling of the brain being too large for the skull and therefore bursting. Vertigo on turning the head, whether lying or standing. Sharp pain in the back of the head on rising in the morning. A feeling of numbness and coldness in or on the side of the head remains for hours after the headache goes.

EYES — Extreme sensitivity to light, with excessive tears.

LARYNX — Sensation of a dry spot in the larynx which causes a dry, hacking cough.

CHEST — Nervous night cough in old people.

BREASTS — Heavy and painful before and during periods. At other times they are lax and shrunken, but may become enlarged and tender, with hard lumps (*see a doctor urgently*).

BLADDER — Frequent urination, sometimes involuntary. The urine flows in fits and starts.

GENITALIA — *Men:* Increased sexual desire but without being able to achieve an erection. Sexual nervousness. Enlarged hard testicles (*see a doctor urgently*).

Women: Itching deep in the vagina, with a discharge about ten days before the period and colic just before it starts. The period is delayed or even suppressed. Sharp ovarian pain (*see a doctor urgently*).

LIMBS — Muscular weakness, especially in the legs.

BETTER

For fasting
In the dark
For letting limbs hang down
For motion
For pressure

WORSE

Lying down
Turning in bed
From celibacy
With physical or mental exertion
Before/during periods
From getting cold

CUPRUM MET

Cuprum metallicum

The patient may show an incoherence of speech, confusion and poor memory.

MAIN MEDICAL USES

Asthma
Catarrh
Cramps and colics
Epilepsy
Facial neuralgia
Gastro-enteritis

Hiccoughs
Muscle cramps
Sinusitis
Vertigo
Whooping cough

MAJOR SYMPTOMS

HEAD — Headache, worse for movement, often accompanied by vomiting and with vertigo on looking up. Sensation of cold water being poured over the head. Catarrhal headache with frontal sinusitis.

FACE — Blue with blue lips (cyanosis). Spasms of the jaw. Facial neuralgia with stinging, burning pain.

MOUTH	Strong metallic taste.
THROAT	Audible gurgling as fluid is swallowed. Spasm of the pharynx and oesophagus produces a paroxysmal cough with intense pain behind the breastbone on swallowing. Hoarseness.
CHEST	Fatiguing, short, violent, dry, spasmodic cough, worse at night (11 p.m.–1 a.m.) and worse when sitting. Respiration may be difficult, with a suffocative loss of breath and palpitations.
STOMACH	Loss of appetite. Hiccoughs with ineffectual retching. Cramp-like pains, with griping and pressure, then vomiting.
ABDOMEN	Tense, hot and tender. Colic and spasm with vomiting. Intense thirst for warm drinks, but better for cold ones.
STOOLS	Violent diarrhoea, watery stools with flakes.
LIMBS	Cramps, convulsive movements, contractions of fingers and toes, clenched thumbs. Force may be needed to open the hand. Shuddering and chilliness, the skin is bluish but not cold. Violent cramps in the calves and feet, especially at night and in elderly people.

BETTER

For drinking cold
water

WORSE

Before the periods
After vomiting
From touch or
pressure

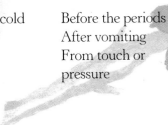

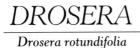

DROSERA
Drosera rotundifolia

MAIN MEDICAL USES

Cough	Osteo-arthritis, especially of the hip and ankle
Laryngitis	Vertigo
Nosebleeds	Whooping cough

MAJOR SYMPTOMS

HEAD	Vertigo, falling to the left, worse outdoors. Cold left side and hot right side of the face.
NOSE	Bleeding brought on by violent coughing.
THROAT	Hoarse and deep voice with a rough, scraping sensation at the back of the throat.
LARYNX	Feels as if being tickled.
CHEST	Violent, dry, tearing, irritating cough in short, frequent bursts, so close that they make breathing difficult. The phlegm is yellow. The cough is worse in bed and after midnight and can lead to chest and abdominal pain, better for firm pressure.
LIMBS	Pain in the hip joint and legs, with stiffness in the ankles and feet. Better for movement.

BETTER

For movement

WORSE

After midnight
Lying down
From a warm bed
From laughing/singing

DULCAMARA
Dulcamara

Typically fat and flabby, the patient may show some confusion.

MAIN MEDICAL USES

Colds	Rheumatism
Diarrhoea	Snuffles in babies
Facial neuralgia	Swollen lymph glands
Hay fever	Warts

MAJOR SYMPTOMS

HEAD	Brown crusts on the scalp, which bleed when scratched.
FACE	Facial neuralgia from being in the cold.
EYES	Profuse, watery discharge during hay fever, which is worse in the open air.
NOSE	Feels blocked when the weather is cold and rainy.
CHEST	Cough, either dry or productive, is worse in cold, wet weather and during the winter. Cough following physical exertion.
STOMACH	Aversion to food and an excessive thirst for cold drinks.
STOOLS	Diarrhoea with mucus in damp, cold conditions. The motion is green-yellow.
BLADDER	Increased urge to pass urine when cold.
PERIODS	Generalized skin rash just before periods.
LIMBS	Muscular rheumatism, worse in the cold damp, may alternate with diarrhoea or follow acute skin eruptions.
SKIN	Itchy, moist skin eruptions, which crust over and bleed if scratched. Swollen lymph glands with the rash. Large, smooth, warty eruptions on the hands and face.

BETTER	**WORSE**
For movement	From damp cold of
For external warmth	any causation
	At night

EUPATORIUM
Eupatorium perfoliatum

There may be sluggishness throughout the body, but the patient may show signs of agitation.

MAIN MEDICAL USES

Bone pain	Hiccoughs
Headache	Influenza

MAJOR SYMPTOMS

HEAD	Throbbing headache on the top and back of the head, with a sensation of pressure.
EYES	With headache, the eyes feel sore.
CHEST	Hoarseness, loose cough and soreness of the chest wall accompany influenza.

| STOMACH | Vomiting of bile with the headache. Great thirst for cold drinks. |
| BACK/ LIMBS | Aching pain in the back and in the limb bones, accompanied by soreness and stiffness. |

BETTER	**WORSE**
No influencing factors	From movement

EUPHRASIA

Euphrasia

This remedy is used almost exclusively for eye complaints.

MAIN MEDICAL USES

Colds	Hay fever
Conjunctivitis	Measles

MAJOR SYMPTOMS

HEAD	Catarrhal headache.
EYES	Profuse discharge, sometimes watery, sometimes thick, but always acrid. The lids burn and swell and the cornea feels as if covered with mucus which obscures the vision. To remove it the patient blinks frequently.
NOSE	Profuse, fluent, bland colds with a loose, hacking cough.
SKIN	Used in the early stages of measles if there are eye symptoms.

BETTER	**WORSE**
In the dark	In sunlight or bright light
For wiping eyes	In warm wind or a warm room

FERRUM MET

Ferrum metallicum

Anaemia is a major feature. Ferrum met individuals are chilly, irritable, cannot accept any opposition and find the slightest noise unbearable. They look pale and any exertion, even speaking, is an effort.

MAIN MEDICAL USES

Diarrhoea	Involuntary urination
Eating disorders (anorexia and bulimia)	Rheumatism
	Toothache
Headache	Vertigo

MAJOR SYMPTOMS

HEAD	Headache after a period; the head feels hot, the feet cold. A hammering, beating, pulsating headache with a hot, red face. Accompanied by vertigo. Vertigo also when looking at flowing water.
MOUTH	Toothache relieved by ice-cold water.
STOMACH	The appetite is variable and can alternate between anorexia and bulimia. Vomiting immediately after eating, or around midnight. Meat and eggs disagree.

STOOLS — Watery and painless with flatulence. Most frequent during or after eating or drinking.

URINE — Involuntary passage of urine, especially in women, when sneezing or coughing.

GENITALIA — Milky, corrosive vaginal discharge with swelling of the vagina and a smarting pain during intercourse.

BACK — Bruised lower-back pain. Soreness in the small of the back on rising.

LIMBS — Shooting, tearing pain from the shoulder down the arm, especially the left. Better for gentle movement. Cramps in the feet and toes.

BETTER	WORSE
For slow walks	For sitting still and immobility
For warmth	From cold (except toothache)
	At night, around midnight

FERRUM PHOS

Ferrum phosphoricum

Nervous, sensitive, anaemic patients with a susceptibility to chest infections. The pulse is rapid and the temperature high with any infection.

MAIN MEDICAL USES

Bronchitis	Conjunctivitis
Colds	Eyeball pain

Feverish illnesses	Rheumatism
Incontinence of urine	Tinnitus (noises in the ear)
Increased heart-rate	Tonsillitis
Indigestion	Vaginal dryness
Middle-ear infection	Whooping cough
Nosebleeds	

MAJOR SYMPTOMS

HEAD — Violent throbbing headache, better after a nosebleed and often occurring just before or during a period. The head and scalp are sore to the touch, better for a cold application.

EYES — Red, burning and painful.

EARS — Ringing and buzzing with deterioration of hearing. Acute infection of the ear with redness and soreness over the mastoid bone.

NOSE — Nosebleeds. Early stages of a cold.

THROAT — Ulcerated sore throat. Acute infection of the tonsils. Sore throat in singers.

CHEST — Acute, short, painful, spasmodic cough, worse in the open air and at night. Sharp stitching pains on deep breathing. Whooping cough, with hoarseness or complete voice loss.

HEART — A full, bounding pulse with a dull, aching pain about the heart, which extends to the spine.

STOMACH — Irregular vomiting of bile-stained fluid, with a poor appetite. Pain in the stomach after eating and from pressure.

URINE — Urine spurts on coughing. Incontinence.

GENITALIA *Men:* A dull ache in the testicles may indicate the start of an inflammation (*see a doctor*). Frequent desire to pass urine, with pain in the urethra.

Women: Dry, sore vagina.

PERIODS Frequent profuse periods with a bearing-down sensation. Ovarian pain.

BACK Stiff neck and shoulder pain.

LIMBS Hot, swollen hands. Rheumatism, especially in the shoulders and hands.

BETTER	WORSE
For cold applications	From movement
For lying down	From 4–6 a.m.

GELSEMIUM
Gelsemium

Patients suffer lassitude, weakness and trembling throughout the body. They are easily fatigued, emotional and jittery, showing anticipatory anxiety, drowsiness and memory failure.

MAIN MEDICAL USES

Apprehension	Influenza
Diarrhoea	Measles
Double vision	Paralysis
Exam nerves	Sore throat
Feverish illnesses	Vertigo
Headaches and migraine	Weakness and trembling

MAJOR SYMPTOMS

HEAD Congestive headache with visual disturbances and pain in the eyes. The head pain may extend to the neck and shoulder muscles.

FACE With fevers the face becomes hot and heavy with a besotted, crimson appearance.

EYES Bloodshot with blurred vision. Pain over the eye with the eyeball itself painful. Weakness of the eye muscles can lead to double vision and vertigo. Drooping of the eyelids.

EARS Pain extends to the ear from the throat, with partial loss of hearing.

NOSE Watery nasal discharge, with sneezing, tingling and a full sensation in the nose. Acute nasal discharge with a sore throat.

MOUTH Numbness of the tongue, which feels thick and makes articulation difficult.

THROAT A sore throat may accompany the period. Difficulty in swallowing.

HEART Feeling that the heart will stop if the patient does not keep moving. Weak, slow pulse in the elderly.

STOOLS Diarrhoea from emotional excitement or fear. Involuntary passage of a stool.

URINE Constant dribbling.

GENITALIA Emission of semen during the night without an erection. The genitals feel cold, with a dragging pain extending to the groin and upper abdomen.

PERIODS Late, with pain and a scanty flow. The pain radiates to the back and hips.

LIMBS Trembling and weakness, especially in the hands and feet.

BETTER

For passing a large quantity of urine
For sitting up or bending forward
In the open air

WORSE

In damp weather and fog
Before a thunderstorm
From excitement or emotional shock

GLONOINE
Glonoinum

This remedy is characterized by familiar things seeming strange and ideas becoming confused.

MAIN MEDICAL USES

Angina
Headache
Menopausal disorders

Palpitations
Sunstroke

MAJOR SYMPTOMS

HEAD Throbbing headache with a red face and a full, quick pulse. Feeling of the blood rushing into the head. Violent, congestive headache following shock, or from excess of sun.

FACE Flushed, hot and sweaty.

EYES The vision becomes dim. Black floating spots are seen when stooping. Neuralgia above the eye.

CHEST Violent heartbeat, with pulsations felt all over the body. Palpitations with a sensation of fullness, heaviness and heat; sharp pains in the heart and shortage of breath.

ABDOMEN Pain before and after defaecation.

RECTUM/ ANUS Constipation, with itching, painful piles, or diarrhoea with copious, black, lumpy stools.

PERIODS May be suppressed.

MENOPAUSE Flushing and feelings of heat.

BETTER

In the open air
When holding the head firmly

WORSE

In sun, bright light or in any heat
For being jarred
For stooping

GRAPHITES
Graphites

Patients are fickle, indecisive, sad and anxious, and often fat, greasy, chilly and constipated. Music may cause tears.

MAIN MEDICAL USES

Asthma
Aversion to intercourse
Constipation
Eczema
Eyelid inflammation
Impetigo

Indigestion
Mouth ulcers
Nosebleeds
Piles
Pre-menstrual symptoms
Sweat rash

MAJOR SYMPTOMS

EYES
Chronic inflammation of the eyelids, with cracked, swollen, ulcerated lids which may stick overnight. Dry scurf in the lashes.

NOSE
Chronic nasal catarrh with an acute sense of smell. Soreness of the nostrils, which are covered with scabs.

MOUTH
Burning blisters on the underside and tip of the tongue. Red or white painful ulcers.

CHEST
Chronic hoarseness associated with skin disease. Cough, worse during periods. Woken by the start of an asthmatic attack.

STOMACH
Aversion to animal foods, the eating of which aggravates many of the symptoms. Sweet foods seem nauseating. Craving for beer, acids and cold drinks. Belches taste of the food eaten several hours after eating. Imperfect, slow digestion. Hunger at the start of and during an asthmatic attack.

ABDOMEN
Clothes have to be loosened because of great distension after eating.

STOOLS
Diarrhoea with undigested food particles, or constipation, with large, difficult stools covered in mucus.

GENITALIA
Men: Lack of ejaculation at intercourse but semen loss can occur without an erection at other times.

Women: Ovarian pain after getting cold or getting the feet wet. Aversion to intercourse.

PERIODS
Often delayed, slow to arrive, scanty and pale; associated with depression and weeping, skin rashes, vertigo and indigestion. Profuse, milky white vaginal discharge, coming in gushes and with back pain, may take the place of the period.

SKIN
Hard and cracked on the hands, it is unhealthy and suppurates easily, the eruptions oozing a thick, honey-like fluid. Smarting and soreness between the thighs and under the breasts. Scaling appears on the scalp and causes itching. Moist, sore areas behind both ears and the fingernails become black, deformed and thickened.

BETTER	**WORSE**
Walking in the open air	From the cold
	During a period

HAMAMELIS
Hamamelis virginica

A bruised soreness is the characteristic of conditions associated with this remedy.

MAIN MEDICAL USES

Bruising	Phlebitis
Chilblains	Piles
Nosebleeds	Varicose veins

MAJOR SYMPTOMS

EYES
Sore and bloodshot.

NOSE
Profuse nosebleed; the blood literally flows away.

ANUS
Piles which are sore and bleed profusely.

GENITALIA   Passive bleed of dark blood between the periods.

LIMBS   Dilated, painful, sensitive varicose veins which may go on to ulcerate or become inflamed (phlebitis).

SKIN   Small bruises, easily caused by quite minor trauma. Bluish chilblains in the winter.

BETTER	WORSE
No influencing factors	From warm, humid conditions
	From movement
	During a period

HEPAR SULPH
Hepar sulphuris calcareum

Typically Hepar sulph patients show mental and physical hypersensitivity, becoming angry at very little. They cannot tolerate pain, touch, draughts or cold and are impossible to please. There is a general tendency for all conditions to become infected and discharge pus.

MAIN MEDICAL USES

Abscesses, particularly dental
Acne
Boils
Bronchitis
Catarrh, chronic
Colds
Conjunctivitis
Corneal ulcers
Croup
Ear infections
Eczema
Erysipelas
Eyelid inflammation
Facial neuralgia
Indigestion
Laryngitis
Mouth ulcers
Pharyngitis
Skin ulcers
Tonsillitis

MAJOR SYMPTOMS

FACE   Cracks in the lower lip. Right-sided facial neuralgia. Blistered skin infections.

EYES   Red, with inflammation, swelling and dislike of light. The lids are sore and tend to stick together overnight. The eye feels bruised if pressed. Pus-like discharge.

EARS   Sharp, sticking pains in the ear on blowing the nose. The external ear is red, hot and itchy. Pus-like discharge.

NOSE   Chronic nasal catarrh with a profuse, green-yellow, offensive discharge. The sense of smell is either hypersensitive or totally lost. Sneezing on exposure to a cold, dry wind.

MOUTH   The saliva is profuse and foul-smelling. White ulcers form on the inside of the lips, the tongue and inner cheek. Offensive bitter taste in the mouth.

THROAT   Splinter-like pains, aggravated by swallowing, extend to the ear on yawning.

CHEST   Three types of cough: a loose cough, worse on deep breathing; a paroxysmal cough, worse for the slightest cold; and a suffocative cough, worse late at night and aggravated by talking and stooping. Asthma, worse in cold, dry weather, better in damp. The head is bent backwards in order to relieve the shortage of breath.

STOMACH — Desire for vinegar and pungent foods, aversion to fat. Morning nausea with frequent, odourless, tasteless belches and vomiting of bile.

ABDOMEN — Pain over the liver, worse from coughing, pressure and walking.

STOOLS — Although the urge is present, there is difficulty in passing even a soft stool. The stool is light-coloured, sticky and some is drawn back each time, i.e. only partially expelled. A sour, light-coloured diarrhoea with undigested food particles in it may also occur.

SKIN — Profuse sour sweat on the slightest exertion. The skin looks yellowish and unhealthy. The slightest injury tends to discharge pus. Spots go on to become boils and abscesses. Soreness and moisture in the skin fold between the scrotum and thigh. Red, itchy spots which become covered with yellow blisters. Cracking and smarting of the hands and feet. Painful skin ulcers which burn, sting and bleed easily.

BETTER

For warmth and warm clothes
In damp weather
For wrapping up the head
After eating

WORSE

In dry, cold air and draughts
For the least touch or least exertion
Lying on the painful side

HYOSCYAMUS

Hyoscyamus

Patients are jealous, suspicious, talkative, quarrelsome, lascivious people, who have a desire to undress and expose themselves. Their hands are in constant motion and they pull at and pull off their bedclothes.

MAIN MEDICAL USES

Delirium
Mania (extreme mood changes with rapid, almost incoherent speech)
Menstrual irregularities

Nymphomania
Plucking at the bedclothes during delirium
Puerperal mania (after childbirth)

MAJOR SYMPTOMS

EYES — Staring, red and wild-looking, with dilated pupils.

MOUTH — The tongue is dry, red, cracked and stiff; speech is impaired because of it.

CHEST — Hoarseness and a frequent dry, hacking, tickling cough, worse at night and lying down, from cold air, eating and drinking, talking, and swimming.

STOMACH — Hiccoughs, belching, nausea, all worse after highly spiced food.

ABDOMEN — Colic with vomiting and screaming.

STOOLS — Involuntary defaecation aggravated by mental excitement and during sleep.

BLADDER — Involuntary urination.

LIMBS | Constant movement, with trembling and twitching of the hands and feet. Constant picking at the bedclothes.

SLEEP | Sleeplessness due to long, continued exhilaration. Restless sleep. In nervous children who cry in their sleep, twitch and tremble, then wake in fright.

BETTER	WORSE
For stooping	At night During a period After eating Lying down

HYPERICUM
Hypericum

MAIN MEDICAL USES

Asthma

Burning, tingling or numbness in the limbs (neuritis)

Cerebro-spinal injury

Coccygeal injury

Crush injuries to the fingers

Eczema

Excessive sweat

Facial neuralgia

Long-term effects of fear/shock

Punctured, incised or lacerated wounds involving nerves and nerve endings

Toothache

MAJOR SYMPTOMS

HEAD | Feels icy cold. The top of the head throbs.

FACE | Right-sided facial neuralgia. Toothache.

CHEST | Asthma, worse in foggy weather and relieved by a profuse perspiration.

BACK | Pain in the neck and lower back. Injury to the coccyx after a fall, with pain radiating up the back and down the legs.

LIMBS | Lancing pains which shoot along injured limbs. Burning, stinging pains in puncture wounds (in this case use Ledum before Hypericum). Tingling, burning, numbness in the limbs (neuritis). Leg cramps.

SKIN | Excessive sweating, worse in the morning after sleep. Eczema of the hands and under the chin.

BETTER	WORSE
For bending the head back	In the cold, in the damp and in the fog From the slightest touch

IGNATIA
Ignatia

Patients are often depressed, cry easily and suffer rapidly changeable moods. Ignatia suits nervous, hysterical people, especially women, who are oversensitive to noise, smells and pain. It is used to treat conditions that occur after suppressed grief or disappointed love.

MAIN MEDICAL USES

Allergy rashes

Anal prolapse

Depression

Emotional shock

Frigidity

Morning sickness in pregnancy

Paradoxical symptoms (i.e. the opposite of what might be expected)

Piles

Sciatica

Sensation of a lump in the throat

Stress-induced illness

Tonsillitis

Urine retention after confinement

Voice loss, hysterical

MAJOR SYMPTOMS

HEAD	Nervous headaches, often confined to one spot, feeling as if a nail is being driven into the brain. Congestive headache associated with a period, or after anger or grief. Worse from smoking or smelling tobacco smoke.
THROAT	Sharp pain, or sensation of a lump in the throat, better for swallowing something solid. Inflamed, swollen tonsils with pain radiating to the ear.
STOMACH	The appetite is very variable but there is a preference for sour, cold foods. Much flatulence.
RECTUM/ ANUS	Frequent sharp, cutting pains shoot up the rectum. Anal prolapse and piles, painful sitting or standing, but eased by walking. There may be bleeding and irritation from them. Painful constriction of the anus after a bowel movement.
STOOLS	Thin, sometimes involuntary, small, frequent stools may alternate with constipation. Emotional diarrhoea caused by worrying about someone else.
BLADDER	Frequent, profuse, watery urine.
PERIODS	Suppressed, or early, either very profuse or very scanty, and black. Urine retention during a period.
PREGNANCY	Morning sickness, with a weak, sinking sensation in the stomach, better for eating. Retention of urine after confinement. Frigidity.

LIMBS	Jerking of the arms when falling asleep. Bruised pain in the back of the thigh, tearing pain in the calf and Achilles tendon. Burning, sciatic pain preceded by coldness, worse at night and from warmth. The patient has to get up and walk to find relief.
SKIN	Itching, allergic rash, very sensitive to cold draughts.

BETTER	WORSE
While eating	In the morning
For change of position	In the open air
	After eating
	From coffee and smoking
	From emotional upsets

IODUM

Iodum

Irritability and sensitivity are key features of this remedy. It is suited to dark-haired people with yellow-tawny skin who are excitable and restless, especially children.

MAIN MEDICAL USES

Angina	Laryngitis
Croup	Liver disorders
Enlargement of lymph glands	Mouth ulcers
Glue ear	Pancreatic disease
Goitre	Raised blood pressure
Headache	Sinusitis
Influenza	Sweaty feet

Tear sac and duct inflammation   Weight loss
Thyroid gland enlargement

MAJOR SYMPTOMS

HEAD   Chronic, congestive headaches in the elderly.

EYES   Pain with violent flow of tears. *See a doctor.*

NOSE   Sudden onset influenza with sneezing. Acrid nasal discharge which corrodes the upper lip. Pain in the nose and frontal sinuses. Loss of sense of smell. The lining membrane of the nose becomes moist and swollen in raised blood pressure.

THROAT   Croup in dark-haired children, aggravated during wet weather. Acute tonsillitis with extension to the ear. Firm enlargement of the thyroid.

LARYNX   Painful laryngitis with a feeling of constriction.

CHEST/   Palpitations from any exertion. The heart feels as if
BREASTS   grasped in an iron fist. Shortage of breath going up stairs and during a period. Shrinkage of the breasts.

STOMACH   Ravenous appetite and thirst, eats well but still loses weight. Excessive flatulence.

ABDOMEN   Liver and spleen enlarged. Pancreatic disease. Jaundice.

RECTUM   Constipation with ineffectual urging.

PERIODS   Irregular, with great weakness during them. Acrid vaginal discharge most abundant during a period.

LIMBS   Pain in the muscles and bones, especially at night. Chronic osteo-arthritis with burning pain in the joints, worse at night. Cold hands and feet. Acrid foot sweat.

BETTER	WORSE
Out of doors	For warmth
In cold air	For wrapping up the
For cold bathing	affected part
	When quiet

IPECAC

Ipecacuanha

This remedy is suited to feeble, fat adults and children, who are miserable and irritable. The face is pale and drawn, and there are blue rings around the eyes.

MAIN MEDICAL USES

Asthma	Morning sickness in
Bleeding (bright red and heavy)	pregnancy
Bronchitis	Nausea and vomiting
Croup	Whooping cough
Diarrhoea	

MAJOR SYMPTOMS

HEAD   Sick headache with bruised pain in the skull. The pain may extend to the tongue.

FACE   Pale.

MOUTH   Profuse salivation; bitter taste but with a clean tongue.

STOMACH   The stomach feels relaxed, as if hanging down. Constant nausea with colicky pains.

ABDOMEN	Griping, colicky pains around the navel and radiating all over the abdomen.
STOOLS	Green, bloody, fermented and with frothy mucus.
CHEST	Dry, spasmodic cough, with shortage of breath on exertion, wheezing and rattling mucus, but little expectoration. In whooping cough the patient loses his breath, goes blue and rigid, with gagging and vomiting. The nose may then bleed.
GENITALIA	All forms of uterine haemorrhage, including heavy periods, bleeding between periods and bleeding with a threatened miscarriage.
SLEEP	The patient sleeps with the eyes half open.

BETTER	WORSE
In the open air	From warmth and damp
	From overeating

IRIS

Iris versicolor

MAIN MEDICAL USES

Diarrhoea	Psoriasis
Eczema	Sciatica
Facial neuralgia	Shingles
Gastro-enteritis	Tinnitus (noises in the ear)
Headache	Vertigo
Migraine	

MAJOR SYMPTOMS

HEAD	Frontal headache accompanied by nausea and a sensation of tightness in the scalp. Migraine comes after relaxing from work (mental or physical) and usually starts with the vision on one side becoming blurred. The pain is frequently in the right temple.
FACE	Pain, which eventually involves the whole face, starts over one eye and comes on after breakfast.
EARS	Tinnitus with roaring, buzzing or ringing in the ears. Deafness and vertigo are often associated.
MOUTH	Feels scalded by the saliva, which is acrid, and from sour, bilious vomiting.
STOMACH	Burning sensation throughout the digestive tract with vomiting. A loss of appetite ensues.
ABDOMEN	Flatulent colic, with soreness and cutting pains over the liver.
STOOLS	Watery, burning, painful, green diarrhoea every night. However, constipation may also occur.
LIMBS	Left-sided sciatica radiates as far as the back of the knee.
SKIN	Shingles associated with gastric disturbance, psoriasis or eczema, which is especially itchy at night.

BETTER	WORSE
From gentle continued movement	In the evening and at night (2–3 a.m.)
From warmth	From rest

KALI BICH
Kali bichromicum

Typical patients are fat, chubby, short-necked children, light-haired catarrhal people who tend to be flabby and lazy, and chilly people who catch cold easily. Ulcers in the mucous membranes are straight-sided, as if made mechanically by a punch, and have a cheesy exudate.

MAIN MEDICAL USES

Bronchitis	Sciatica
Catarrhal affections	Sinusitis
Conjunctivitis	Snuffles
Croup	Ulceration in mucous membranes
Diarrhoea	Urinary tract infections
Eyelid inflammation	Vaginal discharge
Indigestion	Varicose ulcers
Rheumatism	

MAJOR SYMPTOMS

HEAD — Headache, with blurred vision preceding the pain and clearing with the onset of the headache. The scalp and facial bones feel sore. Sinus pain behind and above the eyes.

EYES — Sticky eyes, yellow discharge with excessive tears and dislike of light.

NOSE — Discharges of plugs and tough, ropy, greenish catarrh with pain at the root of the nose. Snuffles in children.

TONGUE — Yellow-coated or smooth, red, shiny, dry and cracked.

THROAT — Inflamed throat with swelling of the uvula and tough, stringy catarrh.

CHEST — Loose, rattling cough with expectoration of tough, stringy mucus.

STOMACH — Gastric disturbances, with flatulence soon after eating. Vomiting of stringy mucus. Likes beer but it produces nausea and vomiting.

URINE — Inflammation in the urinary tract, with stringy, ropy mucus in the urine. Protein in the urine due to kidney disease.

LIMBS — Alternation of gastric symptoms and rheumatism. Rheumatic pains occur in small areas and shift rapidly from place to place, coming and going quickly. Left-sided sciatica.

BETTER	WORSE
For heat	In cold, open air
	When undressing
	Between 2–4 a.m.
	From beer

KALI CARB
Kali carbonicum

Patients are usually dark-haired, have a tendency to obesity and are more likely to be elderly. They are irritable, never contented and never want to be left alone. There is marked prostration, coldness and depression with stitching pains and sensitivity to draughts. Kali carb individuals perspire easily.

MAIN MEDICAL USES

Asthma	Nosebleeds
Bronchitis	Obesity
Fluid retention	Piles
Heavy periods	Pleurisy
Lumbago	Rheumatism

MAJOR SYMPTOMS

HEAD — Headache from a cold wind. Travel nausea. Very dry, loose hair.

FACE/EYES — Puffiness between the upper eyelids and the forehead.

EARS — Itching, pain and ringing noises.

NOSE — Blocked nose in a warm room. Thick, fluent, yellow discharge. Crusting. Nosebleed while washing the face in the morning.

THROAT — Sensation of a fishbone in the larynx. Swallowing is difficult.

CHEST — Dry, paroxysmal cough with vomiting or gagging. Stitching pains in the chest with bronchitis, or pleurisy which more frequently occurs in the lower right lung. Asthma and other chest symptoms are worse at about 3 a.m. and are better for leaning forward.

STOMACH — Distension. Flatulence. Sour belching with nausea, better lying down and worse for cold water.

PERIODS — Weakness and exhaustion before a period, with backache before and during it. The period is either early and profuse, or late, pale and scanty, with soreness of the external genitalia. Delayed first period.

BACK — The small of the back feels weak. Back pain in pregnancy. Lumbago with sharp pain going up the back and down to the thighs. Pain in the pelvic bones, the hip joint and the thighs.

LIMBS — Weakness of the legs.

BETTER	WORSE
During the daytime	In cold weather
From motion	From soup or coffee
In warm, moist weather	About 3 a.m.
	Lying on the left and the painful side
	After intercourse

KALI PHOS

Kali phosphoricum

Typical patients suffer extreme nervous depression – the slightest effort causes mental and physical fatigue. They are anxious, lethargic, shy, dislike meeting people and are disinclined to enter into conversation. This remedy is also suited to young people tired out by learning and examinations.

MAIN MEDICAL USES

Asthma	Headache
Ear infections	Period problems
Fatigue after illness, emotional upsets, mental and physical overwork and sexual excesses	Throat infections
	Tinnitus (noises in the ear)
	Vertigo

MAJOR SYMPTOMS

HEAD	Headache with extreme fatigue, mental or emotional, and an empty feeling in the stomach. Headache at the back of the head, better on rising.
FACE	Sunken, with hollow eyes. Right-sided neuralgia relieved by cold applications.
EARS	Deafness and buzzing in the ears. Vertigo from most movements and when looking upwards.
MOUTH	Offensive breath, with dry, brown-coated tongue, especially in the morning. Toothache with gums that bleed easily.
THROAT	Severe sore throat with laryngitis due to 'paralysis' of the vocal cords.
CHEST	Asthma, worse after eating and on climbing stairs. Cough with yellow sputum.
PERIODS	Loss of periods accompanied by severe depression, or late and scanty periods. Particularly likely to occur in pale, tearful, irritable women.
GENITALIA	*Men:* Nocturnal emissions with impotence. Considerable fatigue after intercourse.

BETTER	WORSE
For warmth	From cold
For gentle motion	In the early morning
	From excitement and worry
	From mental and physical exertion

°LAC CAN

Lac caninum

Patients feel weak, are forgetful, fear their illness is incurable and have attacks of rage and intense despondency. They feel they are walking on air or floating when lying down. The symptoms move across the body, from side to side.

MAIN MEDICAL USES

Backache	Rheumatism
Colds	Sciatica
Heavy periods	Suppression of lactation
Mastitis	Throat infections
Migraine	Tonsillitis

MAJOR SYMPTOMS

HEAD	Headache which moves from side to side and is accompanied by blurred vision, nausea and vomiting. Sensation of floating.
NOSE	One nostril blocked, one free, alternately. The end of the nose becomes sore and cracked.
MOUTH	White tongue with red edges and profuse salivation. The jaw cracks while eating.
NECK	Pain shoots over the head to the forehead.
THROAT	Tonsillitis goes from one side to the other. The throat is sensitive to the touch, feels raw and burned, and swallowing is painful. The pain extends to the ears. Sore throat with each period.
BREASTS	Mastitis, which is worse for the slightest touch.

269

PERIODS	Early, profuse and flow in gushes. The breasts become swollen and sore before the period but better once it starts. A sore throat and cough may accompany the period.
BACK/ LIMBS	The spine is sensitive to touch or pressure. Right-sided sciatica, with the leg feeling numb and stiff. Rheumatic pains in the limbs and back go from side to side. Burning sensation in the soles of the feet and the palms of the hands.

BETTER

For cold and cold drinks

WORSE

During periods

LACHESIS
Lachesis

This remedy is suited to thin, suspicious, loquacious people, who suffer from extremes of mood, going from great mental activity to depression and anxiety in which they become silent and sullen. Their illnesses develop from long-standing grief, sorrow, vexation or jealousy. They are intolerant of anything tight about the neck, abdomen or pelvis. An aggravation of all complaints occurs after sleep, but they feel much better once a discharge appears, for example at the start of a period or when a carbuncle bursts. Complaints tend to occur more on the left side of the body.

MAIN MEDICAL USES

Abscesses	Headache
Asthma	Menopausal problems
Bedsores	Mouth ulcers
Carbuncles	Piles
Croup	Tonsillitis
Erysipelas	Toothache
Facial neuralgia	

MAJOR SYMPTOMS

HEAD	Neuralgic headaches extend to the nose, face, eyes and shoulders. Head pain on waking. Headache from too much sun.
FACE	The skin below the left eye itches at night, reddens and swells the next day with erysipelas. Left-sided facial neuralgia. The face may become purple, mottled and swollen.
MOUTH	Raw, burning ulcers. Trembling, red, burning and dry tongue. Toothache which extends to the ears. Dark, purplish bleeding gums.
THROAT	Tonsillitis starts on the left side, but may go to the right. The throat looks dark purple and is worse after sleep and hot drinks. Swallowing solids is easier than swallowing liquid. The throat is very sensitive to external touch and pressure. Cannot bear tight collars.
CHEST	Asthma after sleep. The patient loosens his clothing and opens the window.
PERIODS	Irregular. Pre-menstrual tension which goes once the period starts.
MENOPAUSE	Hot flushes, perspiration, sleeplessness, palpitations with fainting and other menopausal symptoms.

BACK — Sticking, drawing pains in the spine radiate to the hips and legs. Right-sided sciatica, better lying down. Pain in the coccyx, worse when rising from a seat.

LIMBS — Blue-purple varicose ulcers on legs which exude a thick, dark, offensive, bloody discharge.

SKIN — Hot sweat. All skin infections and ulcerations have a blue-purple appearance.

BETTER	WORSE
In open air	After sleep
For warm applications	From a warm bath
	From pressure or constriction
	From hot drinks
	In the spring

LEDUM

Ledum palustre

There is a general lack of body heat in Ledum patients and they always feel cold. There is a tendency to abuse alcohol. Complaints often alternate, for example rheumatism and facial eczema occur in turn, and symptoms travel diagonally, such as from the right leg to the left arm.

MAIN MEDICAL USES

Acne	Eczema
Anal fissures	Eye injuries, especially a black eye
Carbuncles	
Chronic bronchitis/emphysema	Gout

Insect bites	Rheumatism
Puncture wounds	

MAJOR SYMPTOMS

FACE — Red pimples or eczema-type rash on the forehead and cheeks. Crusty eruption around the nose and mouth.

EYES — Specific for a black eye and injuries to the eyes caused by a soft object.

CHEST — Shortage of breath with a sensation of constriction. Spasmodic cough. Chronic bronchitis and emphysema in the elderly.

RECTUM — Anal fissure and painful piles.

LIMBS — The small joints of the foot become swollen and hot, but are pale, not red. Throbbing pain in the right shoulder, worse for movement and the warmth of the bed. Rheumatism starts in the leg and spreads up the body to other joints. Swollen ankles. The soles of the feet are painful and tender.

SKIN — Acne, especially on the forehead. Facial eczema. Itchy feet and ankles, worse for scratching and the warmth of the bed. Discoloration of the skin through bruising. Puncture wounds and insect bites.

BETTER	WORSE
For cold	From heat
For putting feet in cold water	From the warmth of the bed
	At night

271

LILIUM TIG
Lilium tigrinum

This remedy is characterized by deep depression which is aggravated by consolation. Patients have an aimless, hurried manner and need to be kept busy. Bad-tempered and irritable, they fear insanity, incurable illness and solitude. Complaints tend to be left-sided. There is a feeling of warmth and tiredness in the afternoon.

MAIN MEDICAL USES

Agitation and hurry
Angina
Anxiety and fear about being
  incurable
Depression
Menopausal symptoms

Palpitations
Period problems
Religious mania complicated
  by obscene thoughts
Restless leg syndrome
Vaginal discharge.

MAJOR SYMPTOMS

CHEST — The heart feels as if in a vice. Palpitations or irregular, rapid pulsations are felt all over the body. Pain over the heart radiates to the right arm.

STOMACH — Flatulence and nausea with the sensation of a lump in the stomach. Hunger and thirst, with desire for frequent long drinks.

ABDOMEN — Bearing-down sensation in the lower abdomen, with pressure on the rectum and a feeling that everything is going to drop out of the pelvis.

STOOLS — Frequent defaecation, with early morning urgency.

BLADDER — Constant desire to pass urine, which is milky, scanty and hot.

272

GENITALIA — Acrid, brown vaginal discharge. Pain over the ovaries radiates down the thighs.

PERIODS — Dark, clotted, offensive, delayed and scanty periods which flow only when moving about. Bearing-down sensation, with an urgent desire to defaecate. This 'dropping' sensation is eased by pressing on the vagina with the hand and from resting.

LIMBS — Restless legs. Pains in the ankles and right arm and hip. Pricking sensation in the fingers. The feet and soles burn.

BETTER	WORSE
For fresh open air	From heat
Keeping busy	From consolation
	From standing up

LYCOPODIUM
Lycopodium clavatum

Intellectually keen but physically weak, Lycopodium subjects have sallow, old-looking and lined faces with prematurely greying hair. They are very irritable, cannot bear contradiction and have a great lack of self-confidence. Apprehensive before an event, they nevertheless perform well. Although disliking company, they are unable to tolerate solitude. At a relatively early age they start to deteriorate mentally, becoming forgetful with a lowered capacity for both mental and physical work.
Lycopodium children look old, are bad-tempered and lack confidence.

MAIN MEDICAL USES

Acne
Allergy rashes
Boils
Colds
Cold sores
Constipation
Eczema
Flatulence
Gallstones
Gout, chronic
Hair loss
Headache
Impotence

Indigestion
Leg cramps
Liver disease
Night vision defects
Palpitations
Piles
Sciatica
Snuffles
Styes
Tonsillitis
Toothache
Vaginal discharges
Varicose veins

MAJOR SYMPTOMS

HEAD — Pressure headache, worse lying down and if regular meals are not taken. Coughing produces a throbbing headache. Colds lead to a headache over the eyes. Premature baldness and greying hair. Deep frown lines on forehead and a vertical one above the nose.

FACE — Redness after eating. Scaly cold sores around mouth.

EYES — Redness of lids. Night vision is poor. Styes. The eyes remain half open when asleep.

EARS — Thick, yellow, offensive discharge. Moist eczema behind the ears. Humming and roaring in the ears with deteriorating hearing.

NOSE — Acute sense of smell. Scanty, acrid, burning discharge, but a runny discharge with colds. Nose feels blocked. Snuffles in children, which they wake up with, rubbing their nose. Fan-like movement of the outer ends of the nostrils.

MOUTH — Dry mouth without thirst. Blisters on the tongue, which is dry, cracked and swollen. Toothache relieved by a warm drink.

THROAT — Infections and tonsillitis, with the back of the throat brownish-red and the infection spreading from the right to the left tonsil. Symptoms worse after sleep, but eased by a hot drink.

CHEST — Infections, often right-sided, with rattling mucus, a hollow cough and shortage of breath. The sputum tastes salty. A tickling night cough also occurs. Palpitations at night, worse lying on the left side.

STOMACH — Even if very hungry, a few mouthfuls of food are enough to satisfy. Excessive flatulence, abdominal rumbling and distension after eating are not eased by bringing wind up or down. Great desire for sweet things, an intolerance of starchy food, onions and oysters, which are eaten nevertheless. All food tastes sour. A bruised pain in the liver region makes lying on the right side difficult.

ABDOMEN — Considerable bloating, even after a light meal.

RECTUM — Constipation with ineffectual urging leads to rectal prolapse and painful, aching piles.

BLADDER — Difficulty in starting urination leads to straining or pain at the start (especially in children).

URINE — Either profuse and pale, or it contains a red gritty deposit (urates).

GENITALIA — *Men:* Impotence from previous sexual excesses.

Women: Acrid, milky or red vaginal discharge. A dry vagina makes intercourse painful.

PERIODS — Too early or too late.

BACK | Burning pain between the shoulder blades. Low back pain relieved by passing urine.

LIMBS | Right-sided sciatica. Right foot hot, left foot cold. Numbness and tearing pains in the limbs, worse at rest and at night. The arms feel heavy, the shoulders and elbows painful. Chronic gout. Pain in the heel. Leg cramps at night in bed.

SKIN | The skin is dry, thick and wrinkled, with many freckles and brown spots. Chronic eczema. Violent itching with an allergy rash. Varicose veins. Offensive perspiration of feet and armpits. Acne and small abscesses, worse for warmth.

BETTER	WORSE
For motion	On the right side
After midnight	From 4–8 p.m.
For warm food and drink	From above downwards
For getting cold	From warm applications
For being uncovered	Before periods

MAG PHOS
Magnesia phosphorica

This is suited to thin, highly nervous people with a dark complexion. They develop colic, cramps and darting, spasmodic, boring, lightning-like pains which change location rapidly. These are relieved by warmth and firm pressure. Complaints tend to be right-sided.

MAIN MEDICAL USES

Colic	Period pain
Cramps in pregnancy	Toothache
Headache	Whooping cough
Hiccoughs	Writer's cramp
Laryngitis	

MAJOR SYMPTOMS

HEAD | Severe spasmodic pains, shooting and shifting about the head, always better for the local application of heat. Three types of headache can develop: a dull headache which starts in the neck and runs over the head; a nervous headache with nausea, flatulent colic and increased tears, worse for cold and mental exertion; and a congestive headache with a flushed, red face, worse lying down.

FACE | Facial neuralgia, involving the right upper jaw and teeth, starts around 2 p.m. and may then spread all over right side of the face. It is worse for touch, opening the mouth and cold.

EYES | Pain above the right eye with increased secretion of tears. The eyes feel hot and tired and the lids may twitch.

EARS | Sharp, intermittent pain behind the right ear, worse for cold air and washing in cold water.

MOUTH | Toothache which comes on after going to bed, better for heat and very much worse for cold drinks and cold air.

CHEST | Dry, spasmodic cough with retching and choking, worse in a warm room, better in the open air.

ABDOMEN — Flatulent colic and distension helped by bending double, warmth and rubbing. Persistent hiccoughs may be accompanied by retching.

PERIODS — Painful and early, with a dark, stringy flow. The pain is worse before and better after the flow has started.

BETTER	WORSE
For heat	From cold air
For bending double	From draughts
For pressure	From bathing
For friction	From motion
For rubbing	From touch

MERCURIUS

Mercurius solubilis

Mercurius patients tend to be light-haired with an earthy or dirty yellow complexion. Somewhat slow mentally, they are mistrustful and weary of life. All discharges tend to be acrid and burning.

MAIN MEDICAL USES

Bronchitis, chronic
Catarrhal affections
Cystitis
Diarrhoea and dysentery
Eye infections
Laryngitis
Lymph gland conditions
Mumps

Offensive and excessive sweat
Pus-discharging conditions and superficial ulcerations
Rheumatism, chronic
Teeth and gum disease
Tonsillitis
Vertigo
Whooping cough

MAJOR SYMPTOMS

HEAD — Catarrhal headache, making the head feel as if bound by a tight band. Scalp eruptions sting and burn. Vertigo lying on the back.

FACE — Facial neuralgia from cold air, with tearing, shooting pains, worse at night.

EYES — Acrid, burning discharge containing pus and mucus, with sticky, raw, red lids and marked dislike of light, worse at night.

EARS — Bloody and offensive yellow discharge, with sticking pains, worse at night.

NOSE — Colds with frequent sneezing. Acrid, offensive, thick yellow-green discharge. Sore, raw nostrils. Sneezing from bright lights.

MOUTH — Toothache worse at night. The teeth become decayed and loose. The gums are swollen and separated from the teeth, bleeding at the slightest touch. Spongy, ulcerated gums that discharge pus and hurt when chewing. The tongue is thick, moist and yellow and the upper surface has a lengthways furrow. It is flabby, trembles and has an imprint of the teeth along its edges. Mouth and tongue ulcers, with profuse saliva, bad taste and breath, and sharp sticking pains, worse at night.

THROAT — Redness of the soft palate, the tonsils and the uvula, with ulceration. The tonsils suppurate and develop sharp, sticking pains. Constant desire to swallow.

CHEST — Severe night cough, worse from tobacco smoke and lying on the right side. The phlegm is thick and yellow-green. Whooping cough with a tendency to nosebleeds.

ABDOMEN	Aversion to bread and butter, wine and brandy. Intense thirst for cold drinks. Perpetually hungry. Flatulent distension with griping and a constant urge to defaecate, but little is evacuated. Chronic liver disease with marked tenderness, jaundice and loose, mucous stools.
STOOLS	Diarrhoea in the evening. The stools, green, slimy and acrid with much mucus, may be streaked with blood. Burning and protrusion of the anus after defaecation.
BLADDER	Constant desire to urinate with great urgency, but little is passed. The urethra burns on starting to urinate. It develops a green, painless discharge, worse at night.
GENITALIA	*Men:* Swollen foreskin with blisters and ulcers on the penis. *Women:* Acrid greenish vaginal discharge which causes smarting and a feeling of rawness.
PERIODS	Heavy with abdominal pain.
LIMBS	Destructive and inflammatory changes in bones lead to boring, throbbing pains, worse at night and in damp, stormy weather. Weakness with trembling, especially of the hands, worse at night, from excitement, or from attempting to hold something.
SKIN	Constant, excessive, smelly perspiration. The skin itches when warm.
GLANDS	Any infection in the body leads to swollen lymph glands.

BETTER	WORSE
In moderate temperatures	From draughts and damp weather At night Lying on the right side From sweating In a warm room or warm bed

MERC CORR
Mercurius corrosivus

The action of this remedy is similar to Mercurius, but much more intense. It is particularly useful in treating a continuous or frequently recurring desire to defaecate which is not relieved by defaecation.

MAIN MEDICAL USES

Acute, destructive inflammations, especially of mucous membranes
Cystitis
Dysentery and diarrhoea

Eye infections
Mouth infections
Mouth ulcers
Vaginal discharge

MAJOR SYMPTOMS

HEAD	Acute inflammation of the eyes and lids with swelling, intense pain, dislike of light and excessive acrid tears.
MOUTH	Violent inflammation in the mouth with large ulcers.

THROAT	Rapidly spreading inflammation and ulceration. Any attempt to swallow, even liquids, is painful.
STOOLS	Excessive straining to defaecate with the passage of scanty, slimy stools, mucus-covered and blood-stained, very offensive, with terrible griping pains. Passing the stool does not relieve the straining.
BLADDER	Straining of the bladder often accompanies the rectal straining, with intense burning in the urethra and scanty urine.
GENITALIA	Profuse, yellow-green, acrid vaginal discharge.

MEZEREUM

Mezereum

The Mezereum patient is extremely chilly. This remedy is especially indicated for all pains which are sensitive to cold air.

MAIN MEDICAL USES

Eczema	Pain after shingles,
Facial neuralgia	especially above the
Gastric ulcer	eye and between the ribs.
Impetigo	Sinusitis
Outer-ear infection, chronic	

MAJOR SYMPTOMS

HEAD	Scalp eczema with thick, leathery crusts under which pus collects. Headache, worse from talking.
FACE	Facial neuralgia and sinusitis. Burning pain below the eyes, worse for washing, heat and at night. Numbness frequently follows.
EYES	Severe, sharp pain above the eye after shingles, coming in paroxysms. Worse at night and from warmth.
EARS	Earache, with a sensation of wind blowing in the ear. Chronic outer-ear infection with eczema behind the ear.
NOSE	Sneezing, with a thin, acrid, blood-streaked, yellow discharge.
STOMACH	Burning pain in the upper-middle abdomen evening and night, worse for pressure on the abdomen and relieved by eating.
BACK	Neck and back pain, worse from motion and at night.
LIMBS	Burning pain in long bones, especially the shin, worse for damp and in bed at night.
SKIN	Ulcers, blisters and pustular eruptions, with copious discharge of thick pus. Tough scabs form over the eruptions. The lesions burn and itch so severely that the patient scratches them until they bleed. The irritation is worse at night and from warmth. Neuralgias following shingles, with severe tearing pains, local soreness and numbness.

BETTER	WORSE
For open air	For cold, humid weather
	Washing in cold water
	At night in a warm bed
	From touch
	From motion

277

NAT MUR

Natrum muriaticum

Typical Nat mur patients feel great weariness and weakness, especially before rising in the morning, and tend to catch cold easily. This remedy is useful for illness caused through grief, fright or anger, when the patient becomes depressed, sad, weepy and irritable, but consolation aggravates. There is a tendency to changeable moods, such as tears with laughter. Patients are generally at their worst between 10 and 11 a.m.

MAIN MEDICAL USES

Allergy rashes	Hangnails
Catarrh	Hay fever
Colds	Headache
Constipation	Migraine
Debility	Psoriasis
Depression	Sinusitis
Eczema	

MAJOR SYMPTOMS

HEAD — Throbbing, blinding, beating headache present from sunrise to sunset, particularly in anaemic women and schoolgirls after a period. Also chronic, one-sided, congestive headache with a pale face and nausea or vomiting. Numbness and tingling in the lips, tongue and nose often precede it. Frontal sinusitis.

EYES — Feel bruised and the lids heavy. Letters run together. Burning, acrid tears. Tears stream when coughing.

NOSE — Thin, fluent, watery discharge. After a few days it changes and the nose becomes blocked. Violent sneezing at the start of a cold.

MOUTH — The tongue looks as if a map has been drawn on it and feels dry, with the sensation of a hair on it. The lips and corners of the mouth are dry and cracked, with a deep crack in the middle of the lower lip. Blisters form on the lips and tongue.

STOMACH — Aversion to acid foods, bread, fat or anything slimy. Craving for salt and salted food. Great thirst. Sweats while eating.

STOOLS — Dry and crumbling, causing pain and anal bleeding when passed.

BLADDER — Unable to urinate if others are present.

GENITALIA — Dry vagina.

PERIODS — Profuse and irregular.

BACK — Severe lower-back pain, better for firm support.

LIMBS — The palms are hot and perspiring, but the nails are dry and cracked. Hangnails develop. The legs feel weak, cold and crack on motion. Numbness and tingling in the fingers and legs.

SKIN — Greasy, with dry, crusty eruptions on the hair margin, bends of joints and behind the ears. Warts form on the palms. Raw, red, inflamed eczema, worse for eating salt and at the seaside. Allergy rash, worse after violent exercise.

BETTER	WORSE
In the open air	From noise
For cold bathing	From music
Lying on right side	For warmth
Pressure against the back	From lying down
	At the seashore
For irregular mealtimes	For mental exertion
	For consolation

NAT SULPH
Natrum sulphuricum

Patients suffer mental depression, worse from music, and have a definite suicidal tendency. They are irritable, especially when spoken to, and have an inability to speak. Every change of weather from dry to damp upsets them.

MAIN MEDICAL USES

Acid indigestion	Genital warts
Asthma, especially in children	Head injuries
Catarrh	Hepatitis
Diarrhoea	Nosebleeds
Ear inflammation	Rheumatism
Eyelid inflammation	

MAJOR SYMPTOMS

HEAD Ill-effects of head injuries, even when the injury was years previously.

EYES Inflammation of the eyelids with dislike of bright light.

EARS Earache in damp weather.

NOSE Thick, yellow catarrh.

MOUTH Toothache, better from cold drinks and cold air. Bitter taste. The tongue has a brown coating.

CHEST Shortage of breath in damp weather. Need to hold the chest when coughing. Thick, ropy, greenish mucus. Asthma, worse 4–5 a.m. and occurring whenever the patient catches a cold. Pain in the lower left side of the chest.

STOMACH Acid indigestion with heartburn and flatulence.

ABDOMEN The liver is tender, with sharp, sticking pains, and the patient may become jaundiced. Bilious vomiting. Tight clothing around the waist is unbearable.

STOOLS Diarrhoea on first rising in the morning. Sudden urging with much wind and rumbling, worse after wet weather. Involuntary stools may occur when passing wind.

GENITALIA *Men:* Penile warts.

Women: Tendency to vulval warts.

PERIODS Nosebleeds and laryngitis may occur with the period.

LIMBS Rheumatism in damp, cold weather, especially in the left hip joint, the knees and the limbs, making the patient change position frequently to get comfortable. Swollen feet with itching between the toes, burning soles, and inflammation of nail bed.

SKIN Warty growths on the skin and mucous membranes. Itching when undressing.

BETTER	WORSE
In dry weather	From music
For pressure	Lying on the left side
	From damp housing and weather
	For sea air

NITRIC ACID
Nitricum acidum

This remedy is suited to people of dark complexion, often past middle age. They tend to catch cold easily and have offensive urine, faeces and perspiration. They are vindictive, headstrong and irritable, and have a hopeless despair about their illness or past.

MAIN MEDICAL USES

Anal fissure	Laryngitis
Blackheads	Mouth and tongue
Catarrh, chronic	blisters and ulcers
Chilblains	Nosebleeds
Colds	Piles
Depression	Vulval blisters and ulcers
Hair loss	Warts
Indigestion	

MAJOR SYMPTOMS

HEAD Headache, like a tight band around the head, worse for noise. The hair falls out easily.

EARS Great sensitivity to noise. Hearing is better in a car or train.

NOSE Green crusts are present each morning. Chronic nasal catarrh with a yellow, offensive, acrid, burning nasal discharge. Colds with sore and bleeding nostrils. Nosebleeds with chest infections.

MOUTH Putrid breath. Ulcers in the soft palate, with sharp, splinter-like pains. The teeth become loose and the gums soft, spongy and bleeding.

CHEST Hoarseness or even loss of voice, with a dry cough. Coughing while asleep. Shortage of breath when climbing stairs.

STOMACH Constant hunger. Liking for indigestible things and craving for fat and salt. Indigestion with mental depression.

RECTUM Great straining to defaecate but little passes. The rectum feels torn, becomes fissured and may bleed. Violent cutting pains after stools may last for several hours. Bleeding piles.

URINE Scanty, dark and offensive, feels cold while being passed.

GENITALIA *Men:* Soreness and ulceration of the penis.

Women: Vulval soreness and ulceration. Brown, watery, offensive vaginal discharge. Genital hair falls out.

PERIODS Early and profuse, with pain in the back, hip region and thighs.

LIMBS Smelly foot sweat causes sore toes with prickling pain. Chilblains. Palms and armpits have offensive sweat. The nails are cold and blue.

SKIN   Warts, ulcers and fissures that bleed slightly but easily. Ulcers are painful, with cutting or pricking pains. Blackheads on the face and small pimples on the forehead.

BETTER

When riding in a vehicle

WORSE

For cold
For weather changes
In the evening

NUX VOM

Nux vomica

Suited to exceptionally chilly, thin, irritable, dark-haired people who are quarrelsome, spiteful, malicious and easily offended. They are often sedentary and studious, have sluggish functions and are oversensitive to other people, noise, light, odours and music.

MAIN MEDICAL USES

Constipation
Drug abuse
Flatulent indigestion
Hangover
Headache
Hypochondria
Inflammation of the nasal lining
Insomnia and unrefreshing sleep

Lumbago
Migraine
Nosebleeds
Piles
Snuffles
Stress from overwork, modern living and responsibility
Vertigo

MAJOR SYMPTOMS

HEAD   Headache from over-indulgence in alcohol or food, and from being in the sun. Frontal headache, better for pressure. Headache at the back of the head with vertigo. The head feels sore all over. Vertigo with momentary loss of consciousness, worse in the morning and late evening.

EYES   Dislike of light, worse in the morning. Smarting, dry lids.

EARS   Itching. Earache, worse in bed. Loud noises are painful and annoy.

NOSE   Runny catarrh by day, blocked nose at night. Snuffles in babies and young children after being in cold, dry conditions. Morning nosebleeds.

MOUTH   The tongue is coated and white. Bad taste in the mouth, with nausea in the morning, especially after eating late the night before.

CHEST   Catarrhal hoarseness with scraping in the larynx. Asthma in the morning or after eating. Coughing leads to a bursting headache.

STOMACH   Sensation of fullness and weight, accompanied by nausea and sour belching, about an hour and a half after eating. The patient feels that vomiting would help the nausea. Ravenous hunger on the day before indigestion occurs. A liking for alcohol, spicy foods and coffee, all of which make the patient worse. Enjoyment and tolerance of fats. Indigestion after coffee.

ABDOMEN   Feels bruised. Flatulent distension with colicky pains which produce an urge to defaecate. Tenderness over the liver.

STOOLS   Constipation with a frequent, ineffectual urge to open the bowels. Incomplete and unsatisfactory defaecation. Alternating diarrhoea and constipation (*see a doctor*).

RECTUM   Painful piles, which may bleed, are better after a bowel action.

PERIODS   Irregular and early, with backache and constipation. Profuse and prolonged loss. Pain in the lower back and hips.

BACK   Lumbago, which makes turning over in bed difficult.

SKIN   The whole body feels burning hot but the slightest movement or uncovering produces excessive chilliness.

SLEEP   Drowsiness after eating and in the early evening. Wakefulness after 3 a.m. but followed by a heavy, unrefreshing sleep. Patients improve for an uninterrupted, short sleep.

BETTER	WORSE
After an uninterrupted nap	In the morning
In the evening	From mental exertion
At rest	After eating
In damp, wet weather	From touch
From pressure	After stimulants and narcotics
	In dry weather
	In cold air
	For being uncovered

OPIUM
Opium

There may be complete loss of consciousness, or the patient is unaware of his condition and has no complaints, no pain and asks for nothing. Delirium, with the patient talking insensibly, can also occur. (In the United States this remedy is available only on prescription.)

MAIN MEDICAL USES

Bowel obstruction	Kidney pain
Coma	Picking at the bedclothes
Constipation	Stroke
Cough	Urine retention
Fright-induced ailments	

MAJOR SYMPTOMS

FACE   Red, bloated face with hot sweat, heavy breathing and half-closed eyes. Comatose.

CHEST   Heavy breathing, slow respiration and pulse. Recurring cycle of deep, fast breathing followed by cessation of breathing.

ABDOMEN   Fluid containing faecal material may be vomited when there is an obstruction in the bowel. Kidney colic with intense pain, cold sweat and scanty urine.

STOOLS   Obstinate constipation from impacted faeces. Stools are hard, round, black balls from inactivity of the rectum. Diarrhoea in children. Involuntary stools in brain-damaged patients.

URINE — Retention of urine with a full bladder. Involuntary urination after a fright.

SKIN — Hot, damp, sweating. Hot perspiration over all the body, except the legs.

SLEEP — Drowsiness or sleepy feeling, but inability to fall asleep because of acute sensitivity to noise. Picking at the bedclothes.

BETTER	**WORSE**
For cold	From heat
From walking	During and after sleep

PHOS ACID

Phosphoricum acidum

This remedy is useful for mental and physical debility, especially in rapidly growing young people. It is used after acute diseases, grief, severe emotional upsets, fatigue and loss of body fluids. The patient is apathetic, indifferent, listless and suffers from impaired memory and intellectual slowness.

MAIN MEDICAL USES

Ailments from loss of body fluids	Hair loss (Alopecia)
Debility	Headache
Diarrhoea, chronic	Heartburn
Excessive urination	Impotence
Grief-induced ailments	Indigestion

MAJOR SYMPTOMS

HEAD — Four types of headache can occur: one feels like pressure on the top of the head, another feels as if the temples are being pressed together, a third comes on after coitus and the fourth is due to eye strain. Baldness and premature greying.

EYES — Sunken and surrounded by blue rings.

MOUTH — Dry, cracked lips. The gums bleed. The tongue is swollen, dry and may be bitten during sleep.

CHEST — Weak feeling in the chest from talking and coughing, with pressure behind the breastbone affecting breathing. Dry, tickling cough. Palpitations in fast-growing children and after grief.

STOMACH — Craving for juicy drinks and cold milk. Sour food and drink lead to nausea and discomfort.

ABDOMEN — Distension and fermentation, with loud rumblings and an ache around the navel.

STOOLS — White, watery, involuntary, painless diarrhoea with much wind. The loss does not tire the patient.

URINE — Frequent, profuse urination, especially at night. The urine appears milky.

GENITALIA — Loss of virility. Partial impotence. Scrotal eczema.

LIMBS — The arms and legs feel weak. Cramps in the upper arm and wrists, with scraping pain in the bones at night. Itching between the fingers and in joint folds.

BETTER	**WORSE**
For keeping warm	From exertion
For sleep	From being talked to
	After sexual excesses

283

PHOSPHORUS

Phosphorus

Typical patients are fair-skinned, sensitive people with quick perception, and rapidly growing children who are tall, stoop-shouldered and hollow-chested. Subjects are restless and fidgety, red-haired with a pale yellowish complexion and long, silky eyelashes. They are full of fears, disinclined to both physical and mental exertion, but have occasional bouts of excitement and enthusiasm followed by exhaustion, tears and apathy. Both sexes develop irresistible sexual desires.

MAIN MEDICAL USES

Asthma	Indigestion
Bronchitis	Laryngitis
Dandruff	Nasal polyps
Diarrhoea, chronic	Peptic ulceration
Gastritis	Ulcerative pharyngitis
Gum disorders	Vertigo
Hepatitis	

MAJOR SYMPTOMS

HEAD	Vertigo after getting up, especially in the elderly. Congestive headaches with a sensation of heat in the spine and cold over the back of the head. The skin of the forehead feels tight. The brain feels 'tired', especially in public speakers who have to 'think on their feet'. Dandruff and itching of the scalp.
EYES	Partial visual loss while reading. Distant objects appear only dimly, and shading the eyes with the hand makes them easier to see. Misting or veiling of vision, or the appearance of coloured lights or haloes require *urgent* medical attention.
EARS	Hearing becomes dulled and sounds re-echo.
NOSE	Swollen, dry and painful to touch. Internal inflammation may lead to a slow bleed. Nasal polyps, which may bleed profusely, interfere with breathing. Chronic catarrh with a bloody, green-yellow discharge can lead to ulcers inside the nostril.
MOUTH	The gums become inflamed, bleed easily, ulcerate and separate from the teeth. The tongue is chalky white with a red line down the centre. Saliva runs from the mouth during sleep.
THROAT	Sore, painful on swallowing, with a burning, raw, scraping feeling. The tonsils and soft palate are dark red and small ulcers with yellow centres form in the pharynx. Swallowing saliva is painful. A sensation of tickling in the throat produces a cough, which is worse in cold air and from talking, laughing, or going from a warm room to a cold one.
CHEST	Painful hoarseness and laryngitis, worse in the evening, makes talking difficult because of the pain. A hard, dry, racking cough with burning chest pain, tightness across the chest and sweet-salty expectoration lead to difficult and fatiguing breathing, worse if lying on the left side.
STOMACH	Ravenous nocturnal appetite for acidic and spicy foods and an unquenchable thirst for cold water, which is vomited up as soon as it warms in the stomach. Nausea, with belching of food, and vomiting associated with tenderness and distensions, occur at night. Stomach pains relieved by cold food and ices. Sour taste and sour belching after eating.

ABDOMEN	Empty, weak sensation with distension. Tenderness over the liver with jaundice.
RECTUM	Smarting during, and burning after, bowel movements. Urge to defaecate on rising in the morning.
STOOLS	White-grey, long and hard, or hard, small and dark, or soft with lumps of white mucus, all signify liver or pancreatic disease. Painless, debilitating, chronic diarrhoea, worse in hot weather and from cold drinks.
PERIODS	Early and scanty, but last too long. Occasional vaginal discharge instead of a period.
BACK/ LIMBS	Weakness and trembling of the arms and legs from the least exertion. Burning sensation between the shoulder blades.
SKIN	Bruising and bleeding from wounds, both readily occurring.

BETTER	**WORSE**
In the dark	In the evening
Lying on the right side	Lying on the left or painful side
For cold food and drink	From thunderstorms and weather changes
During rest and after sleep	From mental and physical exertion

PHYTOLACCA
Phytolacca decandra

Patients may show an indifference to life and not care whether they live or die. Complaints tend to be right-sided.

MAIN MEDICAL USES

Breast disorders	Rheumatism
Conjunctivitis	Sciatica
Eczema	Teething children
Mastitis in pregnancy	Tonsillitis
Piles	

MAJOR SYMPTOMS

EYES	Feeling of sand in the eye. Excessive hot tears.
MOUTH	Teething children who clench their teeth.
THROAT	The tonsils and palate are dark purple and swollen. The throat feels sore and dry and pain shoots to the ears on attempting to swallow. Tonsillitis accompanied by pus often occurs with backache, dark, scanty urine, a heavily coated tongue and a high fever. Worse from hot drinks.
BREASTS	Swollen, hard, painful breasts with sore nipples. *See your doctor urgently.* Pain radiates from the nipples all over the body when breast-feeding.
NECK/ BACK	Stiffness in the morning on waking. Shooting pain in the lower-back area extends down the outside of the hip to the foot.
LIMBS	Rheumatic pains in the arms and legs, notably below the elbows and knees. Burning pains shoot, like

electric shocks, down the bone, are worse at night and during stormy weather, and fly from one part to another. Severe pain in the heel is better by keeping the heel higher than the body.

MUSCLES   Aching, bruised soreness in all the muscles, worse for movement but must move nevertheless.

BETTER	WORSE
For rest	For damp, cold
In warm, dry	weather
weather	At night

PLANTAGO
Plantago major

This remedy is associated with depression and insomnia in heavy smokers.

MAIN MEDICAL USES

Allergy rashes	Diarrhoea
Bed-wetting	Earache
Chilblains	Insomnia
Dental conditions, including	To stop smoking by causing
toothache	an aversion to tobacco

MAJOR SYMPTOMS

FACE   Recurrent facial pain, worse from 7 a.m. to 2 p.m., accompanied by excessive tears and dislike of light. The pain radiates to the temples and lower part of the face.

EYES   Pain associated with toothache or middle-ear infection.

EARS   Severe earache which seems to go through the head to the opposite ear. Toothache often accompanies the earache. Hearing becomes acute and noises painful.

MOUTH   Profuse salivation. The teeth are sensitive and painful when touched. The toothache is better while eating and worse for direct contact with anything cold.

RECTUM   Painful piles make even standing unpleasant.

STOOLS   Frequent desire to defaecate, but inability to pass a stool. Watery brown diarrhoea.

BLADDER   Profuse flow of urine, leading to bed-wetting at night.

SKIN   Itching, burning eruptions.

BETTER	WORSE
For sleeping and	At night in a warm
eating	room

PLUMBUM
Plumbum metallicum

Typical subjects are apathetic, irritable and over-concerned about their health. They suffer memory loss, an inability to find the correct word when speaking, great lassitude and show rapid emacitation. There is a fear of being assassinated.

MAIN MEDICAL USES

Colic	Recurrent miscarriages
Constipation	Spasms and cramps
Dry skin	Tinnitus (noises in the ear)
Emaciation	Vaginal spasms
Impotence	Vertigo
Jaundice	Wrist drop

MAJOR SYMPTOMS

HEAD Aching, with a heaviness and throbbing. Tearing pain accompanied by vertigo and tinnitus.

FACE Sunken cheeks with greasy, shiny, pale skin.

MOUTH Trembling of the tongue makes talking difficult. A blue line develops along the gum margins, the breath is fetid and the gums swollen.

BREASTS Shrinkage occurs.

STOMACH Hiccoughs with belching and almost constant vomiting. Sudden, severe stomach pain, better for hard pressure.

ABDOMEN Severe colic radiating to all parts of the body. The abdominal wall feels as if pulled in towards the back.

STOOLS Constipation, with hard, lumpy, black stools, urging and anal spasm.

URINE Continual urging with scanty urine.

GENITALIA *Men:* Impotence.

Women: Vaginal spasm (vaginismus) and constipation. Tendency to miscarriages.

BACK/ LIMBS Neuralgic pains in the spine extending to the back of the head. Cutting pain in the lumbar region radiates to the hips and legs and is better for pressure and rubbing. Trembling of the hands and legs, spasmodic contraction of joints, worse at night. Pains in the thigh muscles, acute cramps and pains in the legs.

SKIN Very dry, yellow or dark brown skin with almost no sweating.

BETTER	WORSE
For pressure	At night
For physical exertion	For motion
For rubbing	

PODOPHYLLUM

Podophyllum

This remedy is suited to depressed, bilious and sluggish individuals.

MAIN MEDICAL USES

Diarrhoea	Piles
Gastro-enteritis	Prolapse, especially after
Liver disease	pregnancy
Ovarian pain	Teething disorders

MAJOR SYMPTOMS

HEAD Dull, pressure headache, worse in the morning, alternates with diarrhoea. The head feels hot and the patient rolls it from side to side.

MOUTH The patient grinds his teeth while asleep at night. Desire to press the gums together.

287

STOMACH | Heartburn, with continual gagging and nausea, especially when pregnant.

ABDOMEN | Distension. Tenderness over the liver, which feels better for rubbing.

STOOLS | Acute and long-standing diarrhoea early in the morning, during teething, from acid fruits and in hot weather. Green, watery, fetid, profusely gushing and painless diarrhoea. Constipation, with clay-coloured, hard, dry, difficult stools, may alternate with diarrhoea. *See a doctor for diagnosis.* Dentition diarrhoea in children who become pale with a puckered mouth just before the stool is passed.

GENITALIA | Pain in the right ovary. Prolapse after childbirth.

PERIODS | Suppressed in girls with constipation.

PREGNANCY | Piles with anal prolapse.

BETTER

Lying on the abdomen

WORSE

In the early morning
In hot weather
When teething

PSORINUM

Psorinum

There is extreme sensitivity to cold, a disagreeable smell to the body and the patient looks thin and emaciated. Psorinum individuals become very depressed and anxious about their future.

MAIN MEDICAL USES

Acne rosacea	Eye inflammation, chronic
Asthma	Hay fever
Bronchitis, chronic	Migraine
Constipation in young children	Offensive perspiration
Eczema	Outer-ear inflammation

MAJOR SYMPTOMS

HEAD | Wakeful during the night with a severe headache and ravenous hunger.

EYES | Recurrent infections, with red lids which stick together overnight.

EARS | Offensive, scabby, discharging eczema around the ears, with intolerable itching. Chronic infection of the external ear.

CHEST | Asthma, worse sitting up, better lying down with the arms outspread. Chronic bronchitis recurring each winter. Hay fever. Periodic nasal colds/sore throats.

STOMACH | Belching like bad eggs. Continual hunger, particularly in the middle of the night.

RECTUM/ANUS | Constipation in pale, sickly children.

SKIN | Coarse, dry, dirty-looking skin or excessively greasy skin both lead to intolerable itching, worse for the heat of the bed or washing. Dry, scaly, crusty eruptions on the scalp and in the bend of joints.

BETTER

For heat and warm clothing

WORSE

For weather changes
For any cold or draught

PULSATILLA
Pulsatilla

This remedy is suited to highly emotional individuals who are timid, irresolute, weep easily, like sympathy and caresses, and are often blue-eyed, blonds with pale faces. Of mild, gentle, yielding disposition, they are changeable and contradictory. They always feel better in the open air and are inevitably thirstless.

MAIN MEDICAL USES

Allergy rashes
Bed-wetting
Bronchitis, chronic
Catarrh, acute and chronic
Chilblains
Colds
Diarrhoea
Ear infections
Eye complaints (conjunctivitis, eyelid inflammation, granular lids, inflammation of the tear ducts, styes)
Facial neuralgia
German measles
Indigestion and flatulence
Lack of periods

Measles
Mumps
Painful periods
Piles
Rheumatism
Senses of smell and taste reduced
Stress incontinence (leak of urine when coughing or laughing)
Testicle and spermatic cord inflammation
Toothache
Vaginal discharges
Varicose veins and ulcers

MAJOR SYMPTOMS

HEAD
Headache from overwork, the pain extending to the face and teeth. Neuralgia starting in the right temple, with scalding, excessive tears on that side.

FACE
Right-sided neuralgia with excessive tears. Swollen lower lip with a central crack.

EYES
Burning and itching, inflammation on the margins of the lower lids, the lids stick together overnight. Thick, profuse, yellow, bland discharge.

EARS
Feel as if stuffed, which affects hearing. Inflammation of the external ear with a thick, pus-like discharge. Inflammation of the middle ear with darting, tearing pains relieved by cold applications.

NOSE
Colds. Nose feels blocked in the late evening and discharges thick, yellow, opaque mucus in the morning. Sneezing discharge of green, offensive mucus. Lost sense of smell and taste, with slight bleeding.

MOUTH
Dry but without thirst. Toothache better for cold mouthwashes. The tongue is covered with a tenacious mucus. Loss or alteration of taste. Bread tastes bitter.

CHEST
Tickling and scraping in the larynx with excessive tears, hoarseness and dry cough, all worse at night and better sitting up. Palpitations after a heavy meal, with anxiety and shortage of breath made worse by lying on the left side.

STOMACH
Belches taste of food and bile. Nausea and vomiting with chilliness, gnawing discomfort and a feeling of having eaten too much. Aversion to fats, pastries and warm food and drink. Craving for fruits and acidic foods. Pain about one hour after eating.

ABDOMEN
Distension after eating, with intermittent colic and rumbling, worse in bed. Wind moves around the

abdomen, and there are griping, pinching pains and frequent diarrhoea.

RECTUM — Painful, protruding, bleeding piles, worse in the evening, with much itching.

GENITALIA — Creamy, burning vaginal discharge, worse on lying down.

PERIODS — None occur, or they are suppressed and late. Period pain after getting feet wet, when run down or after anger.

LIMBS — Pains in the legs with restlessness, sleeplessness and chilliness. Rheumatic pains shift rapidly from joint to joint. Varicose veins and varicose ulcers with smarting, itching and chilliness, but warmth aggravates.

SKIN — Allergy rash with diarrhoea after rich food. Measles. Acne at puberty.

SLEEP — Difficult to get off, then sleep may be restless. Children often sleep with their hands above their heads.

BETTER

In the open air
For movement
For cold applications
For cold food and drink

WORSE

From heat
From rich, fat food
After eating
In the evening
In a warm room
Lying on the left or painless side
When allowing the feet to hang down

RANUNC BULB
Ranunculus bulbosus

This remedy acts especially on the muscular tissues and skin, particularly the chest wall. It may also be useful in treating the effects of excess alcohol.

MAIN MEDICAL USES

Alcoholism	Pain between the ribs
Hay fever	Rheumatism
Headache	Shingles

MAJOR SYMPTOMS

HEAD — Severe neuralgic headache in the forehead and top of the head, which seems to go to the eyes. Worse in the evening and on going in to a warm room.

EYES/NOSE — Hay fever with acrid tears and nasal discharge. At other times the nostrils feel dry and blocked.

CHEST — Feels sore and bruised. Walking outside leads to a feeling of chilliness in the chest wall. Shooting and stitching chest wall pains, worse in damp weather.

SKIN — Burning sensation with intense itching. Shingles with bluish blisters. Cold sores with much itching.

BETTER

No influencing factors

WORSE

In open air
From movement and contact
From wet and stormy weather
In the evening

RHODODENDRON
Rhododendron

Patients dread storms and have a great fear of thunder; in fact, any illness they have is much worse before stormy weather. Their rheumatism is paradoxical (odd) because it is worse during hot weather. They are often unable to sleep unless their legs are crossed, and have a tendency to be forgetful.

MAIN MEDICAL USES

Facial neuralgia

Gout

Headache

Hydrocele (fluid in the sac surrounding the testicle)

Rheumatism

Summer diarrhoea

Testicle inflammation (orchitis)

Toothache

MAJOR SYMPTOMS

HEAD — Tearing, boring headache in the forehead, spreading to the temples; worse from wine, wind and cold, wet weather.

FACE — Violent jerking pain, better for warmth and from eating. The pain is felt from the temple to the lower jaw and chin.

EYES — Burning pain in the eye, worse before a storm, better after the storm breaks.

EARS — Pain in the outer ear. Humming, buzzing and ringing in the ear after being up and out of bed for a few hours. Hearing is always much better in the morning.

TEETH — Drawing, cutting pains in the teeth in damp, windy weather and before a storm. The gums may become swollen and the teeth loose.

STOOLS — Diarrhoea in damp weather and from eating under- or over-ripe fruit. Relieved by eating.

GENITALIA — Inflammation, enlargement and drawing pain in the testicle, especially the right. The pain radiates up into the abdomen and down the thigh. (*Medical help is essential for these symptoms.*)

BACK — Drawing, tearing, sprained pain in the bones of the lumbar region, worse from rest and in rainy weather.

LIMBS — Bruised, cramp-like pain in the long bones. Neck stiffness in bed in the morning and after rising. Gout in the right big toe. Rheumatic pain in all the limbs is described as 'tearing'. It occurs more often on the right side of the body and is worse at rest.

BETTER	WORSE
After the storm breaks	At the approach of a storm
For warmth (not heat)	In rough, cold, windy weather
For eating	

291

RHUS TOX

Rhus toxicodendron

Patients show extreme restlessness, apprehension and depression, all of which are much worse at night. Any fever is very weakening and may lead to a mental stupor or even mild delirium. They dream of being involved in acts which require great exertion.

MAIN MEDICAL USES

Agitation and
  restlessness
Allergy rashes
Blistery skin eruptions
Cellulitis (diffuse inflammation
  of the skin)
Cold sores
Eczema
Erysipelas

Influenza
Lumbago
Muscular strains
Rheumatism
Sciatica
Shingles
Sprains and pulled muscles
Swelling due to fluid
  retention

MAJOR SYMPTOMS

FACE	Swelling and redness from erysipelas spreading from the left to the right. Pain in the jaw joint.
EYES	Infected lids with profuse yellow pus and dislike of light.
MOUTH	The corners may ulcerate, cold sores develop and the lips have dried brown crusts on them.
TONGUE	The tongue is coated white, except for a triangular, red tip. It feels dry and sore.
CHEST	Dry, tickling cough, worse after midnight, occurs when any part of the body gets cold.
STOMACH	Unquenchable thirst, especially for milk, but no appetite.
STOOLS	Loose, with blood, slime and brown mucus. Frothy, painless, offensive and involuntary, passed while asleep. They lead to great exhaustion.
BACK	Pain and stiffness in the small of the back, better for moving about or lying on something hard.
LIMBS	Rheumatic pains with hot, swollen joints which are sore to the touch and develop marked stiffness from overuse. They are painful on starting to move, improve with continued movement but become painful again from excessive movement. The limbs feel stiff and paralysed. Numbness and trembling after overwork and exposure to cold, damp conditions. With all symptoms there is marked restlessness, anxiety and apprehension, and the patient changes position frequently to obtain relief.
SKIN	Red, swollen and intensely irritable. In eczema the surface is raw and develops a thick crust which oozes pus. Small blisters which easily discharge pus.

BETTER	WORSE
In warm, dry weather	During sleep
	In cold, wet, rainy weather
From changing position	At night, after midnight
	During rest
For rubbing	From getting wet
For warm applications	after over-heating
	Lying on the back or the right side

RUTA
Ruta graveolens

Patients can experience a feeling of great lassitude, weakness and despair. All parts of the body may feel painful, as though badly bruised, but in spite of this and the lassitude, the patient feels very restless and cannot settle.

MAIN MEDICAL USES

Constipation	Sciatica
Eye strain	Sprains and lameness
Ganglia (cystic swelling around a tendon)	Strained tendons
	Tennis elbow
Hangover	Mechanical injuries to bones causing bruised pains

MAJOR SYMPTOMS

HEAD　　Hangover headache.

EYES　　Red, hot and painful from overuse or very close work. Often leads to a headache.

RECTUM　　Prolapse after defaecation and after confinement.

STOOLS　　Difficult faeces, much straining required to move them. Constipation alternating with frothy, mucous stools. Bleeding with defaecation. *See a doctor.*

BLADDER　　Constant urge to urinate; the bladder feels perpetually full.

LIMBS　　The bones and back feel bruised and stiff. Tendons, especially those in the thigh, are painful and tender, worse on stretching. Pain and stiffness in the wrists and hands, weakness in the hips and legs. Sciatica.

BETTER	WORSE
For movement	Lying down
	In cold, wet weather

SABADILLA
Sabadilla

Patients are nervous and easily startled. They develop weird imaginary illnesses, such as believing the limbs are twisted or one part of the body is shrunken and too small. In women imaginary pregnancies may occur.

MAIN MEDICAL USES

Colds	Sore throat
Hay fever	Tonsillitis

MAJOR SYMPTOMS

HEAD　　Headache and sleeplessness due to endless thoughts. Vertigo with a sensation of fainting. Frontal headache with colds.

EYES　　Red, burning eyelids with excessive flow of tears.

EARS　　Deteriorating hearing.

NOSE　　Spasmodic sneezing with a runny nose. The nasal discharge is copious and watery.

THROAT　　Soreness starts on the left side and goes to the right. Sensation of something in the throat, producing a constant desire to swallow. Warm food and drink relieve the sore throat.

293

STOMACH	Spasmodic pain associated with dry cough. Thirst is absent. Dislike of strongly flavoured foods but a great desire for hot, sweet foods.
PERIODS	Often late, stopping and starting within a period.
SKIN	Dry, with deformed and thickened nails.

BETTER	WORSE
For warm food and drink	From cold of any sort
For being well wrapped up	At the full moon

SABINA

Sabina

Often depressed, Sabina types find music insufferable and become nervous and anxious with it.

MAIN MEDICAL USES

Arthritis	Tendency to miscarriage
Gout	Uterine and ovarian
Heavy periods	affections
Increased sexuality	Vaginal discharge
Piles	Warty growths

MAJOR SYMPTOMS

| HEAD | Bursting headache with sudden onset and sudden cessation. |
| MOUTH | Toothache when chewing, and pain in the chewing muscles. |

STOMACH	Craving for lemonade, which causes heartburn and bitter taste.
RECTUM	Piles which bleed easily and copiously. The blood is bright red.
GENITALIA	*Men:* Penile warts with difficulty in retracting the foreskin. Increased sexuality.
	Women: An acrid, burning, offensive discharge after the period. Increased sexuality. Recurrent miscarriage and threatened miscarriage. Pain runs from the lower back to the pubis and from below it shoots up the vagina.
PERIODS	Bright red and profuse, with pain extending into the thighs.
LIMBS	Arthritic joint pains. Gout, worse in the warmth. The thighs feel bruised and there are shooting pains in the heels and feet.
SKIN	Itching, burning, warty growths develop.

BETTER	WORSE
In cool, fresh air	From the slightest movement
	From heat

SANGUINARIA
Sanguinaria

Complaints tend to be on the right side of the body. Diarrhoea often follows the cessation of catarrh anywhere in the respiratory tract.

MAIN MEDICAL USES

Acne
Asthma
Bronchitis
Colds
Croup
Diarrhoea
Headache and migraine

Inflammation of the nose
  lining, chronic
Menopausal problems
Polyps in the nose, ear,
  uterus and bladder
Rheumatism

MAJOR SYMPTOMS

HEAD   Pain starts at the back of the head and runs over the top to settle above the eyes, especially the right. The headache recurs at regular intervals (often every seven days), and may be accompanied by vomiting. It also returns at the menopause when it is accompanied by hot flushes and red, flushed cheeks. Better when lying down and from sleep, worse in the sun.

FACE   Facial neuralgia starts in the upper jaw and radiates in all directions.

NOSE   Profuse, yellow, offensive nasal catarrh. Colds followed by diarrhoea, and chronic nasal inflammation, with dry, congested nostrils.

CHEST   Dry, hacking cough interferes with sleep as it is worse lying down. Also a spasmodic cough after influenza or whooping cough. Asthma with a cough, associated with gastric disturbances, better after belching or passing wind. Burning soreness in the right chest radiates to the right shoulder. Acute chest infections with severe shortage of breath, a feeling of constriction, offensive breath and pus-like sputum.

LIMBS   Rheumatism in the right arm and shoulder makes raising the arm painful, worse at night. Palms of the hands and soles of the feet both feel hot and burning.

SKIN   Acne associated with scanty periods. The cheeks have a well-defined red flush.

BETTER	WORSE
When quiet	From sweets
In the dark	For movement
For sleep	From a jar or touch

SEPIA
Sepia

Typically a remedy for female complaints, Sepia may nevertheless be used by men. The patients are thin, weak and worn out through overwork. They have a sallow complexion, are often sad and depressed, dread being alone but develop an indifference to their family. Consolation makes them worse and they become weepy when talking of their illness. They are very chilly people and often have a yellow, saddle-like discoloration over the nose and cheeks.

MAIN MEDICAL USES

Bed-wetting

Constipation in pregnancy

Depression

Genital itching

Headache

Heavy periods

Lack of periods

Menopausal complaints

Morning sickness

Nasal polyps

Painful periods

Premenstrual syndrome (PMS)

Prolapse

Sweaty feet

MAJOR SYMPTOMS

HEAD
Headache associated with a period, especially when the loss is scanty. The top of the head feels cold to the patient. Hair loss and pimples along the hair margin.

FACE
Red, rough and yellow-brown spots on the neck and face.

EYES
Redness, with burning, smarting and swelling on waking. Feeling of grit in the eye.

NOSE
Feels stuffed and dry, and may become inflamed, swollen and scabby. Nasal polyps and dry, chronic nasal catarrh both occur.

STOMACH
There is an empty, 'all gone' sensation with great hunger, a craving for vinegar and sour foods and an aversion to meat. Nausea, better for eating, comes in the morning and evening. Vomiting during pregnancy with an empty nauseous feeling. Acid indigestion with sour belches, bloated abdomen, nausea, vomiting and diarrhoea.

ABDOMEN
Tenderness over the liver, relieved by lying on the right side.

RECTUM
Constipation, especially in pregnancy, with hard stools like small balls.

URINE
Appears reddish and contains a sand-like deposit. Involuntary urination during the first sleep. Frequent urge to urinate.

GENITALIA
The vagina and vulva feel dry and cause discomfort when walking. Yellow acrid discharge before a period. The womb feels as if it is going to drop out. Some prolapse may be present.

PERIODS
Too early or too late, and may be very scanty. Lack of periods is accompanied by flushes of heat, indigestion, nausea and vomiting (better for eating and lying down) and a longing for acidic foods. Discharge with lack of periods and also with painful periods.

MENOPAUSE
Chills and hot flushes, irregular periods with great variations in the amount of loss, pain in the lower back, worse standing, better lying down. Tremulous feeling around the heart, unrefreshing sleep, cold, damp feet and a neuralgic headache.

BACK/
LIMBS
Weakness and pain in the small of the back, coldness between the shoulder blades and restlessness in all limbs.

SKIN
Red roughness on the face, round, red spots on the hands, small, red blisters above the hips and on the side of the neck. Brown or brown-yellow areas on the elbows, neck, back and abdomen. Itching is not relieved by scratching. The feet are sweaty and smelly.

BETTER	WORSE
In the warmth of the bed	From cold air and cold weather
For hot applications	Before thunderstorms
For violent exercise	
For warmth	From washing

SILICA
Silicea

Typical Silica patients are very sensitive to noise and become very anxious when subjected to it. They are easily startled, gloomy, irritable, peevish, lachrymose people, who lack ambition and 'grit' both mentally and physically. They are always very chilly and every injury tends to become infected and discharge pus. As children they have large, sweaty heads and big abdomens, weak ankles and are late to walk. They fear pointed objects, such as pins.

MAIN MEDICAL USES

Abscesses	Nail deformities
Anal fissure	Nasal catarrh
Asthma	Neck, hip, lumbar and coccygeal pain
Boils	
Carbuncles	Offensive sweats
Constipation	Piles
Discharge of pus	Sleep-walking
Eczema	Styes
Gum disease (pyorrhoea)	Tear-duct obstruction
Headache	Vaginal discharge
Ingrowing toenails	Vertigo

MAJOR SYMPTOMS

HEAD — Headache which starts in the neck and goes over the head to the eyes, producing a bruised feeling which is aggravated by opening the eyes. A throbbing, bursting headache better for lying down and binding the head tightly. Headaches associated with nervous exhaustion. Vertigo on looking up.

EYES — Red rims and an aversion to light. Styes. Obstruction of the tear duct leads to excessive watering of the eyes.

EARS — Thin, watery ear discharge. Soreness over the mastoid bone, with a sharp, sticking pain, worse for cold and pressure. Roaring noises in the ear.

NOSE — Blood-stained mucous discharge. The nose feels dry and sore.

MOUTH — Root abscesses in the teeth and gum disease (pyorrhoea).

CHEST — Morning hoarseness with a tickle in the larynx. Cough with pus-like sputum which is coughed up in lumps.

STOMACH — Dislike of meat and warm food.

RECTUM — Stinging, cutting pains with an ineffectual desire to defaecate. The rectum feels paralysed, with no power to expel the stool fully and some slips back. Sticky moisture with itching is felt around the anus, with sensitive internal piles.

GENITALIA — *Men:* Itching with scrotal swelling. Violent erections with nocturnal emission of semen.

Women: Itching during a period with soreness and eruptions on the inner side of the thighs. Bearing-down vaginal pains with a white watery discharge. Labial abscesses. An acrid, burning discharge associated with heavy periods leads to irritability and weakness. Constipation always occurs before and during a period.

BACK/ LIMBS Stiffness and chilliness in the neck, pain in the coccyx after prolonged sitting, and a bruised pain in the hips and lumbar region at night. The fingernails become deformed. The feet are icy cold and sweaty. Ingrowing toenails.

BETTER	WORSE
For warmth	In the morning
For wrapping up the head	From washing
	During a period
In the summer	From uncovering
	Lying down and lying on the left

SPIGELIA
Spigelia

In many cases Spigelia types fear sharp, pointed objects. They feel chilly and this causes them to shudder frequently. Symptoms are chiefly left-sided.

MAIN MEDICAL USES

Angina	Pain between the ribs
Facial neuralgia	Palpitations
Nasal catarrh, chronic	Toothache

MAJOR SYMPTOMS

HEAD Burning, tearing pains in the head extend to the eye, especially the left. Worse in the evening and from motion, jarring and walking.

FACE Recurrent facial neuralgia.

EYES Pain on moving the eyes. Severe pain in and around the eye extends deep into the socket.

MOUTH Foul breath and toothache, worse from cold water.

CHEST Cutting pains beneath the left nipple area extend to the left upper arm, worse on deep breathing. Violent palpitations with anxiety, worse sitting down and bending forward. Pain over the heart, worse for movement. Extreme shortage of breath on exertion.

BETTER	WORSE
Lying on the right side with the head high	For touch, motion, noise and washing
	In cold, damp, stormy weather

SPONGIA
Spongia tosta

The patient is often a child or young woman with a fair complexion. Both suffer from anxiety and many fears.

MAIN MEDICAL USES

Bronchitis, chronic and acute	Inflammation of the testicle and spermatic cord
Croup	
Hiccoughs	Laryngitis

Swollen glands
Thyroid enlargement

Whooping cough

MAJOR SYMPTOMS

THROAT
Constant clearing of the throat. Sore throat, worse after eating sweets. The thyroid gland may become enlarged.

LARYNX
Pain when singing, with a scraping, burning, constrictive sensation in the larynx; dry and hoarse.

CHEST
Both whooping cough and croup are worse before midnight. A dry cough both day and night, and all the air passages from the throat downwards feel dry. The patient wakes after midnight with pain in the chest and a sense of suffocation. Bronchitis with wheezing and coughing, better after eating and drinking, but worse for cold air and in a stuffy room.

STOMACH
Great thirst and perpetual hunger. Unable to wear tight clothing around the abdomen. Hiccoughs.

GENITALIA
Swelling of the spermatic cord and testicle with pain and tenderness. *Urgent medical advice needed.*

PERIODS
Palpitations before a period. The patient may be woken with shortage of breath during a period.

GLANDS
Swollen lymph glands, especially in the neck.

BETTER

Lying down
For warm food and drinks

WORSE

In cold, dry winds
On awakening
From exertion

STAPHYSAGRIA
Staphysagria

Very easily offended, Staphysagria patients are continually peevish and have a violent temper. Illnesses often follow some emotional upset. They tend to dwell on sexual matters. There is perpetual worry about the future and what other people think of them.

MAIN MEDICAL USES

Constipation
Cystitis
Dental conditions
Eczema
Eyelid cysts
Gum diseases
Injuries caused by sharp objects, and incised wounds

Irritable bladder
Pain relief after abdominal surgery
Piles
Prostate enlargement
Sexual disorders
Styes
Warts

MAJOR SYMPTOMS

EYES
Recurrent styes and cysts on the lids. The eyes appear sunken and have dark (blueish) rings around them.

THROAT
A sharp pain radiates to the left ear on swallowing.

MOUTH
Toothache during a period. The teeth look black and crumble. The gums become spongy and bleed easily.

STOMACH
Tremendous hunger, even when full. Desire for stimulants.

ABDOMEN
Colic when angry. The abdomen becomes swollen with wind, especially in children. Wind feels warm

299

when being passed. Pain relief after abdominal surgery.

STOOL Diarrhoea after taking cold drinks. Constipation may also occur and it leads to piles.

GENITALIA *Men:* Emission of semen leads to backache and a feeling of weakness. Shortage of breath after intercourse. Frequent masturbation leads to a feeling of guilt.

Women: The external genitalia are very sensitive, worse when sitting down.

BLADDER Cystitis and ineffectual urging to pass urine, especially in young women. The bladder feels incompletely emptied and there is a sensation of urine being continually passed. Burning sensation in the urethra both when passing urine and when not.

BACK/ LIMBS Backache, at its worst in the morning before rising. The arms and legs feel bruised and painful and the joints stiff.

SKIN Eczema with thick scabs which are very itchy. The rash appears mainly on the head, ears, face and body. Scratching leads to the itch appearing elsewhere on the body. Warty growths with a stalk.

BETTER	**WORSE**
After breakfast	From emotional
For warmth	upsets and anger
For rest at night	From sexual
	excesses
	From tobacco
	From the slightest
	touch on any
	affected part of
	the body

SULPHUR
Sulphur

Patients tend to be irritable, depressed, thin and weak, very selfish, lazy, untidy and dirty. Hasty-tempered, they revel in arguing and philosophizing and are chronic grumblers. They cannot stand for long and hate bathing. Any illness they have constantly relapses. All the body orifices, such as the nose, anus and ears, look red.

MAIN MEDICAL USES

Asthma	Hot flushes
Bed-wetting	Indigestion
Conjunctivitis	Insomnia
Constipation	Lack of periods
Diarrhoea	Nasal catarrh, chronic
Erysipelas	Painful periods
Eyelid inflammation	Skin conditions
Gastritis	Vaginal discharge
Gout	

MAJOR SYMPTOMS

HEAD A dry, itchy scalp with hair loss. The top of the head feels hot to the patient. A sick headache recurs periodically.

EYE Redness during the day, itching at night, with a sensation of grit under the lids. Redness and burning of the lids, which stick overnight. Marked dislike of light and of getting the lids wet.

NOSE Soreness, itching and burning of the nostrils, especially at the opening of the nose. Nasal catarrh with dry scabs and some bleeding.

MOUTH — The lips are red and dry, the tongue coated yellow-white and dry, and the palate dry. Saliva tastes bitter and coppery, especially in the morning on waking.

CHEST — A cough with rawness in the larynx, shooting chest pains and a hot head with cold hands. Dry cough in the evening which may cause the patient to be woken with breathlessness during the night. A feeling of pressure on, and burning in, the chest is associated with anxiety. Green, pus-like sputum rattles in the chest and is easy to cough up.

STOMACH — Ravenous hunger, but the appetite goes at the sight of food. Headache and lassitude if the hunger is not relieved. Sour belches tasting of bad eggs during the day, worse after eating. Nausea in the morning and with a faint, empty feeling before meals and around 11 a.m. Full feeling after eating very little. Milk and cereal products can cause indigestion.

ABDOMEN — Constant gurgling, with offensive wind and griping before and during defaecation.

RECTUM — Sticking pain, worse in the evening, and cutting pains during defaecation. Painful, ineffectual straining to defaecate on waking, followed by a copious, watery stool causes the patient to dash out of bed. Itching, burning and sore piles. Constipation with hard, knotty stools, painful to pass, may alternate with diarrhoea. Redness of the anal orifice.

STOOLS — Fluid, frequent and fetid in the morning.

BLADDER — Frequent urination, especially at night. The urine feels hot and burns when being passed.

GENITALIA — Redness, itching and burning of the external genitalia in both sexes. Women may experience an acrid, burning vaginal discharge.

MENOPAUSE — Frequent hot flushes.

LIMBS — Hot, sweaty hands. Burning in the hands and feet at night, better for putting the legs out of bed. Patients may be stoop-shouldered.

SKIN — Itching anywhere burns after being scratched. Water aggravates all skin conditions. The skin is dry, scaly, unhealthy and burns. Any injury tends to become infected and discharge pus. Pimples, pustules, abrasions in the skin folds and itching all occur. The body is hot and has a foul-smelling sweat. Frequent flushing.

SLEEP — In catnaps. Disturbed by the slightest noise. Restless sleep and difficulty in sleeping between 2 and 5 a.m.

BETTER	WORSE
In dry, warm weather	At rest and when standing
Lying on the right side	From the warmth of the bed
	For washing and bathing
	At 11 a.m.
	From alcoholic drinks

THUJA
Thuja occidentalis

Easily exhausted and emaciated, Thuja patients often have weird ideas, such as believing they are made of glass and will break easily, or that there is something alive in the abdomen, such as an animal or a pregnancy. Emotionally sensitive, music causes tears and trembling. They may become depressed and weary of life.

MAIN MEDICAL USES

Anal fissure and warts	Laryngitis, chronic
Asthma in children	Mouth ulcers
Brittle nails	Nasal catarrh, chronic
Carbuncles	Nasal polyps
Constipation	Polyps
Diarrhoea	Sinusitis
Effects of previous vaccination	Styes
Eyelid cysts	Vaginal discharge
Gum disease (pyorrhoea)	Vertigo
Hair loss	Warts and wart-like growths
Headaches	on the skin and mucous
Insomnia	membranes

MAJOR SYMPTOMS

HEAD — Chronic headache, like a nail driven into the skull, usually left-sided. Dandruff and dry hair which falls out easily.

EYES — The lids stick together overnight and are dry and scaly. Styes and eyelid cysts develop.

EARS — Buzzing, roaring and creaking sounds. Polyps in the canal and a putrid, smelly discharge.

NOSE — Chronic, thick green catarrh with mucus, pus or blood (or any combination). The nose feels dry. Ulceration with scabs just inside the nostril. The frontal sinuses are painful.

MOUTH — The tip of the tongue is painful and the mouth filled with blisters. Retraction of the gums.

CHEST — Short, dry, hacking cough. Asthma, especially in children. Chronic laryngitis.

ABDOMEN — Flatulent distension with rumblings and colic, and sensation of something moving within the abdomen.

RECTUM — Constipation with rectal pain, the stool recedes after partial expulsion. Painful and swollen piles, worse after sitting down. Anal fissure and anal warts.

STOOLS — Chronic diarrhoea, sudden, copious and explosive, worse after breakfast.

BLADDER — Frequent and urgent desire to urinate, often associated with prostate enlargement.

GENITALIA — *Men:* Itching and intermittent burning under the foreskin. Penile warts.

Women: Itching of the vulva during and after urination. Burning pain in the vagina when walking and sitting. Yellow-green vaginal discharge. Vulval warts.

SKIN — Appears dirty and the nails are brittle. Brown spots on the skin. Eruptions, mainly on parts that are covered, are sensitive to touch and worse after scratching. The perspiration is sweet and strong and occurs when asleep, either only on uncovered parts, or all over the body, except for the head.

SLEEP — Persistent insomnia.

BETTER	WORSE
On the left side	At night from the heat of the bed At 3 a.m. or 3 p.m. From cold, damp air After breakfast, alcohol, vaccination, fat and coffee

URTICA
Urtica urens

This remedy is said to antidote the ill-effects of eating shellfish. Symptoms tend to return at the same time each year.

MAIN MEDICAL USES

Allergy rashes	Gout, acute
Burns and scalds	Lactation failure
Chicken-pox	Rheumatism
Eyelid inflammation	Stings, especially bee
Genital irritation	stings

MAJOR SYMPTOMS

HEAD	Headache, with pain felt in the left upper part of the abdomen at the same time. Extreme vertigo with a tendency to fall forward.
EYES	Stinging eyelids with a sensation of grit in the eye.
THROAT	Burning pain in the throat makes the patient feel nauseous.

CHEST/BREASTS	The chest feels as if bruised. Failure in milk secretion in lactating mothers.
GENITALIA	*Men:* Itching of the scrotum, which may become swollen, interferes with sleep. *Women:* Extreme irritation of the external genitalia with stinging, itching and swelling.
LIMBS	Pain and stiffness, mainly in the right shoulder, arms, wrists, knees and ankles. Rheumatism alternates with a burning, stinging skin eruption. Acute gout.
SKIN	Violent itching blotches and wheals, allergy rash with burning and stinging.
SLEEP	Patients may fall asleep while reading.

BETTER	WORSE
No influencing factors	From contact with water In a cool, damp atmosphere

VERATRUM ALB
Veratrum album

In typical patients sullen indifference alternates with violent excitement, anger and rages. Destructive moods occur in which they cut and tear clothes, but they may also have bouts of depression and stupor. Typical symptoms include collapse with extreme coldness, weakness, cold sweat, violent vomiting and purging, and cramps in the limbs.

MAIN MEDICAL USES

Bronchitis, acute and
  chronic
Diarrhoea
Collapse
Colic
Constipation, particularly
  in babies
Convulsions

Headache
Night cramps
Palpitations
Period pain
Rheumatism
Sciatica
Vertigo
Whooping cough

MAJOR SYMPTOMS

HEAD
Persistent vertigo, with a cold sweat on the forehead and great weakness, even fainting. Neuralgic headache, either with a sensation of ice on the top of the head, or a headache with vomiting and pains like shocks on raising the head, better for pressure on top of the head.

FACE
Ice-like coldness of the nose and face. In collapse the face is very pale, blue and cold.

CHEST
Acute and chronic bronchitis (especially in the elderly), with hard-to-raise sputum and a loud, barking cough, worse on entering a warm room after being in cold air. Drinking cold water can bring on the cough. Involuntary urination occurs with the coughing. Palpitation accompanied by anxiety and rapid audible breathing may develop.

STOMACH
Ravenous appetite and thirst for cold water; the latter is vomited as soon as swallowed. Craving for fruit, fruit juices and cold food. Nausea and vomiting, worse for drinking and the slightest movement.

ABDOMEN
Colic and swelling, sensitive to pressure, accompany a cold, sinking feeling. Pain just before defaecation.

STOOLS
Constipation from rectal inactivity, accompanied by a headache. Constipation in babies. The stool is large and requires much straining to pass it, which leads to exhaustion and a cold sweat. Painful and watery diarrhoea also leads to extreme exhaustion.

PERIODS
Profuse, early and exhausting, with pain, coldness and diarrhoea before they start. Sexuality is greatly increased just before a period.

LIMBS
Sciatica, with the pain shooting down the leg like an electric shock. Cramps in the calves, worse in bed.

SKIN
Blue, cold and clammy. Cold sweat. The skin of the hands and feet becomes wrinkled.

BETTER	WORSE
For walking	At night
For warmth	In wet, cold weather

ZINC MET

Zincum metallicum

Patients are physically and mentally broken down, with little vitality. They dislike noise very much, repeat everything said to them and appear lethargic and stupid. Trembling develops, especially with chronic disease. Moods are variable and may alternate between depression and elation. They are much better after any potential discharge starts to flow and also when any latent rash comes out.

MAIN MEDICAL USES

Back pain	Restless leg syndrome
Chilblains	Sensation of a lump in the throat
Colic	Sleep-walking
Conjunctivitis	Stress incontinence
Headaches	Teething difficulties
Indigestion	Varicose veins
Migraine	Vertigo
Premenstrual syndrome (PMS)	Violent erections

MAJOR SYMPTOMS

HEAD Headache, from even a minute amount of wine, is worse in the open air and from washing in cold water. Vertigo, preceded by sharp pain at the root of the nose and followed by nausea, faintness, hand trembling and severe headache, makes the patient fall to the left. A severe headache in the afternoon from too much study or lack of sleep comes on with visual disturbance, dislike of light and tiredness.

EYE Red, inflamed conjunctiva, worse on the inner side of the eyeball. Blurring of half the vision precedes a migraine. The lids become sore and itchy.

MOUTH The lips are pale, cracks develop in the corners of the mouth, the gums bleed and the teeth are loose. Slow, painful teething in children is accompanied by rolling of the head, boring the head into the pillow, constant motion of first one foot, then the other. Weakness and coldness.

THROAT Sensation of constriction in the oesophagus when attempting to swallow.

STOMACH Ravenous hunger around 11 a.m. Burning indigestion from sweets and eating too quickly.

ABDOMEN Distension, pain, flatulent colic and griping after a meal. The abdominal wall does not relax between bouts of colic.

STOOLS Hard, small, constipated stool, or diarrhoea with green, watery stools (especially in children).

BLADDER Hysterical retention of urine, passed only when the patient is sitting and bent backwards. Involuntary urine loss when walking, coughing or sneezing.

GENITALIA Violent erections, nightly emissions of semen and retraction of the testicles.

PERIODS Left ovarian pain. The periods come late and the loss is greatest at night. The breasts are painful, the nipples sore. Restlessness, depression, coldness, spinal tenderness and restless feet accompany all symptoms. A dry cough may develop before the period starts.

BACK/ LIMBS Burning pain along the back when sitting or walking, and great aversion to it being touched. Dull ache in the lower back. The neck becomes sore after being bent for a long time, such as when writing. Weakness and trembling in the limbs. The feet and legs are being moved about constantly. Large varicose veins on the legs. The soles of the feet become sore.

BETTER	WORSE
While eating	From cold
	After mental or physical exertion
	From wine
	From touch
	Between 5 and 7 p.m.

305

BIBLIOGRAPHY

The following titles have been particularly helpful during the writing of this book.

Anatomy, Descriptive and Applied, 25th edition, Dr Henry Gray (Longman, Green & Co., London, UK, 1932)

Children's Types, Dr Douglas M. Borland (British Homeopathic Association, London, UK)

Classical Homeopathy, Dr Marjory Blackie, ed. Dr Charles Elliot and Dr Frank Johnson (Beaconsfield Publishers, Beaconsfield, UK, 1986)

Digestive Drugs, Dr Douglas M. Borland (British Homeopathic Association, London, UK)

The Essentials of Homeopathic Materia Medica, Dr Jacques Jouanny (Laboratoire Boiron, France, 1980)

The Essentials of Homeopathic Therapeutics, Dr Jacques Jouanny (Laboratoire Boiron, France, 1980)

Everyday Homeopathy, Dr David Gemmell (Beaconsfield Publishers, Beaconsfield, UK, 1987)

Homeopathic Drug Pictures, Dr Margaret L. Tyler (Health Science Press, Sussex, UK, 1970)

Homeopathic Medicine, Dr Trevor Smith (Thorsons Publishers Ltd, Wellingborough, UK, 1982)

Homeopathic Prescribing, Dr Noel Pratt (Beaconsfield Publishers, Beaconsfield, UK, 1980)

Homeopathy in Practice, ed. Dr Kathleen Priestman (Beaconsfield Publishers, Beaconsfield, UK, 1982)

Homeopathy: Medicine for the 21st Century, Dana Ullman (North Atlantic Books, Berkeley, California, USA, 1988)

Keynotes of Leading Remedies, 2nd edition, Dr H.C. Allan (Bhattacharyya Publications, Calcutta, India, 1968)

Lectures on Homeopathic Materia Medica, 2nd edition, Dr James Tyler Kent (Boericke & Tafel, Philadelphia, USA, 1911)

Lectures on the Theory and Practice of Homeopathy, Dr R.E. Dudgeon (Jain Publishing, New Delhi, India, 1978)

Materia Medica of New Homeopathic Remedies, Dr O.A. Julian, trans. Virginia Munday (Beaconsfield Publishers, Beaconsfield, UK, 1979)

The Merck Manual of Diagnosis and Therapy, 15th edition, ed. Dr Robert Berkow (Merck Sharp & Dohme Research Laboratories, Rahway, New Jersey, USA, 1977)

The Organon of Medicine, Dr Samuel Hahnemann, 5th edition, trans. R.E. Dudgeon, with additions by William Boericke (Roy Publishing House, Calcutta, India, 1970)

The Organon of Medicine, Dr Samuel Hahnemann, 6th edition, trans. J. Kunzli, A. Naude and P. Pendleton (Tarcher Publications, Los Angeles, USA, 1982)

The Patient, Not the Cure, Dr Marjory Blackie (Macdonald & Jane's, London, UK, 1976)

Pocket Manual of Homeopathic Materia Medica, 9th edition, Dr W. Boericke (Boericke & Tafel, Philadelphia, USA, 1927)

Practical Homeopathic Therapeutics, 2nd edition, Dr W.A. Dewey (Boericke & Tafel, Philadelphia, USA, 1914)

A Primer of the Materia Medica, Dr T.F. Allen (Boericke & Tafel, Philadelphia, USA, 1892)

Repertory of the Homeopathic Materia Medica, 6th US edition, 1st Indian edition, Dr James Tyler Kent (Sett Dey & Co., Calcutta, India, 1961)

Towards Earlier Diagnosis, Dr Keith Hodgkin (E. & S. Livingstone Ltd, Edinburgh, UK, 1963)

World Index with Rubrics of Dr Kent's Repertory, 3rd edition, Dr R.P. Patel (Sai Homeopathic Book Corporation, Kerala, India, 1986)

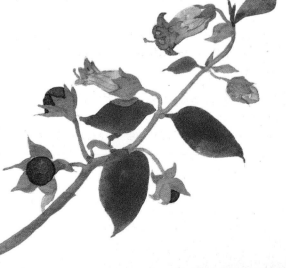

FURTHER READING

Once their interest in homeopathy has been kindled, many people want to deepen their knowledge of this fascinating form of treatment. With this in mind, and purely to start you off, the following are a few of the many books available.

A Brief Study Course in Homeopathy, 3rd edition, Dr Elizabeth Wright-Hubbard (Formur Inc., St Louis, USA, 1983)

A slim volume which explains the principles of homeopathy in simple terms.

Children's Types, Dr Douglas M. Borland (British Homeopathic Association, London, UK)

A booklet (56 pages) of very useful information for treating children constitutionally.

The Handbook of Homeopathy, Gerhard Koehler (Thorsons Publishing Group, UK and USA, 1986)

The principles and practice of homeopathy presented in a clear, well-structured manner. Recommended for serious further study.

Homeopathic Drug Pictures, Dr M.L. Tyler (Health Science Press, Rushington, Sussex, UK, 1989)

A bulky but easy-to-read book (868 pages) which will extend and deepen your knowledge of the major homeopathic remedies.

Homeopathy: Medicine for the 21st Century, Dana Ullman (North Atlantic Books, Berkeley, California, USA, 1988)

An interesting book which looks at the historical background of homeopathy, especially in the USA, and discusses its place in modern medicine. It also contains a good deal of valuable information about homeopathic treatment.

Introduction to Homeopathic Medicine, 2nd edition, Hamish W. Boyd (Beaconsfield Publishers, Beaconsfield, UK, 1990)

A systematic introduction to homeopathic medicine with information about the theory and principles, case-taking, diagnosis, and the application of remedies. It also contains some materia medica.

Materia Medica with Repertory, William Boericke (Boericke & Runyon, Philadelphia, USA, and the Homeopathic Book Service, Kent, UK, 1990)

This is essentially a reference book for use in the practice of homeopathy at a serious and professional level. It is used throughout the English-speaking world.

The Patient, Not the Cure, Dr Marjory Blackie (Macdonald & Jane's, London, UK, 1976)

A very readable introduction to the whole of homeopathy, full of interesting anecdotes and help in remedy selection.

Samuel Hahnemann, Trevor M. Cook (Thorsons Publishers Ltd, Wellingborough, UK, 1981)

A biography of the founder of homeopathic medicine.

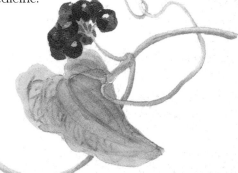

USEFUL ADDRESSES

UK Homeopathic organizations

To obtain the names of qualified homeopathic doctors and further information about homeopathy, contact one of the following organizations.

British Homeopathic Association
27a Devonshire Street
London W1N 1RJ
Tel: 071-935 2163

Faculty of Homeopathy
Royal London Homeopathic Hospital
Great Ormond Street
London WC1N 3HR
Tel: 071-837 9469

The Hahnemann Society
2 Powis Place
London WC1N 3HT
Tel: 071-837 2495

Homeopathic Development Foundation
9 Cavendish Square
London W1M 9DD
Tel: 071-629 3205

To obtain the names of non-medically qualified homeopaths contact:

Society of Homeopaths
2 Artizan Road
Northampton NN1 4HU
Tel: (0604) 21400

Homeopathic hospitals (NHS)

You can be referred to any of these by your GP.

Bristol Homeopathic Hospital
Cotham Road
Bristol BS6 6JU
Tel: (0272) 731231

Glasgow Homeopathic Hospital
1000 Great Western Road
Glasgow G12 0NR
Tel: 041-339 2786

Mossley Hill Hospital
Department of Homeopathic Medicine
Park Avenue
Liverpool L18 8BU
Tel: 051-724 2335

Royal London Homeopathic Hospital
Great Ormond Street
London WC1N 3HR
Tel: 071-837 8833

Tunbridge Wells Homeopathic Hospital
Church Road
Tunbridge Wells
Kent TN1 1JU
Tel: (0892) 42977

Homeopathic pharmacies

Although most pharmacists can obtain homeopathic medicines to order, it is wisest to obtain them from specialized pharmacies which carry a full range and are conversant with the correct handling and dispensing of homeopathic remedies. Most also have a mail-order service.

Ainsworths Homeopathic Pharmacy
38 New Cavendish Street
London W1M 7LH
Tel: 071-935 5330

Buxton and Grant
176 Whiteladies Road
Bristol BS8 2XU
Tel: (0272) 735025

Freeman's
7 Eaglesham Road
Clarkston
Glasgow G76 7BU
Tel: 041-644 4640

Galen Homeopathics
Lewell Mill
West Stafford
Dorchester
Dorset DT2 8AN
Tel: (0305) 263996

Helios Homeopathic Pharmacy
92 Camden Road
Tunbridge Wells
Kent TH1 2QP
Tel: (0892) 26393

P.A. Jansenn
The Pharmacy
28 Amptill Road
Bedford MK42 9HG
Tel: (0234) 53484

Jolleys Pharmacy
36 Witton Street
Northwich
Cheshire CW9 5AH
Tel: (0606) 331552

Nelson's Homeopathic Pharmacy
73 Duke Street
London W1M 6BY
Tel: 071–629 3118

Weleda UK Ltd
Heanor Road
Ilkeston
Derbyshire DE7 8DR
Tel: (0602) 309319

US Homeopathic organizations

Those with 800 numbers may be dialled free of charge within the United States.

Homeopathic Educational Services
2124 Kittredge Street
Berkeley
CA 94704
Tel: (510) 649 0294; orders (800) 359 9051
This organization sells homeopathic books, tapes, software, medical kits and medicines. It also has a general information service.

Homeopathic Pharmacopeia Convention
P.O. Box 174
Norwood
PA 19074
Tel: (215) 461 7380
Will supply a list of manufacturers of homeopathic medicines.

International Foundation for Homeopathy
2366 Eastlake Avenue E. #329
Seattle
WA 98102
Tel: (206) 324 8230
The foundation promotes the teaching of classical homeopathy to health professionals.

National Center for Homeopathy
801 N. Fairfax #306
Alexandria
VA 22314
Tel: (703) 548 7790
The major organization for homeopathy in the USA, it publishes a monthly newsletter, has training courses for health professionals and educational programmes for the general public.

Homeopathic pharmacies/manufacturers

Although American interest in homeopathy is steadily growing, there are still very few homeopathic pharmacies in the USA. However, those that do exist generally offer a mail-order service (as do manufacturers), so you can obtain remedies within a few days. (Those with 800 numbers may be dialled free of charge.)

Biological Homeopathic Industries
11600 Cochiti S.E.
Albuquerque
NM 87123
Tel: (800) 621 7644

Boericke & Tafel
2381 Circadian Way
Santa Rosa
CA 95407
Tel: (707) 571 8202; orders (800) 876 9505

Boiron-Borneman Inc
1208 Amosland Road
Norwood
PA 19074
Tel: (215) 532 2035; orders (800) 258 8823

Boiron-Borneman Inc
98c W. Cochran
Simi Valley
CA 93065
Tel: (805) 582 9091

Dolisos America Inc
3014 Rigel Avenue
Las Vegas
NV 89102
Tel: (702) 871 7153; orders (800) 365 4767

Longevity Pure Medicines
9595 Wilshire Boulevard #502
Beverly Hills
CA 90212
Tel: (310) 273 7423; orders (800) 327 5519

Luyties Pharmacal
4200 Laclede Avenue
St Louis
MO 63108
Tel: (314) 533 9600; orders (800) 325 8080

Standard Homeopathic Company
154–210 W. 131st Street
Los Angeles
CA 90061
Tel: (213) 321 4284; orders (800) 624 9659

INDEX

Figures in **bold** indicate main entries.
Figures in *italic* indicate illustrations.

Abdominal cavity *127*
Abies can: cravings (pregnancy) 175
palpitations 125
Abies nig: cravings (pregnancy) 175
indigestion 144
loss of appetite 139
rapid heart-rate 125
Abrasions and grazes **16**
Abscess or gumboil **110**
children 43
Abscesses, boils and carbuncles **204–5**
Absent-mindedness 51–2
irritability and 64
moodiness and 66
shyness/timidity and 70
Absinthium: hallucinations 60
Absinth: memory loss 65
Acetabulum *187*
Acetic acid: backache and lumbago 189
belching/flatulence 139
fainting 19
swelling/fluid retention 212
Acne 205
Aconite 221–2
acute and chronic bronchitis 130
angina 121
anxiety 53
asthma 128
backache and lumbago 189
Bell's palsy 72
breast conditions, including mastitis 162
burns and scalds 18
chest pain 132
chicken-pox 44
clinical depression 57
coating/discoloration of tongue 107
cold feet 192
cold hands 195
colds and influenza 95, 133
children 29
coughs 134
children 32
cramps after swimming 213
croup 33
cuts, lacerations, incised wounds 19
diarrhoea 151
children 34

discoloration of face 73
earache without discharge 89
children 37
emotional states 59
fainting 19
fears and phobias 59
fractures 21
gout 193
heart attack 22, 124
heavy bleeding 17
hoarseness and voice loss 114
insomnia 63
measles 46
miscarriage 179
nasal blockage/snuffles 98
nightmares 40
nosebleeds 101
children 41
pain in face 74
palpitations 125
panic attacks 24
preparing for labour 178
rapid heart-rate 125
red hands 196
restlessness 67
shock and collapse 25
sleep problems (children) 41
sore throat 116
stroke 26
sudden chills (holiday) 216
sunburn and overheating (holiday) 215
toothache and teething problems 42
urine retention 159
weak legs and ankles 197
Actaea racemosa *see* Cimicifuga
Actea spic: rheumatism and arthritis 199
weak hands 196
Adenoids *113*, 114
nasal polyps and 100
Adonis ver: palpitations 125
Adrenal gland *155*
Aesculus 222–3
backache/lumbago/muscle pains 174, 189
coating/discoloration of tongue 107
jaundice 145
piles 152
red hands 196
Aethusa: feeding problems 38
palpitations 125
restlessness 67
sore throat 116
sweat rash 212
vomiting (children) 43
Agaricus: burning sensation in face 73
chilblains 207
discoloration of face 73
eye strain 83

genital irritation (female) 64
mouth ulcers 106
pain in face 75
palpitations 125
restlessness 67
Agnus: frigidity 163
impotence 183
itching of the eyes 84
rapid heart-rate 125
Agraphis: adenoids 114
Air hunger 17, 25, 27
Alcoholism: and indolence 63
jaundice with 146
Aletris: backache and muscle pains 174
heavy periods 167
indigestion 144
Alfalfa: cravings (pregnancy) 176
Allergy rashes 206
with insect stings and bites 24
Allium cepa 223
colds and influenza 95, 133
children 29
earache without discharge 89
children 37
hay fever 96
nasal discharge 99
Allium sat: deafness 88
Aloe 223–4
backache and lumbago 189
cracked lips and mouth 105
incontinence 157
piles 152
prostate disorders 185
stomach upsets (holiday) 215
Alumen: difficulty with stools 153
hair loss/baldness 75
Alumina 224–5
anal itching 150
bleeding gums 110
conjunctivitis 80
constipation 151
children 31
disorders of nails 198
hair loss/baldness 76
loss of appetite 139
restlessness 67
sense of smell disorders 101
urine retention 159
vaginal discharge 172
Alvioli *127*
AMA: and homeopathy 11
Ambra: excessive sexual desire (female) 171
genital irritation (female) 164
hand and arm cramp 191
palpitations 125
restlessness 67
senility 69
shyness and timidity 70
Ambrosia: itching of the eyes 84

Amenorrhoea *see* Periods: absence of
American Institute of Homeopathy 11
Ammon carb 225–6
blue hands 194
decreased sexual desire (male) 185
emotional states 59
genital irritation (female) 164
heartburn 143
indigestion 144
nasal blockage/snuffles 98
palpitations 125
toothache 111
Ammon caust: hoarseness and voice loss 114
Ammon iod: Ménière's disease 92
Ammon mur: backache and lumbago 189
dandruff and eczema of the scalp 72
sciatica 201
Ammon phos: gout 193
Amnesia *see* Memory loss
Amyl nit: menopause 166
Anacardium: absent-mindedness 51
allergy rashes 206
clinical depression 57
difficulty with stools 153
eczema 208
gastric and duodenal ulcers 146
hallucinations 60
headache 76
increased sexual desire (male) 186
indigestion 144
lack of confidence 55
palpitations 126
senility 69
sense of smell disorders 101
Anaemia: discoloration of face and 74
excessive sensitivity and 69
fainting with 19
with palpitations 126
Aneurysms 123
dissecting 132
Anger and its effects **52–3**
and miscarriage 179, 180
Angina (Angina pectoris) **121–2**
raised blood pressure and 122
see also Chest pain
Ankles: rheumatism and arthritis in 200
see also Legs and ankles
Anorexia nervosa *see* Eating disorders
Ant carb: hair loss/baldness 75

Ant crud 226–7
acne 205
allergy rashes 206
anal itching 150
anger and its effects 52
belching/flatulence 139
bleeding gums 110
coating/discoloration of tongue 107
colitis 141
corns and calloses 190
cracked lips and mouth 105
digestive upsets (children) 35
disorders of nails 198
eating disorders 58
eczema 208
loss of appetite 139
moodiness 66
toothache 111
vomiting (children) 43
weak hands 196
Ant tart 227–8
acute and chronic bronchitis 130
asthma 128
cellulitis/erysipelas/impetigo 210
chicken-pox 44
confusion of mind 56
coughs 134
children 32
fainting 19
suffocation 27
whooping cough 49
Anthemis: chilblains 207
Anus *see* Rectum and anus
Anvil (incus) *86*
Anxiety 53–4
allergy rash from 206
and angina 121
and colitis 141
and insomnia 63
and irritability 64
diarrhoea with 151
during menopause 166
indifference and 62
palpitations with 125, 126
raised blood pressure and 12
sleep problems with (children) 41, 42
with asthma 129
children 130
with bronchitis 130
with coughs (children) 32
with depression 57
with diarrhoea (children) 34
with feeling of suffocation 136
with heart attack 22, 124
with hysteria 61
with restlessness 67, 68
with shock and collapse 25
with stroke 26
with vomiting 43

Aorta *119*, *155*
see also Chest pain
Apathy *see* Indifference
Aphasia *see* Speech disorders
Apis 228–9
cellulitis/erysipelas/impetigo 210
clumsiness 55
coating/discoloration of tongue 108
conjunctivitis 80
cravings (pregnancy) 176
earache without discharge 90
children 37
emotional states 59
eyelids turning in or out 83
incontinence 157
indifference 62
insect bites and stings 23, 214
painful intercourse 165
scarlet fever 48
shingles 48
styes 84
suffocation 27
swelling of eye/eyelids 85
swelling/fluid retention 212
Apis mel: rheumatism and arthritis 199
Apocynum can: restlessness 67
swelling/fluid retention 212
Appendix *137*
Appetite, loss of **139**
see also Digestive upsets (children)
Aqueous humour *79*
Aragallus: confusion of mind 56
restlessness 67
Aralia: asthma 128
Aranea: heel pain 196
restlessness 67
Arelia: coughs 134
Arg met: hand and arm cramp 191
hoarseness and voice loss 114
inflammation of eyelids 82
weak legs and ankles 197
Arg nit 229
absent-mindedness 52
angina 121
anxiety 53
belching/flatulence 140
bleeding gums 110
coating/discoloration of tongue 108
colitis 141
conjunctivitis 80
cravings (pregnancy) 176
digestive upsets (children) 35
discharge from the eye 81
emotional states 59
eye strain 83
fears and phobias 59

gastric and duodenal ulcers
146
headache 76
impotence 183
insomnia 63
palpitations 126
panic attacks 24
sensations in throat 115
sleep problems (children) 41
sore throat 116
children 42
swelling of eye/eyelids 85
toothache 111
Arms: bones of *187*
eczema on (children) 37, 38
Arms, pains in: angina and
121
backache and lumbago and
190
breast conditions and 163
cramp **191**
heart attack and 22, 124
Arnica 230
abscesses, boils and
carbuncles 204
after-pains (childbirth) 174
anger and its effects 52
angina 121
black eye 80
bruises 18
chest pain 132
cuts, lacerations, incised
wounds 19
discoloration of face 74
fractures 21
gout 193
head injuries and concussion
21
headache 39
heart attack 22, 124
heavy bleeding 17
injuries and accidents
(holiday) 214
injuries to the ear 91
miscarriage 179
nosebleeds 101
children 41
preparing for labour 178
restlessness 68
rheumatism and arthritis 199
shock and collapse 25
sinusitis 102
sprains and strains 26
stroke 26
whooping cough 49
Arrogance 54
Ars alb 230–1
abscesses, boils and
carbuncles 204
allergy rashes 206
anal burning 149
anxiety 53

asthma 129
clinical depression 57
colds 95
colds and influenza 95, 133
children 29
dandruff and eczema of the
scalp 72
diarrhoea 151
children 34
digestive upsets (children) 35
earache with discharge 88
children 35
eczema 208
fainting 19
feeling of suffocation 136
gastric and duodenal ulcers
147
hallucinations 60
hay fever 97
heavy bleeding 17
indigestion 144
insomnia 63
irritability 64
mouth ulcers 106
nasal blockage/snuffles 98
palpitations 126
panic attacks 24
piles 152
psoriasis 210
restlessness 68
shingles 48
shock and collapse 25
stomach upsets (holiday) 215
swelling of eye/eyelids 85
swelling/fluid retention 212
vaginal discharge 172
vomiting (children) 43
Ars brom: rosacea 211
Ars iod: chronic catarrh 94
nasal discharge 99
nasal irritation/itching 100
psoriasis 211
Arteries, hardening of the 123
and raised blood pressure 122
see also Aorta
Arteriosclerosis *see* Arteries,
hardening of the
Arthritis *see* Rheumatism and
arthritis
Arum triph: colds and
influenza 133
children 29
cracked lips and mouth 105
hay fever 97
hoarseness and voice loss 114
nasal blockage/snuffles 98
nasal discharge 99
Arundo 231–2
burning feet 192
burning hands 195
cracks and fissures 207
hay fever 97
irritation in mouth 105

sweaty feet 193
Asafoetida: hysteria 61
Asphyxia *see* Suffocation
Asterias: increased sexual
desire (male) 186
Asthma 128–30
cardiac 129
raised blood pressure and
122
in children 130
with angina 121
with feeling of suffocation 136
with hardening of arteries 123
Aurum met 232
absent-mindedness 52
bad breath 103
clinical depression 57
emotional upsets (during
pregnancy) 176
hardening of the arteries 123
quarrelsomeness 67
raised blood pressure 122
sinusitus 102

Back and limbs 187–202
see also Arms; Legs and ankles
Backache and lumbago
189–90
during labour 178
during miscarriage 179, 180
kidney stones and 158
menopause and 166
on holiday 214
with excessive sexual desire
171
with heavy periods 167, 168
with impotence 183
with irregular periods 168
with prostate disorders 185
Bad breath 103–4
palpitations with 126
with bleeding gums 110, 111
Badiagia: dandruff and eczema
of the scalp 72
Baldness *see* Hair loss/baldness
Baptisia 232–3
coating/discoloration of
tongue 108
confusion of mind 56
sore throat 116
stomach upsets (holiday) 215
Bar mur: asthma 129
Baryta carb 233–4
cold feet 192
decreased sexual desire (male)
186
glandular fever 46
hardening of the arteries 123
impotence 183
lack of confidence 56
memory loss 65
prostate disorders 185

raised blood pressure 122
senility 69
sore throat (children) 42
tonsillitis 118
toothache 111
Bed-wetting (children) **28–9**
Bee sting 23
Belching/flatulence **139–40**
raised blood pressure and 122
with angina 121
with asthma 129
with colic 140, 141
children 30, 31
with colitis 141, 142
with gall-bladder problems
143
with heartburn 143
with hysteria 61
with indigestion 144
with ulcers 146, 147
with vomiting 43
see also Disgestive upsets
(children)
Belladonna 234–5
abscess or gumboil 110
abscesses, boils and
carbuncles 204
absence of periods 167
acute and chronic bronchitis
131
bed-wetting 28
breast conditions, including
mastitis 162
cellulitis/erysipelas/impetigo
210
chicken-pox 44
coating/discoloration of
tongue 108
cold feet 192
coughs 134
children 32
discoloration of face 74
earache with discharge 88
children 36
glandular fever 46
gout 193
hallucinations 60
headache 76
children 39
heatstroke 23
heavy bleeding 17
heavy periods 167
hoarseness and voice loss 114
insect bites and stings 214
lactation problems 178
miscarriage 179
mumps 47
nightmares 40
pain in face 75
painful intercourse 165
painful periods 169
palpitations 126
restlessness 68
rheumatism and arthritis 199

rosacea 211
scarlet fever 48
sleep problems (children) 41
sore throat 116
children 42
stammering 115
temperature fits 20
tonsillitis 118
urine retention 159
whooping cough 49
Bellis 235
after-pains (childbirth) 174
breast conditions, including
mastitis 162
hysteria (children, holiday)
216
menopause 166
muscle aches and pains
(holiday) 214
varicose veins and varicose
ulcers 202
during pregnancy 181
Bell's palsy 72
Benzoic acid: bed-wetting 28
bunions 190
cystitis 156
nappy (diaper) rash 40
rheumatism and arthritis 199
Berberis 236
acne 205
anal fissure 149
cystitis 156
gallstones and gall-bladder
disease 143
kidney stones 158
salivation problems 107
Berberis aquifol: psoriasis 211
Berberis vulg: frigidity 163
Bilious attacks, with jaundice
146
Bismuth: hand and arm cramp
191
toothache 111
Bladder *155*, *160*, *173*, *182*
irritation with heavy periods
167
kidney stones and 159
paralytic *see* Incontinence
prostate disorders and 185
Bleeding: after intercourse 165
and suffocation 27
between irregular periods 169
between periods 164, 165
indifference and 62
reducing during labour 178
with anal fissure 149
Bleeding, heavy 16–17
from piles 153
with cuts, lacerations, incised
wounds 19
with miscarriage 179, 180
Blepheritis *see* Eyelids:
inflammation of
Blisters: on lips and mouth 105

with eczema 209
with infected skin conditions
210
see also Shingles
Blood pressure, raised **122–3**
hardening of the arteries and
123
with stroke 26
Blood vessels *203*
see also individual types
Boils *see* Abscesses, boils and
carbuncles
Bone *109*, *160*, *182*
broken *see* Fractures
Borax 237
abscess or gumboil 110
anxiety 53
bad breath 103
chilblains 207
eyelids turning in or out 83
mouth ulcers 106
psoriasis 211
Bovista: allergy rashes 206
clumsiness 55
stammering 115
suffocation 27
weak hands 196
Bowel, large *182*
Bowels *see* Rectum and anus
Brachycardia 125
Brain 50
Breast conditions, including
mastitis **162–3**
frigidity and 163
genital irritation and 164
with irregular periods 168
see also Lactation problems
Bronchioli *127*
Bronchitis, acute and chronic
130–1
Bronchus: right and left *127*
Bruises 18
on holiday 214
on the ear 91
reducing during labour 178
sensation of with backache
and lumbago 189
with cuts, lacerations, incised
wounds 19
with mastitis 162
see also Black eye
Bryonia 238–9
acute and chronic bronchitis
131
backache and lumbago 189
backache and muscle pains
174
breast conditions, including
mastitis 162
coating/discoloration of
tongue 108
confusion of mind 56
constipation 151
children 31

coughs 134
  children 32
cracked lips and mouth 105
eating disorders 58
fainting 19
gastric and duodenal ulcers 147
gout 193
headache 76
heatstroke 23
indigestion 144
irritability 64
measles 47
rheumatism and arthritis 200
sinusitis 102
sore throat 116
sprains and strains 26
toothache and teething problems 42
Bufo: impotence 183
  premature ejaculation 184
Bulimia nervosa *see* Eating disorders
Bunions 190
Burns and scalds **18**
  on holiday 214
Bursitis *see* Housemaid's knee

Cactus 239
  angina 121
  chest pain 132
  cold hands 195
  hardening of the arteries 123
  heart attack 22, 124
  palpitations 126
  restless legs 198
  urine retention 159
Cadmium sulph: Bell's palsy 72
  nasal polyps 100
Caecum *137*
Caladium: asthma 129
  cravings (pregnancy) 176
  impotence 183
  vaginal itching during pregnancy 181
Calc ars: anger and its effects 52
  confusion of mind 56
Calc carb 240–1
  absence of periods 166
  allergy rashes 206
  bleeding gums 110
  breast conditions, including mastitis 162
  chilblains 207
  cold feet 192
  coughs 134
  cramps (pregnancy) 175
  earache with discharge 89
    children 36
  eczema 208

excessive sexual desire (female) 171
fears and phobias 59
feeding problems 38
genital irritation (female) 164
heartburn 143
heavy periods 167
impotence 183
increased sexual desire (male) 186
inflammation of eyelids 82
lactation problems 179
loss of appetite 139
nasal polyps 100
palpitations 126
premature ejaculation 184
rheumatism and arthritis 200
toothache 111
vaginal discharge 172
Calc fluor: abscess or gumboil 110
  backache and lumbago 189
  cracks and fissures 207
  deafness 88
  heavy periods 167
  sore throat 116
  varicose veins and varicose ulcers 202
Calc iod: varicose veins and varicose ulcers 202
Calc phos 241
  adenoids 114
  colic 140
  cravings (pregnancy) 176
  excessive sexual desire (female) 171
  fractures 21
  tooth decay 112
Calc sil: irregular periods 168
  irritability 64
  lack of confidence 56
Calc sulph: burning feet 192
  discharge from the eye 81
Calcarea: anxiety 53
  cravings (pregnancy) 176
  restlessness 68
Calendula 242
  abrasions and grazes 16
  cuts, lacerations, incised wounds 19
  deafness 88
Calendula cream: injuries and accidents (holiday) 214
Calloses *see* Corns and calloses
Camphor 242
  cold feet 192
  increased sexual desire (male) 186
  shock and collapse 25
Canine *109*
Cantharis 242–3
  burning feet 192
  burning sensation in face 73
  burns and scalds 18

cellulitis/erysipelas/impetigo 210
cystitis 156
discoloration of face 74
excessive sexual desire (female) 171
fair skin 216
heavy periods 167
increased sexual desire (male) 186
insect bites, stings 23
mouth ulcers 106
restlessness 68
sore throat 116
sunburn and overheating (holiday) 215
Capsicum: cold sores 104
  cravings (pregnancy) 176
  discoloration of face 74
  piles 152
  sore throat 116
    children 42
Carb acid: leg cramp 191
  sense of smell disorders 101
Carb sulph: indolence 63
  irritability 64
  memory loss 65
  noises in ear 90
  sciatica 201
Carbo an: blue hands 194
  chilblains 207
  clinical depression 57
  rosacea 211
Carbo veg 243–4
  acute and chronic bronchitis 131
  asthma 129
  belching/flatulence 140
  bleeding gums 110
  coating/discoloration of tongue 108
  cravings (pregnancy) 176
  digestive upsets (children) 35
  discoloration of face 74
  eating disorders 58
  heavy bleeding 17
  indifference 62
  involuntary passing of stools 154
  memory loss 65
  mouth ulcers 106
  nasal irritation/itching 100
  shock and collapse 25
  suffocation 27
  sunburn and overheating (holiday) 215
  sweaty feet 193
  varicose veins and varicose ulcers 202
  whooping cough 49
Carbolic acid: indigestion 144
  insect bites, stings 23
Carbuncles *see* Abscesses, boils and carbuncles

Carduus: jaundice 145
  varicose veins and varicose ulcers 202
Carotid artery *119*
Carpus *187*
Cataracts: senility and 69
Catarrh: and obstruction of the eustachian tube **87**
  from colds and influenza (children) 29, 30
  hair loss and 76
  noises in the ear and 90
    see also Deafness
  with colds and influenza 133
  with whooping cough 49
Catarrh, chronic 94–5, 98
  and sense of smell 101
  nasal polyps and 100
  sinusitis and 102
Caulophyllum 244
  after-pains (childbirth) 174
  false labour 177
  heavy periods 167
  miscarriage 180
  painful periods 169
  preparing for labour 178
Causticum 244–5
  bed-wetting 28
  Bell's palsy 72
  catarrh/obstruction of eustachian tube 87
  clinical depression 57
  coughs 134
  deafness 88
  eye strain 83
  hoarseness and voice loss 114
  incontinence 157
  indigestion 144
  inflammation of eyelids 82
  noises in ear 90
  restless legs 198
  restlessness 68
  rheumatism and arthritis 200
  senility 69
  sweat rash 212
  urine retention 159
Cellulitis 209–10
Cenchris: moodiness 66
Cerebellum *71*
Cerebrum (brain) *71*
Cereus serp: anger and its effects 52
Cervix *160*
Chamomilla 245–6
  anger and its effects 52
  coating/discoloration of tongue 108
  colic 140
    children 30
  diarrhoea 152
    children 34
  earache with discharge 89
    children 36
  irritability 64

miscarriage 180
painful periods 169
preparing for labour 178
restlessness 68
rheumatism and arthritis 200
sleep problems (children) 41
temperature fits 20
toothache and teething problems 43, 111
  during pregnancy 181
  on holiday 216
'Change of life' (female) 165
Chelidonium 246–7
  acute and chronic bronchitis 131
  backache and lumbago 189
  coating/discoloration of tongue 108
  cold hands 195
  discoloration of face 74
  gallstones and gall-bladder disease 143
  indolence 63
  jaundice 145
Chenopodium: deafness 88
  Ménière's disease 92
Chest pain 132–3
  raised blood pressure and 122
  with angina 121
  with bronchitis 131
  with coughs 134
    children 32, 33
  with heart attack 22, 124
  with rapid heart-rate 125
Chicken-pox 45
  see also Shingles
Chilblains 207
  on hands 194
Childbirth *see* After-pains
Children's ailments 28–43
Chills, on holiday **216**
Chimaphila: prostate disorders 185
  urine retention 159
Chin sal: Ménière's disease 92
  noises in ear 90
Chin sulph: noises in ear 90
China 247–8
  asthma 129
  belching/flatulence 140
  colitis 142
  diarrhoea 152
    children 34
  discoloration of face 74
  gallstones and gall-bladder disease 143
  headache 76
  heavy bleeding 17
  indifference 62
  shock and collapse 25
  toothache 111
Chlorum: memory loss 65
Choroid *79*
Chrysarobinum: psoriasis 211

Cicuta 248–9
  head injuries and concussion 21
Ciliary muscle *79*
Cimicifuga 249
  after-pains (childbirth) 174
  backache and lumbago 189
  false labour 177
  headache 76
  heavy periods 167
  irregular periods 168
  menopause 166
  migraine 78
  miscarriage 180
  painful periods 169
  rheumatism and arthritis 200
  sciatica 201
Cina 249–50
  eye strain 83
  irritability 64
  nasal irritation/itching 100
  worms 250
Cinchona 8–9
  see also China
Circulatory system 119–26
Cistus can: cracks and fissures 208
  sensations in throat 115
Clavicle (collar bone) *187*
Clematis: conjunctivitis 80
  sweat rash 212
  varicose veins and varicose ulcers 202
Clitoris/clitoral hood *160*
Clumsiness 54–5
  indifference and 62
Coca: restlessness 68
  tooth decay 112
Cocculus 250–1
  after-pains (childbirth) 174
  backache, lumbago and muscle pains 175, 189
  cold hands 195
  emotional states 59
  excessive sensitivity 69
  headache 76
  loss of appetite 139
  painful periods 169
  travel sickness 92, 216
Coccus cacti: coughs 134
  whooping cough 49
Coccyx *182, 187*
Cochlea *86*
Coffea 251
  hyperactivity 61
  insomnia 64
  palpitations 126
  raised blood pressure 122
  restlessness 68
  sleep problems (children) 41
  toothache 111
Coitus: palpitations during 126
Colchicum: cold feet 192
  cravings (pregnancy) 176

disorders of nails 198
eating disorders 58
gout 194
rheumatism and arthritis 200
toothache 111
Cold sores 104
see also Herpes
Colds and influenza 133–4
and eyes 81
and the nose 95–7
asthma with 129
children 29–30
sinusitis after 102
tonsillitis after 118
Colic 140–1
anger and 52, 53
children 30–1
difficulty with stools and 154
on holiday 214
restlessness and 68
sleep problems with (children) 41
with belching/flatulence 140
with diarrhoea (children) 34
see also Colitis
Colitis 141–2
Collagen fibres 203
Collapse, from shock *see* Shock and collapse
Collinsonia: chronic catarrh 94
constipation and piles during pregnancy 181
piles 153
Colocynth 251–2
anger and it effects 52
colic 140
children 30
colitis 142
cramps (pregnancy) 175
diarrhoea 152
children 34
painful periods 169
sciatica 201
stomach upsets (holiday) 215
toothache 111
Colon 137
Concentration, lack of 55
memory loss and 65
Concha 86
Concussion *see* Head injuries
Confidence, lack of 55–6
Confusion of mind 56
Conium 252–3
absent-mindedness 52
breast conditions, including mastitis 162
conjunctivitis 81
coughs 134
during pregnancy 181
hardening of the arteries 123
heartburn 143
increased sexual desire (male) 186
jaundice 145

prostate disorders 185
shyness and timidity 70
Conjunctiva 79
Conjunctivitis 80–1
see also Eyes
Constipation 151
anal itching with 150
children 31
difficulty with stools and 154
during pregnancy 181
on holiday 215
with allergy rash 206
with colic 141
children 30
with gall-bladder problems 143
with piles 153
with vaginal discharge 172
Convallaria: genital irritation (female) 164
Convulsions (children) *see* Fits, temperature
Coordination, impaired 52
Copaiva: allergy rashes 206
genital irritation (female) 164
nasal discharge 99
Cornea 79
Corns and calloses 190–1
see also Verrucae
Coronary artery: right and left 119
Coronary thrombosis *see* Heart attack
Coughs 134–5
children 32–3
see also Whooping cough
during pregnancy 181
involuntary urination with 157, 158
with asthma 128, 129
children 130
with bronchitis (children) 130, 131
with feeling of suffocation 136
with hoarseness and voice loss 115
with measles 46, 47
with sore throat (children) 42
Cracks and fissures, skin 207–8
Cramps: abdominal: with weak legs and ankles 197
after swimming 213
anxiety and 53
during pregnancy 175
leg 191
raised blood pressure and 122
sweaty feet with 193
with angina 121
with heatstroke 23
with painful periods 169, 170
Cranium (skull) 71, 187
Crataegus: hardening of the arteries 123

Crocus: anger and its effects 52
bad breath 103
hysteria 61
weak legs and ankles 197
Crotalus: moodiness 66
palpitations 126
Croton tig: genital irritation (female) 164
Croup (children) 33
Crown (tooth) 109
Cullen, Professor 8–9
Cuprum ars: leg cramp 191
Cuprum met 253–4
angina 121
asthma 129
coughs 134
children 32
cramps (pregnancy) 175
feeling of suffocation 136
heatstroke 23
stammering 115
Cuts, lacerations and incised wounds 19
on holiday 214
Cyclamen: hiccoughs during pregnancy 181
Cypripedium: sleep problems (children) 41
Cystitis 156–7

Dandruff and eczema of the scalp 72–3
Deafness 88
catarrh and 87
noises in the ear and 90
see also Menière's disease
Debility 52
Dementia: with memory loss 65
Dentine 109
Depression, clinical 56–8
and emotional upsets during pregnancy 176, 177
and frigidity 163
and impotence 183
hallucinations with 60
indifference and 62
indigestion with 145
with confusion of mind 56
with impotence 183
with indolence 63
with irritability 65
with lactation problems 179
with raised blood pressure 122
with restlessness 68
with shyness and timidity 70
Diabetes 150
and genital irritation 164
Diaper rash *see* Nappy (diaper) rash
Diaphragm 127
Diarrhoea 151–2
after asthma attack 129

anal itching with 150
and suffocation 27
anxiety and 53
children 34
emotional states and 59
fear and 59
indifference and 62
on holiday 214
with allergy rash 206
with colitis 141, 142
with flatulence 140
with loss of appetite 139
with piles 152
with vomiting 43
Digestive system 137–47
Digestive upsets (children) 35
Digitalis: chest pain 132
cystitis 156
heart attack 22, 124
palpitations 126
prostate disorders 185
Dioscorea: angina 121
belching/flatulence 140
colic 141
difficulty with stools 154
Dreams and dreaming:
moodiness and 66
restlessness and 67
see also Nightmares/Night terrors
Dropsy *see* Swelling/fluid retention
Drosera 254
asthma 129
coughs 135
children 32
whooping cough 49
Drugs: and suffocation 27
Duboisis: absent-mindedness 52
Dulcamara 255
acute and chronic bronchitis 131
allergy rashes 206
cold sores 104
colds and influenza 95, 133
children 29
difficulty with stools 154
discharge from the eye 81
hay fever 97
nasal blockage/snuffles 98
rheumatism and arthritis 200
sore throat 116
children 42
stuffy nose/sore eyes (holiday) 216
Dysmenorrhoea *see* Periods: painful
Dyspepsia *see* Indigestion

Ear drum *see* Tympanic membrane

Earache: with discharge 88–9
children 36
with sore throat (children) 42
without discharge 89–90
children 37
Ears 86, 86–92
injuries to the 91
noises in 90–1
see also Catarrh; Deafness; Eczema; Menière's disease
Eating disorders 58
Echinacea: abscesses, boils and carbuncles 204
insect bites and stings 214
Ectropion *see* Eyelids: turning in or out
Eczema 208–9
anal fissure with 149
and deafness 88
and eyelid inflammation 82, 85
and hair loss 76
children 37–8
cracks and fissures with 208
of the ears 91
of the scalp *see* Dandruff and eczema of the scalp
on weak hands 196
scrotal 75
Ejaculation, premature 184
impotence and 183
Elaps: bad breath 104
blue hands 194
chronic catarrh 94
colds and influenza 133
children 29
fainting 20
Emergencies and first aid 15–27
Emotional and nervous disorders 50–70
Emotional states 59
upsets during pregnancy 176–7
Enamel (tooth) 109
Entropion *see* Eyelids: turning in or out
Epidermis 203
Epiglottis 113, 137
Epistaxis (children) *see* Nosebleeds (children)
Equisetum: bed-wetting 28
cystitis 157
Erysipelas 209–10
Eucalyptus: asthma 129
nasal blockage/snuffles 98
salivation problems 107
sinusitis 102
Euonymus: memory loss 65
migraine 78
Eupatorium 255–6
coating/discoloration of tongue 108

Euphorbium: cellulitis/erysipelas/impetigo 210
Euphrasia 256
colds 95
conjunctivitis 81
discharge from the eye 81
hay fever 97
measles 47
nasal discharge 99
swelling of eye/eyelids 85
Eustachian tube 86, 93
obstruction of 87
see also Deafness
External auditory canal 86
Eye strain 83–4
Eyelashes, loss of 83
Eyelids 79
inflammation of 82
see also Styes; Conjunctivitis
neuralgia with toothache 112
swelling of, and eye 85
turning in or out 83
Eyes 79, 79–85
black 80
colds and 95, 96
discharge from 81–2
hay fever and 97, 98
itching of the 84
hay fever and 97, 98
migraine and 78
swelling of, and eyelids 85
see also Cataracts; Conjunctivitis; Eye strain

Face: burning sensations in 73
discoloration of 73–4
pain in 74–5
see also Head
Faculty of Homeopathy 11
Fagopyrum: genital irritation (female) 164
itching of the eyes 84
Fainting 19–20
confusion of mind and 56
from blood loss 17
indifference and 62
with angina 121
with hysteria 61
with irregular periods 168
with periods: palpitations with 126
Fallopian tubes 160
Family doctor: referring illnesses to 13
Fat and subcutaneous tissue 160, 173, 203
Fauces 103
Fears and phobias 59–60
and colitis 141
emotional upsets during pregnancy and 177
rapid heart-rate and 125

sleep problems with (children)
41, 42
with bronchitis 130
with depression 57
with palpitations 125
see also Sensitivity, excessive
Febrile convulsions see
Fits, temperature
Feeding problems (children)
38–9
Feet: burning 192
cold 192–3
cramp in 191
crushed toes on holiday 214
restless: with varicose veins
202
rheumatism and arthritis in
199
sciatica and 201
sweaty 193
see also Ankles; Chilblains;
Corns and calloses
Female health 160–72
Femoral artery 119
Femur 187
Ferrum met 256–7
absence of periods 167
discoloration of face 74
headache (children) 39
indigestion 144
toothache 111
Ferrum phos 257–8
earache with discharge 89
children 36
excessive sensitivity 69
heavy bleeding 17
incontinence 158
noises in ear 90
nosebleeds 101
children 41
Ferrum pic: corns and calloses
191
Fibroids 167
bleeding 17
Fibrositis 189
Fibula 187
Fingers see Chilblains
First aid see Emergencies and
first aid
Fits, temperature 20–1
Flatulence see Belching/
flatulence
Flu see Colds and influenza
Fluid retention see Swelling/
fluid retention
Fluoric acid: chronic catarrh
94
disorders of nails 198
excessive sexual desire
(female) 171
hair loss/baldness 76
increased sexual desire (male)
186
tooth decay 112

varicose veins and varicose
ulcers 202
Foetus 173
Food poisoning: diarrhoea
with (children) 34
Formica: nasal polyps 100
Fractures 21
Fragaria: allergy rashes 206
Fright, anger after 52
severe 24
shock and collapse with 25
with diarrhoea (children) 34
Frigidity 163–4

Gall bladder 137
Gallstones and gall-bladder
disease 143
with jaundice 145
Gelsemium 258–9
Bell's palsy 72
coating/discoloration of
tongue 108
colds and influenza 96, 133
children 29
earache without discharge 90
children 37
emotional states 59
fears and phobias 59
hand and arm cramp 191
hay fever 97
headache 77
children 39
inflammation of eyelids 82
involuntary passing of stools
154
measles 47
nasal irritation/itching 100
pain in face 75
panic attacks 24
sore throat 116
sunburn and overheating
(holiday) 215
Genital irritation: from
infected skin conditions 210
Genital irritation, female 164
excessive sexual desire and
171
with heavy periods 168
with vaginal discharge 172
Genital irritation, male:
with increased sexual
desire 186
German measles 45
Gingivitis see Teeth and gums:
bleeding
Glands, swollen: with infected
skin conditions 210
with infectious illness 46
with scarlet fever 48
see also Mumps
Glandular fever 45–6
Glandular fever nosode 46
Glans penis 182

Glonoine 259
angina 121
confusion of mind 56
fainting 20
headache 77
children 39
heatstroke 23
sunburn and overheating
(holiday) 215
temperature fits 20
toothache 111
Gnaphalium: backache and
lumbago 189
sciatica 201
Gnat bite 23
Gout 193–4
with bunions 190
Graphites 259–10
anal fissure 149
aversion to intercourse (male)
184
bad breath 104
breast conditions, including
mastitis 162
catarrh/obstruction of
eustachian tube 87
cellulitis/erysipelas/impetigo
210
colitis 142
constipation 151
children 31
cracks and fissures 208
discoloration of face 74
disorders of nails 198
eczema 208
children 37
of the ear 91
frigidity 163
gastric and duodenal ulcers
147
glandular fever 46
indolence 63
inflammation of eyelids 82
piles 153
premature ejaculation 184
sensations in throat 115
shyness and timidity 70
sweat rash 212
swelling of eye/eyelids 85
styes 84
vaginal discharge 172
Gratiola: anal burning 149
Guaiacum: gout 194
rheumatism and arthritis 200
sore throat 116
tonsillitis 118
Gumboil see Abscess or
gumboil
Gums see Teeth and gums

Haemorrhage: intestinal 17
post-partum 17
shock and collapse with 25

see also Bleeding, heavy
Haemorrhoids see Piles
Hahnemann, Dr Samuel 8–9,
11
Hair loss/baldness 75–8
eczema and 208
Hair/hair follicle 203
Halitosis see Bad breath
Hallucinations 60–1
Hamamelis 260–1
chilblains 207
heavy bleeding 17
nosebleeds 101
children 41
piles 153
varicose veins/ulcers 202
Hamamelis cream: injuries
and accidents (holiday) 214
Hammer (malleus) 86
Hands and fingers: blue 194
with shock and collapse 25
burning 195
cold 195
with cold feet 193
with sweaty feet 193
cracks and fissures on 207,
208
crushed, on holiday 214
eczema on 208, 209
children 37, 38
numbness of and clumsiness
55
palpitations and 125
red 196
rheumatism and arthritis in
199
weak 196
see also Cramps;
Phalanges; Wrists
Hay fever: and irritation in
mouth 105
and the nose 96–8
asthma with 129
see also Nasal blockage/
snuffles
Head 71, 71–8
eczema on 208, 209
infected skin conditions on
210
psoriasis on 211
Head injuries 21
headache with (children) 39
Headache 76–8
absence of periods and 166,
167
after head injury 21
and confusion of mind 56
and discoloration of face 74
and hair loss 75
children 39
during menopause 166
during miscarriage 179

from sunburn and overheating
215
from travel sickness 216
'hangover' 77
hardening of the arteries and
123
indifference and 62
indigestion with 145
raised blood pressure and 123
sinusitis and 102
with anger 52
with backache and lumbago
189
with chicken-pox 45
with chronic catarrh 94
with coughs (children) 32
with hay fever 96
with heartburn 144
with heatstroke 23
with heavy periods 168
with infected skin conditions
210
with irritability 64
with jaundice 146
with loss of appetite 139
with mastitis 162
with Menière's disease 92
with painful periods 169, 170
with palpitations 125
with PMS 170, 171
with raised blood pressure 122
with restlessness 67
with tonsillitis 118
with travel sickness 92
see also Migraine
Heart 119
atria and ventricles 119
Heart attack 22, 124
see also Chest pain
Heart pain see Angina
Heart-rate: rapid 125
'fluttery' 170
Heartburn 143–4
with indigestion 145
with palpitations 126
Heatstroke 23
Heels: calcaneal spur 196
cracks and fissures on 207
pain in 196
Hekla lava: abscess or gumboil
110
heel pain 196
toothache 111
tooth decay 112
Helleborus: cracked lips and
mouth 105
Helonias: irritability 64
Hepar sulph 261–2
abrasions and grazes 16
abscesses, boils and
carbuncles 204
allergy rashes 206
asthma 129
bleeding gums 110

colds 96
conjunctivitis 81
coughs 135
children 32
cravings (pregnancy) 176
croup 33
earache with discharge 89
children 36
genital irritation (female) 164
hoarseness and voice loss 115
injuries to the ear 91
mouth ulcers 106
nasal discharge 99
punctured wounds 24
sensations in throat 115
sore throat 117
children 42
tonsillitis 118
Hepatitis 145
acute 146
Herpes: on mouth 105
see also Cold sores
Herpes zoster see Shingles
Hiatus hernia see Indigestion
Hiccoughs: during pregnancy
181
with belching/flatulence 140
with indigestion 145
Hippocrates 9
Hives see Allergy rashes
Hoarseness see Throat
Holiday remedies 213–16
Homeopathic medicines: how
to take them 221
manufacture of 218
origins of 218
potencies 218
choosing the right one
219–20
storing remedies 221
types of preparation 219
Homeopathy: and orthodox
medicine 9–10
around the world 10–11
discovery of 8–9
research in 10
Royal Family's interest in 11
'Honeymoon' cystitis 157
Hormone Replacement
Therapy (HRT) 166
Horsefly bites 215
Hot flushes (menopausal) 166
and indifference 62
Housemaid's knee 197
Humerus 187
Hydrastis: backache and
lumbago 189
catarrh/obstruction of
eustachian tube 87
deafness 88
gallstones and gall-bladder
disease 143
indigestion 144
sinusitis 102

vaginal discharge 172
Hyoscyamus 262–3
belching/flatulence 140
colic 141
excessive sexual desire
(female) 171
nightmares 40
sleep problems (children) 41
Hyperactivity 61
Hypericum 263
abrasions and grazes 16
asthma 129
cravings (pregnancy) 176
cuts, lacerations, incised
wounds 19
injuries and accidents
(holiday) 214
insect bites, stings 23
punctured wounds 24
toothache 111
Hyperkinesis see Hyperactivity
Hypertension see Blood
pressure, raised
Hypochondria 52
with depression 57
Hysteria 61–2
children, on holiday 216
with emotional upsets during
pregnancy 177
with fainting 20
with palpitations 126

Iberis: palpitations 126
rapid heart-rate 125
Ichthyolum: itching during
pregnancy 181
lack of concentration 55
Ignatia 263–4
anal itching 150
anger and its effects 52
clinical depression 57
colitis 142
coughs 135
cravings (pregnancy) 176
emotional states 59
emotional upsets (during
pregnancy) 177
excessive sensitivity 69
frigidity 163
headache 77
hysteria 61·
insomnia 64
loss of appetite 139
moodiness 66
piles 153
quarrelsomeness 67
sensations in throat 115
sore throat 117
toothache 112
Ilium 187
Immunization after-effects
213
against whooping cough 49

Impetigo 210
Impotence 183–4
and memory loss 65
see also Ejaculation, premature
Incisor 109
Incontinence 157–8
prostate disorders and 184
Indifference 62
emotional upsets during
pregnancy and 177
with restlessness 68
Indigestion 144–5
absence of periods and 166
heavy periods and 167
nervous 51
with belching/flatulence 140
anal itching with 150
with heartburn 143
Indolence (aversion to work)
63
Infectious diseases 44–9
temperature fits with 21
Infectious mononucleosis see
Glandular fever
Influenza see Colds and
influenza
Injuries and accidents, holiday
214
Insect bites and stings 23–4
on holiday 214
on the ear 91
Insomnia 63–4
during pregnancy 181
with restlessness 68
Intercourse: abhorrence of
(female) see Frigidity
Intercourse: aversion to (male)
184
see also Ejaculation,
premature; Impotence
painful 165
frigidity and 163
Intestine 137, 148, 173
Iodum 264–5
jaundice 145
raised blood pressure 122
rapid heart-rate 125
restlessness 68
sweaty feet 193
Ipecac 265–6
acute and chronic bronchitis
131
coughs (children) 33
eating disorders 58
feeling of suffocation 136
headache 77
inflammation of eyelids 82
morning sickness 180
vomiting (children) 43
Iridium: lack of concentration
55
Iris 266
headache 77
children 39
pain in face 75

Iris (eye) 79
Irritability 64–5
and indolence 63
and miscarriage 180
anger and 53
depression and 58
menopause and 166
painful periods and 169
with eczema 208
with frigidity 164
with hallucinations 60
with morning sickness 180,
181
with PMS 170
with restlessness 67
with travel sickness 216
see also Quarrelsomeness
Ischium 187
Itching: anal 149
chronic catarrh and 95
during pregnancy 181
eyelids 82
eyes 84
facial 73
frigidity and 163
hair loss and 76
mouth irritation and 105
nose: colds and 97
hay fever and 98
with allergy rash 206
with burning hands 195
with chicken-pox 45
with chilblains 207
with eczema 208, 209
with hay fever 98
with psoriasis 210, 211
with restlessness 67
with shingles 48, 49
with varicose veins 202
see also Genital irritation

Jaundice 145–6
indolence and 63
with gall-bladder problems
143
Jugular vein 119

Kali bich 267
acute and chronic bronchitis
131
asthma 129
catarrh/obstruction of
eustachian tube 87
chronic 94
coating/discoloration of
tongue 108
coughs 135
children 33
earache with discharge 89
children 36
inflammation of eyelids 82
measles 47

nasal blockage/snuffles 98
nasal discharge 99
sciatica 201
sense of smell disorders 101
sinusitis 102
sore throat 117
vaginal discharge 172
Kali brom: 205
absent-mindedness 52
allergy rashes 206
cough during pregnancy 181
decreased sexual desire (male)
186
impotence 183
restlessness 68
Kali carb 267–8
acute and chronic bronchitis
131
asthma 129
backache, lumbago and
muscle pain 175, 189
digestive upsets (children) 35
fears and phobias 60
heartburn 143
heavy periods 168
indigestion 144
jaundice 146
palpitations 126
preparing for labour 178
sensations in throat 115
swelling of eye/eyelids 85
Kali iod: colds 96
hay fever 97
nasal discharge 99
rosacea 211
sciatica 201
sinusitis 102
Kali mur: catarrh/obstruction
of eustachian tube 87
dandruff and eczema of the
scalp 72
eczema 209
housemaid's knee 197
mouth ulcers 106
sore throat 117
tonsillitis 118
Kali perm: nasal irritation/
itching 100
Kali phos 268–9
asthma 129
backache and lumbago 190
coating/discoloration of
tongue 108
excessive sensitivity 69
hysteria 61
incontinence 158
irritability 64
shyness and timidity 70
toothache 112
Kali sil: shyness and timidity
70
Kali sulph: dandruff and
eczema of the scalp 72

Kalmia: palpitations 126
rapid heart-rate 125
Kidney 119, 155
Kidney stones 158–9
'Kissing disease' 45–6
Knees: gout in 194
see also Housemaid's knee
Kreosote: bed-wetting 29
bleeding gums 111
genital irritation (female) 164
heavy periods 168
painful intercourse 165
tooth decay 112
toothache and teething
problems 43
vaginal discharge 172

Labia: minora and majora 160
Labour: false 177
preparing for 178
Lac can 269–70
coating/discoloration of
tongue 108
cracked lips and mouth 105
feeding problems 38
Lac deflor: lactation problems
179
Lacerations see Cuts,
lacerations and incised
wounds
Lachesis 270–1
abscesses, boils and
carbuncles 204
anxiety 53
asthma 129
bleeding gums 111
cellulitis/erysipelas/impetigo
210
chest pain 132
clinical depression 57
cravings (pregnancy) 176
fainting 20
heart attack 22, 124
indolence 63
menopause 166
mouth ulcers 106
noises in ear 90
pain in face 75
palpitations 126
premenstrual syndrome 170
raised blood pressure 122
sciatica 201
sensations in throat 115
sore throat 117
children 42
tonsillitis 118
toothache 112
Lactation problems 178
Lactiforous sinus 160, 173
Laryngitis: with asthma 129
see also Throat: hoarseness
and voice loss
Larynx 113, 127

Lathyrus: leg cramp 191
Latrodectus: angina 121
chest pain 132
heart attack 22, 124
weak legs and ankles 197
Lauroceraseus: suffocation 27
Ledum 271
acne 205
backache and lumbago 190
bruises 18
black eye 80
gout 194
injuries to the ear 91
insect bites, stings 23, 214
punctured wounds 24
rheumatism and arthritis 200
Ledum tincture: injuries and
accidents (holiday) 214
Legs: restless 68, 198
with burning feet 192
sciatica in 201
see also Cramps
Legs and ankles 187
eczema on (children) 38
weak 197
see also Feet
Lens 79
Lilium tig 272
angina 121
chest pain 132
clinical depression 57
difficulty with stools 154
fainting 20
heart attack 22, 124
indifference 62
vaginal discharge 172
Limbs: feeling of suffocation
and 136
see also Arms; Back and limbs;
Legs
Lips 103, 113
see also Mouth, tongue and
lips
Lithium carb: heartburn 143
Liver 137
disease see Jaundice
Lobelia inf: asthma 129
deafness 88
heartburn 143
Lobules 160, 173
Lumbago see Backache and
lumbago
Lungs 127
see also Chest pain
Lycopodium 272–4
absent-mindedness 52
arrogance 54
belching/flatulence 140
burning feet 192
clinical depression 57
coating/discoloration of
tongue 108
constipation 151
children 31

corns and calloses 191
cracked lips and mouth 105
cravings (pregnancy) 176
digestive upsets (children) 35
discoloration of face 74
eating disorders 58
excessive sensitivity 69
frigidity 163
gastric and duodenal ulcers 147
hair loss/baldness 76
impotence 183
indigestion 144
inflammation of eyelids 82
styes 84
insomnia 64
irritation in mouth 105
kidney stones 158
lack of confidence 56
nasal blockage/snuffles 99
palpitations 126
piles 153
prostate disorders 185
raised blood pressure 122
rheumatism and arthritis 200
sense of smell disorders 101
sore throat 117
stomach upsets (holiday) 215
sweaty feet 193
toothache 112

Mag carb: constipation 151
children 31
cravings (pregnancy) 176
feeding problems 38
heavy periods 168
palpitations 126
restlessness 68
rheumatism and arthritis 200
toothache 112
during pregnancy 181
Mag phos 274–5
angina 121
belching/flatulence 140
colic 141
children 30
coughs 135
earache without discharge 90
children 37
eye strain 83
hand and arm cramp 191
painful periods 169
toothache 112
weak hands 196
Male health 182–6
Manganum: cellulitis/erysipelas/impetigo 210
eczema 209
Mastitis see Breast conditions
Mastoid process 86
Measles 46–7
and deafness 88

bronchitis after 131
Medicine chest, homeopathic 220
Medorrhinum: burning feet 192
burning hands 195
chronic catarrh 95
coating/discoloration of tongue 108
dandruff and eczema of the scalp 72
impotence 183
lack of concentration 55
nappy (diaper) rash 40
prostate disorders 185
restless legs 198
Memory, poor 52
Memory loss 65
moodiness and 66
see also Mind, confusion of
Menarche 161
Ménière's disease 88, 90, **92**
Menopause, the 165–6
and eczema 209
and indifference 62
and painful intercourse 165
raised blood pressure at 122
Menorrhagia see Periods: heavy
Mental fatigue: with infectious diseases 46
Merc corr 276–7
colitis 142
cystitis 156
discoloration of face 74
sore throat 117
swelling of eye/eyelids 85
Merc sol: toothache and teething problems 43
Mercurius 275–6
abscesses, boils and carbuncles 204
absent-mindedness 52
acute and chronic bronchitis 131
anger and its effects 52
bad breath 104
bleeding gums 111
coating/discoloration of tongue 108
colds and influenza 96, 133
children 30
colitis 142
discharge from the eye 82
hair loss/baldness 76
jaundice 146
memory loss 65
mouth ulcers 106
mumps 47
salivation problems 107
scarlet fever 48
sore throat 117
tonsillitis 118
tooth decay 112

vaginal discharge 172
Metacarpus 187
Mezereum 277
eczema 209
children 37
pain in face 75
shingles 48
tooth decay 112
Migraine 78–9
and eye strain 83
emotional states and 59
with frigidity 163
Milk intolerance (children) 38, 39
Millefolium: piles during pregnancy 181
varicose veins and varicose ulcers 202
Mind, confusion of **56**
head injuries and 21
Miscarriage 179–80
bleeding from 17
Molars 109
Mononucleosis, infectious see Glandular fever
Mons 160
Moodiness 66
Morning sickness 180–1
Morphinum: rapid heart-rate 125
urine retention 159
Moschus: fainting 20
hysteria 61
increased sexual desire (male) 186
Mouth 86, 127, 137
Mouth, tongue and lips 93, 103–8, 113
acne and 205
Bell's palsy and 72
coating/discoloration of tongue **107–8**
with mumps 47
colitis and 141
cracked **104–5**
with colds and influenza 134
children 29, 30
eczema around 208
irritability and 64
irritation in **105**
salivation problems **107**
swollen: suffocation and 27
with scarlet fever 48
ulcers and 147
see also Bad breath; Cold sores; Teeth and gums
Multiple sclerosis: and urine retention 159
Mumps 47
Murex: clinical depression 57
excessive sexual desire (female) 171
irregular periods 168

Muriatic acid: anal itching 150
involuntary passing of stools 154
piles 153
during pregnancy 181
Muscle 203
Muscle aches and pains: on holiday **214**
with gout 194
with rheumatism and arthritis 200, 201
see also Pregnancy and labour
Myocardial infarction see Heart attack
Myrica: jaundice 146

Nails: cracks and fissures on 208
disorders of 198–9
Naja: angina 121
asthma 129
Nappy (diaper) rash 40
Nasal cavity 127
Nat ars: conjunctivitis 81
Nat carb: belching/flatulence 140
feeding problems 38
indifference 62
indigestion 145
restlessness 68
sunburn and overheating (holiday) 215
weak legs and ankles 197
Nat mur 278–9
allergy rashes 206
anal fissure 149
anger and its effects 53
anxiety 54
clinical depression 57
cold sores 104
cracked lips and mouth 105
cravings (pregnancy) 176
eczema 209
eye strain 83
hay fever 97
headache 77
heartburn 143
incontinence 158
indifference 62
irregular periods 168
nasal blockage/snuffles 99
palpitations 126
premenstrual syndrome 170
rapid heart-rate 125
sensations in throat 115
sinusitis 102
weak legs and ankles 197
Nat phos: cold feet 192
discoloration of face 74
heartburn 143
Nat sal: confusion of mind 56
deafness 88
Ménière's disease 92

Nat sulph 279–80
asthma 129
clinical depression 57
colitis 142
head injuries/concussion 21
indigestion 145
involuntary passing of stools 154
jaundice 146
nasal discharge 99
Nausea: anxiety and 53
children see Digestive upsets
confusion of mind and 56
raised blood pressure and 123
with anxiety 53
with emotional upsets during pregnancy 177
with hardening of the arteries 123
with headache 77
with heartburn 143
with heavy periods 168
with jaundice 145, 146
with kidney stones 159
with loss of appetite 139
with PMS 170
with sunburn/overheating 215
with travel sickness 21
with ulcers 147
see also Digestive upsets; Eating disorders; Morning sickness
Neck: backache and lumbago and 189
'Nerve rash' 206
Nerves/nerve fibres 50, 203
Nervous disorders see Emotional and nervous disorders
Nervous system: role of 50–1
Nettle rash 206
Neuralgia: and discoloration of face 74
facial **74–5**
tooth decay and 112
with abscess 110
with toothache 111, 112
with earache (children) 37
with indolence 63
with restlessness 67
with shingles 48
NHS: and homeopathy 11
Niccolum: indigestion 145
migraine 78
Nightmares/night terrors: children 40
emotional upsets during pregnancy and 176
with hysteria 61
with restlessness 67, 68
Nipples see Breast conditions
Nitric acid 280–1
anal fissure 149
bleeding gums 111

blue hands 194
chronic catarrh 95
irritability 64
nasal discharge 99
sensations in throat 115
sore throat 117
children 42
Nocturnal enuresis see Bed-wetting (children)
Nose and sinuses 93, 93–102
blockage/snuffles **98–9**
in fat babies 94
on holiday **216**
chronic catarrh and 94
discharge from **99**
infected skin conditions 210
irritation/itching **100**
rosacea on 211
sense of smell disorders **101**
see also Catarrh; Colds; Hay fever; Itching; Polyps; Sinusitis
Nosebleeds 17, **101**
after facial injury 101
children **41**
nasal polyps and 100
raised blood pressure and 122
sinusitis and 102
Nostril 93
Nuphar luteum: decreased sexual desire (male) 186
Nux moschata: absent-mindedness 52
cravings (pregnancy) 176
indigestion 145
irregular periods 168
moodiness 66
toothache 112
during pregnancy 181
Nux vom 281–2
after-pains (childbirth) 174
anal itching 150
anger and its effects 53
asthma 129
backache and lumbago 190
belching/flatulence 140
bleeding gums 111
burning sensation in face 73
coating/discoloration of tongue 108
colds and influenza 96, 133
children 30
colic 141
children 30
constipation 151
children 31
cramps: after swimming 213
during pregnancy 175
difficulty with stools 154
digestive upsets (children) 35
excessive sensitivity 69
fainting 20
gastric/duodenal ulcers 147
hay fever 98

headache 77
heavy periods 168
indigestion 145
insomnia 64
irregular periods 168
irritability 64
leg cramp 191
morning sickness 181
mouth ulcers 106
piles 153
quarrelsomeness 67
sore throat 117
stomach upsets (holiday) 215
vomiting (children) 43
Nymphomania see Sexual desire: excessive (female)

Ocimum can: kidney stones 159
Oesophagus 113, 127, 137
Oleander: absent-mindedness 52
eczema of the ear 91
Onosmodium: cravings (pregnancy) 176
decreased sexual desire (male) 186
eye strain 83
frigidity 163
impotence 183
lack of concentration 55
Opium 282–3
constipation 151
children 31
coughs 135
difficulty with stools 154
involuntary passing of 154
lack of concentration 55
panic attacks 24
stroke 26
suffocation 27
urine retention 159
Optic nerve 79
Otitis externa/otitis media 88, 114
Ovary 160
Overeating: children: colic after 30
vomiting and 43
fainting after 19
Overheating see Sunburn and overheating
Oxalic acid: angina 121
backache and lumbago 190
palpitations 126
Oxytropis: decreased sexual desire (male) 186

Paeonia: anal burning 149
anal fissure 149
Palate 93, 103, 113
Palpitations 125–6

absence of periods and 166, 167
and angina 121
and discoloration of face 73
anxiety and 53
chest pain with 132
during menopause 166
heartburn with 143
nervous 126
raised blood pressure and 122
with asthma 129
with feeling of suffocation 136
with hardening of the arteries 123
with heart attack 22, 124
with hysteria 61
with PMS 170
with restlessness 67
Pancreas 137
Panic attacks 24, 59
Paralysis: and urine retention 159
Pareira brava: cystitis 157
Passiflora: restlessness 68
Patella (kneecap) 187
Penis 182
Perineum 160
Periods: absence of 166–7
and acne 205
and eczema 109
and excessive sensitivity 69
excessive sexual desire and 171
frigidity and 164
genital irritation and 164
headache with 77
heavy 167–8
irregular 168–9
joint pains between 189
painful 169–70
palpitations before/during 126
rosacea and 211
tender/swollen breasts before 162
toothache before 111
toothache during 112
vaginal discharge before 172
Petroleum: anal itching 150
chilblains 207
cracks and fissures 208
eczema 209
children 37
of the ear 91
eyelids turning in or out 83
psoriasis 211
quarrelsomeness 67
sweat rash 212
travel sickness 92, 216
Pertussin: whooping cough 49
Phalanges (fingers/toes) 187
Pharynx 103
Phlebitis: with varicose veins 202
Phobias see Fears and phobias

Phos acid 283
backache/muscle pains 175
bleeding gums 111
cracked lips and mouth 105
diarrhoea 152
children 34
headache (children) 39
impotence 183
indifference 62
palpitations 126
premature ejaculation 184
Phosphorus 284–5
acute/chronic bronchitis 131
anxiety 54
backache and lumbago 190
belching/flatulence 140
bleeding gums 111
coating/discoloration of tongue 108
coughs 135
children 33
dandruff and eczema of the scalp 72
difficulty with stools 154
eating disorders 58
emotional upsets (during pregnancy) 177
excessive sensitivity 69
eye strain 84
fears and phobias 60
feeling of suffocation 136
gastric/duodenal ulcers 147
heavy bleeding 17
hoarseness and voice loss 115
jaundice 146
nasal polyps 100
palpitations 126
restlessness 68
sleep problems (children) 42
sore throat 117
children 42
vomiting (children) 43
Physalis: absent-mindedness 52
Phytolacca 285–6
breast conditions, including mastitis 163
coating/discoloration of tongue 108
earache without discharge 37, 90
lactation problems 179
restlessness 68
sciatica 201
sensations in throat 115
sore throat 117
children 42
tonsillitis 118
Picric acid: conjunctivitis 81
loss of appetite 139
Piles 152–3
anal itching with 150
bleeding 17
during menopause 166

during pregnancy 181
on holiday 214
Pilocarpus: eye strain 84
mumps 47
Pinna 86
Pituitary gland 71
Placenta 173
Plantago 286
earache without discharge 90
children 37
toothache and teething problems 43, 112
Platina: arrogance 54
excessive sexual desire (female) 171
heavy periods 168
pain in face 75
painful intercourse 165
Pleura 127
Plumbum 286–7
colic 141
children 30
hallucinations 60
memory loss 65
PMT see Premenstrual syndrome
Pneumothorax, spontaneous 132
Podophyllum 287–8
belching/flatulence 140
diarrhoea 152
children 34
piles and prolapse during pregnancy 181
Polyps: and heavy periods 167
bleeding 17
nasal 100
adenoids and 114
with chronic catarrh 95
Pore 203
'Post-nasal drip' 32
Pothos: asthma 130
Pregnancy and birth 173–81
after-pains 174
backache and muscle pains 174–5, 189
cravings 175–6
cystitis in 157
lactation problems 178–9
occasional problems of 181
toothache during 111, 112
varicose veins in 202
see also Cramps; Emotional states; Labour; Morning sickness
Premenstrual syndrome (PMS) 170–1
Pre-molars 109
Prickly heat 216
Primula veris: migraine 78
Prolapse: anal: during pregnancy 181
incontinence with 157
rectal 149

Prostate disorders 185
and impotence 183
and urine retention 159
incontinence with 157
Prostate gland 182
Pruritis ani see Itching: anal
Pruritis vulvae see Genital irritation, female
Psoriasis 210–11
sweat rash with 212
Psorinum 288
asthma 130
earache with discharge 89
children 36
eczema 209
children 38
Ptelea: salivation problems 107
Puberty: female 161
Pubis 187
Pulmonary artery 119
Pulmonary vein 119
Pulp (tooth) 109
Pulsatilla 289–90
absence of periods 167
allergy rashes 206
anxiety 54
backache/muscle pains 175
bad breath 104
bed-wetting 29
chilblains 207
clinical depression 57
coating/discoloration of tongue 108
colds and influenza 96, 134
children 30
colic 141
children 31
conjunctivitis 81
coughs (children) 33
cystitis 157
deafness 88
digestive upsets (children) 35
discharge from the eye 82
earache with discharge 89
children 36
emotional states 59
emotional upsets (during pregnancy) 177
fears and phobias 60
gastric and duodenal ulcers 147
headache 77
indigestion 145
lactation problems 179
loss of appetite 139
measles 47
moodiness 66
mumps 47
nasal blockage/snuffles 99
nightmares 40
painful periods 169
premenstrual syndrome 170
restless legs 198
restlessness 68

rheumatism and arthritis 200
sense of smell disorders 101
shyness and timidity 70
sinusitis 102
styes 84
toothache 112
vaginal discharge 172
Pupil 79
Pyorrhoea see Teeth and gums: bleeding

Quarrelsomeness 66–7
travel sickness and 216
Quinn, Dr Frederick 11

Radius 187
Ranunc bulb 290
corns and calloses 191
rheumatism and arthritis 200
shingles 48
Ranunc sceleratus: corns and calloses 191
Rashes: with asthma 129
with scarlet fever 48
see also Allergy rash; Nappy (diaper) rash; Sweat rash
Ratanhia: anal burning 149
anal fissure 150
Rectum and anus 137, 148–54, 182
burning 149
with constipation (children) 31
with diarrhoea (children) 34
with piles 152
female 160, 173
anal canal 148
fissure 149–50
itching 149, 150
during pregnancy 181
with piles 153
painful during pregnancy 181
pains in after childbirth 174
see also Constipation; Diarrhoea; Piles; Stools
Reilly, Dr D. T. 10
Reproductive system: female 161
Respiratory system 127–36
Restless leg syndrome 198
Restlessness 67–8
and bed-wetting (children) 28
and indolence 63
and nightmares (children) 40
anxiety and 53
diarrhoea with 151
emotional upsets during pregnancy and 176
menopause and 166
with allergy rash 206
with anxiety 53
with asthma 128

with bronchitis 130
with colic 140
    children 30
with coughs (children) 32
with depression 57
with diarrhoea (children) 34
with earache (children) 36
with palpitations 125
with panic attack 24
with shock and collapse 25
see also Hands: burning;
    Insomnia
Retina 79
Rheumatism and arthritis
199–201
and headache 77
and weak hands 196
belching/flatulence with 140
in the neck *see* Spondylitis
indigestion with 145
raised blood pressure with 122
with backache/lumbago 190
Rhododendron 291
rheumatism and arthritis 200
toothache 112
Rhus aromat: incontinence
    158
Rhus tox 292
abscesses, boils and
    carbuncles 205
allergy rashes 206
backache, lumbago and
    muscle pains 175, 190
burning hands 195
cellulitis/erysipelas/impetigo
    210
chicken-pox 44
clinical depression 57
coating/discoloration of
    tongue 108
cold sores 104
eczema 209
    children 38
genital irritation (female) 164
mouth ulcers 106
mumps 47
muscle aches and pains
    (holiday) 214
palpitations 126
restlessness 68
rheumatism and arthritis 200
scarlet fever 48
sciatica 201
shingles 49
sprains and strains 26
Rhus ven: chilblains 207
swelling of eye/eyelids 85
Ribs *187*
Ricinus comm: lactation
    problems 179
Ringworm 150
Robinia: heartburn 144
Rosacea 211
318 **Rubella** *see* German measles

Rumex: coughs 135
    jaundice 146
    nasal discharge 99
Ruta 293
    backache and lumbago 190
    housemaid's knee 197
    injuries and accidents
        (holiday) 214
    rheumatism and arthritis 200
    sprains and strains 26
    weak legs and ankles 197

Sabadilla 293–4
    disorders of nails 198
    hay fever 98
    inflammation of eyelids 82
    nasal discharge 99
    shyness and timidity 70
Sabal serr: incontinence 158
    prostate disorders 185
Sabina 294
    after-pains (childbirth) 174
    excessive sexual desire
        (female) 171
    gout 194
    heavy bleeding 17
    miscarriage 180
Sacrum *187*
Salicylic acid: confusion of
    mind 56
    noises in ear 90
Sambucus: asthma 130
    blue hands 194
    feeling of suffocation 136
'Sand': red 158
    with gout 194
Sanguinaria 295
    acne 205
    chronic catarrh 95
    cravings (pregnancy) 176
    headache 77
    menopause 166
    mouth ulcers 106
    nasal polyps 100
    noises in ear 90
    pain in face 75
    rheumatism and arthritis 201
    rosacea 211
Sanicula: cracks and fissures
    208
    dandruff and eczema of the
        scalp 72
Sarsaparilla: excessive
    sensitivity 69
    moodiness 66
    mouth ulcers 106
Scalds *see* Burns and scalds
Scalp *71, 71–8*
    and hair loss 76
    eczema/dandruff of *72–3,*
        208, 209
    in children 37
    infected skin conditions 210

psoriasis on 211
Scapula (shoulder blade) *187*
Scarlet fever 48
Scarletina *see* Scarlet fever
Sciatica 201
Scrotum *192*
Scutellaria: migraine 78
Sebaceous gland *203*
Secale: coating/discoloration of
    tongue 108
    cold feet 192
    cold hands 195
    hardening of the arteries 123
    involuntary passing of stools
        154
    irregular periods 169
    miscarriage 180
    palpitations 126
    restlessness 68
    senility 69
Selenium: impotence 183
Semicircular canal *86*
Seminal vesicles *182*
Senega: hoarseness and voice
    loss 115
    Bells' palsy 72
Senile dementia: hardening of
    the arteries and 123
Senility 69
    and memory loss 65
Sensitivity, excessive 59,
    69–70
Sepia 295–7
    absence of periods 167
    after-pains (childbirth) 174
    allergy rashes 206
    backache and lumbago 190
    chronic catarrh 95
    clinical depression 58
    coughs 135
    cravings (pregnancy) 176
    discoloration of face 74
    eating disorders 58
    emotional upsets (during
        pregnancy) 177
    fainting 20
    frigidity 163
    genital irritation (female) 164
    headache 77
    indifference 62
    indigestion 145
    indolence 63
    irregular periods 169
    irritability 65
    kidney stones 159
    menopause 166
    miscarriage 180
    morning sickness 181
    nasal discharge 99
    painful intercourse 165
    palpitations 126
    premenstrual syndrome 170
    psoriasis 211
    rosacea 211

travel sickness 216
    vaginal discharge 172
Septum *93*
Sexual desire: decreased
    (male) 185–6
    excessive (female) 171
        before painful periods 170
    increased (male) 186
    strong (male): with impotence
        183
Shingles 48–9
Shock and collapse 25
    from blood loss 17
    from cuts, lacerations, incised
        wounds 19
    from suffocation 27
Shyness and timidity 70
Sickness *see* Nausea; Vomiting
Silica 297–8
    abscesses, boils and
        carbuncles 205
    anal fissure 150
    bad breath 104
    breast conditions, including
        mastitis 163
    cold feet 192
    constipation 151
        children 31
    discoloration of face 64
    disorders of nails 198
    earache with discharge 36, 89
    feeding problems 39
    headache 77
    immunization after-effects
        213
    nasal irritation/itching 100
    punctured wounds 24
    rheumatism and arthritis 201
    sinusitis 102
    styes 84
    sweaty feet 193
Sinapsis nig: bad breath 104
Sinuses *see* Nose and sinuses
Sinusitis 102
Skatol: lack of concentration 55
Skin 203–12
Sleeping problems: children
    41–2
        on holiday 214
    with bronchitis 131
    with indifference 62
    with raised blood pressure 122
    see also Insomnia
Slipped disc 189
Smell, disorders of sense of *see*
    Nose and sinuses
Smoking: and indigestion 144
    and rapid heart-rate 125
    and sore throat 116, 117
Snuffles *see* Nose and sinuses:
    blockage/snuffles
Spartium: raised blood

pressure 122
Speech disorders: memory loss
    and 65
    see also Stammering
Sphincter *148, 182*
'Spider veins' 202
Spigelia 298
    angina 121
    bad breath 104
    cravings (pregnancy) 176
    headache 78
    nasal discharge 99
    pain in face 75
    palpitations 126
    toothache 112
Spinal cord *50, 71*
Spine *160, 173, 182*
    injury to and urine retention
        159
    see also Vertebrae
Spleen *see* Jaundice
Spondylosis: and headache 77
Spongia 298–9
    angina 121
    coughs 135
        children 33
    croup 33
    discoloration of face 74
    hoarseness and voice loss 115
    palpitations 126
Sprains and strains 26
Squilla: cold feet 193
    cold hands 195
    coughs 135
Stammering 115
Stannum met: colic 141
    vaginal discharge 172
Staphysagria 299–300
    anger and its effects 53
    bleeding gums 111
    colic 141
    cuts, lacerations, incised
        wounds 19
    cystitis 157
    prostate disorders 185
    styes 85
    toothache 112
Sternum (breastbone) *187*
Sticta: confusion of mind 56
    coughs (children) 33
    housemaid's knee 197
Stomach *137, 148*
Stomach upsets and pains:
    and headache 77
    belching/flatulence with 140
    on holiday **215**
    ulcers and 146, 147
    with asthma 129
    with bronchitis 131
    with coughs 135
    with heartburn 143
    with palpitations 125
    with sore throat 117

with swelling/fluid retention
    212
    see also Colic
Stools: difficulty with **153–4**
    during colitis 141, 142
    involuntary passing of **154**
        with piles 153
    with anal fissure 149, 150
    with jaundice 145, 146
    see also Constipation;
        Diarrhoea
Strains *see* Sprains and strains
Stramonium: asthma 130
    feeling of suffocation 136
    hallucinations 60
    stammering 115
'Strawberry' tongue 48
Stroke 26
    and discoloration of face 74
Strontia: burning sensation in
    face 73
    hardening of the arteries 123
    loss of appetite 139
    nasal irritation/itching 100
    raised blood pressure 123
Strophanthus: asthma 130
    hardening of the arteries 123
    palpitations 126
Strychninum: irritation in
    mouth 105
    stroke 26
Styes 82, 84–5
Suffocation 27
Suffocation, feeling of 136
    with angina 121
    with asthma 129
        children 130
    with heart attack 124
Sulph acid: chilblains 207
Sulphur 300–1
    abscesses, boils and
        carbuncles 205
    acne 205
    acute/chronic bronchitis 131
    adenoids 114
    anal burning 149
    anal itching 150
    burning feet 192
    burning hands 195
    clinical depression 58
    coating/discoloration of
        tongue 108
    colitis 142
    constipation 151
        children 31
    cravings (pregnancy) 176
    discoloration of face 74
    eczema 209
        children 38
    fainting 20
    genital irritation (female) 164
    heartburn 144
    impotence 183